RADIATION IN TISSUE BANKING

Basic Science and Clinical Applications of Irradiated Tissue Allografts

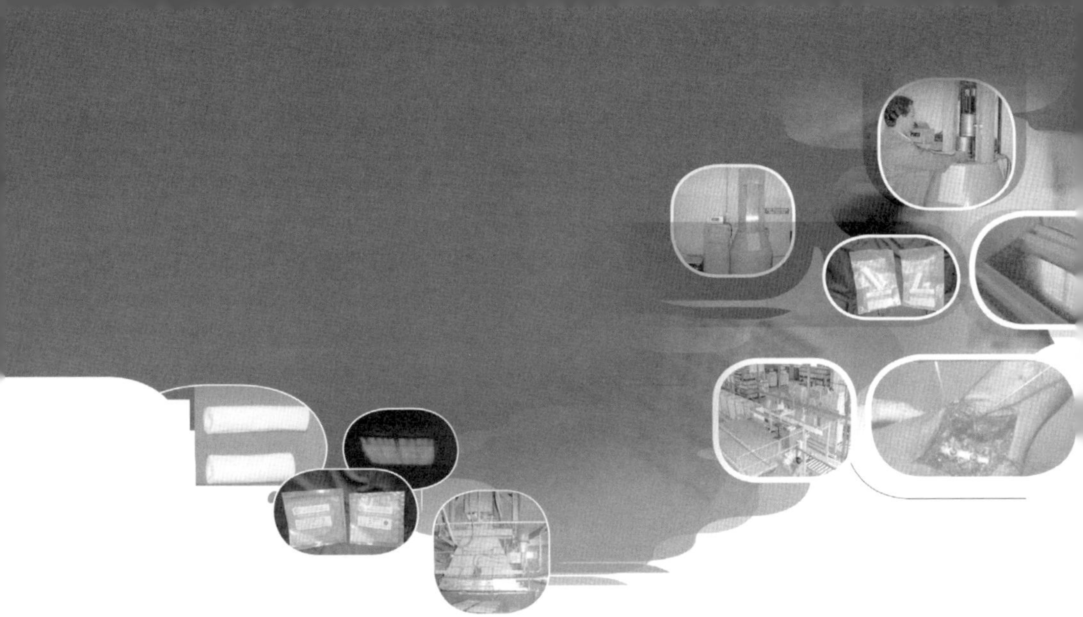

RADIATION IN TISSUE BANKING

Basic Science and Clinical Applications of Irradiated Tissue Allografts

Editors

Aziz Nather
National University of Singapore, Singapore

Norimah Yusof
Malaysian Nuclear Agency, Malaysia

Nazly Hilmy
BATAN Research Tissue Bank, Indonesia

World Scientific

NEW JERSEY • LONDON • SINGAPORE • BEIJING • SHANGHAI • HONG KONG • TAIPEI • CHENNAI

Published by

World Scientific Publishing Co. Pte. Ltd.
5 Toh Tuck Link, Singapore 596224
USA office: 27 Warren Street, Suite 401-402, Hackensack, NJ 07601
UK office: 57 Shelton Street, Covent Garden, London WC2H 9HE

British Library Cataloguing-in-Publication Data
A catalogue record for this book is available from the British Library.

RADIATION IN TISSUE BANKING
Basic Science and Clinical Applications of Irradiated Tissue Allografts

ISBN-13 978-981-270-590-7
ISBN-10 981-270-590-2

Typeset by Stallion Press
Email: enquiries@stallionpress.com

Printed in Singapore by B & JO Enterprise

Foreword from the Chairman of the National Nuclear Energy Agency of Indonesia (BATAN)

First, I would like to congratulate the authors and editors of this book for their excellent work in promoting the application of nuclear technology in tissue banking. I believe that this book will contribute significantly in meeting the need for relevant, qualified applications of irradiated tissue allografts in response to the increasing worldwide demand.

Increasing demands for surgical allografts such as bone, amnion, fascia, tendon, skin, and cardiovascular tissue have to be supported by the increasing quality and safety of these products for safe clinical use. The quality, sterility, and safety aspects of tissue bank products are analogous with the preparation of pharmaceuticals and medical devices in the manufacturing industry. The elimination of disease transmission from donor to recipient, especially the diseases caused by viruses, necessitates thorough donor screening, although (1) viruses at the window period and new emerging viruses may not be detected and (2) several diseases can still be transmitted through transplantation. These phenomena were reported by the Centers for Disease Control and Prevention (CDC) in the USA in 2003. The implementation of a quality system in tissue banking activities and the radiation sterilization of end products have been proven by several researchers around the world to be beneficial in overcoming these problems.

Radiation technology for the sterilization of healthcare products was first utilized in 1956 in the UK and Australia, and has since been followed by other countries such as the USA, Scandinavian countries, and other European countries. At present, more than 200 gamma irradiators of cobalt-60 and about 10 electron beam machines have been installed to sterilize around 40% of disposable healthcare products around the world.

In 1983, an Asia-Pacific regional project on the Radiation Sterilization of Tissue Grafts (RAS/7/003) was established by the International Atomic Energy Agency (IAEA), followed by a program on the Implementation of

Quality Systems in the Radiation Sterilization of Tissue Grafts for safe clinical use (RAS/7/008). Under the IAEA project (INT/6/052), two valuable standards were published: the IAEA International Standards for Tissue Banks (2002), and the IAEA Code of Practice for the Radiation Sterilization of Tissue Allografts (2004). May I take this opportunity to thank the IAEA for its efforts to establish several tissue banks in some countries in the Asia-Pacific region, as well as for carrying out training for potential users of tissue allografts and conducting diploma courses for tissue bankers that complete and enhance tissue banking activities in developing countries.

This book is certainly very useful to support one of the main pillars — the application of isotope and radiation technology — being developed by BATAN to enhance the contribution of nuclear techniques in health. I am confident that this book will also contribute to achieve one of the main millennium development goals, i.e. health, which is of paramount importance especially for countries in the Asia-Pacific region.

Professor Soedyartomo Socntono, MSc, PhD
Chairman
National Nuclear Energy Agency of Indonesia (BATAN)
Jakarta, Indonesia
December 2006

Foreword from the Director-General of the Malaysian Nuclear Agency (NM)

Radiation technology plays a vital role in the healthcare industry, with gamma irradiation used worldwide to sterilize more than 45% of all disposable medical products and devices. The radiation sterilization of tissue allografts — which was promoted by the International Atomic Energy Agency (IAEA) through regional and interregional programs from the 1990s to the early 2000s — highlights the peaceful use of nuclear technology in the health sector. In Malaysia, the Malaysian Nuclear Agency (or Nuclear Malaysia, NM) has played a big role in the establishment of the National Tissue Bank at the University of Science Malaysia and bone banks at several hospitals. NM also assists in radiation-sterilizing allografts processed by these banks as well as those from neighboring countries.

At a regional level, most of the tissue banks in the Asia-Pacific region have chosen gamma irradiation to sterilize their tissues. The supply of radiation-sterilized tissue allografts has met the expectations of end-users and clinicians. However, the sustainability of the supply of quality tissues is very much dependent on the availability of trained manpower to continue with the operation of tissue banks and ensure that the products are clinically safe. The availability of reading materials and textbooks is undoubtedly important in the training of manpower. Therefore, this publication is timely by helping readers keep abreast with the most recent developments in tissue banking. I hope that this book will serve as a useful reference, since it is authored by those who have been actively involved in tissue banking for many years.

May I congratulate the authors and editors for their dedicated effort in publishing this book. I am sure the book will not only be useful for operators in tissue banking, but will also be a good and handy reference for young clinicians who intend to know more about the potential use of tissue grafts.

Daud Mohamad, PhD
Director-General
Malaysian Nuclear Agency (NM)
Ministry of Science, Technology and Innovation
Bangi, Selangor, Malaysia
December 2006

Preface

AZIZ NATHER

NUH Tissue Bank
Department of Orthopaedic Surgery
Yong Loo Lin School of Medicine
National University of Singapore
Singapore

At present, gamma irradiation has yet to be used in the processing of tissue allografts by all tissue banks. The Massachusetts General Hospital Tissue Bank in Boston — set up in 1990 by the pioneer Dr Henry J. Mankin — is still a surgical tissue bank employing sterile procurement and processing techniques, but not gamma irradiation (Mankin was succeeded by Dr William Tomford). Similarly, in Latin America, the Musculoskeletal Tissue Bank in Latin Hospital, Buenos Aires, Argentina, set up by another famous pioneer Dr Ottolenghi (now run by Dr Musculo), is also a surgical tissue bank. In Europe, the largest tissue bank, the DIZG Tissue Bank, set up by Dr von Versen, employs only chemical processing and does not use radiation.

In Singapore, Dr Nather started a surgical tissue bank at the National University Hospital (NUH) in 1988, and converted to using radiation in 1992 upon joining the International Atomic Energy Agency (IAEA) Program RAS 7/008: "Radiation Sterilization of Tissue Grafts". In the Asia-Pacific region, several tissue banks (e.g. in Korea and Japan) started likewise as surgical tissue banks, but were required to employ radiation as the end-processing sterilization step upon joining RAS 7/008. There is no doubt that the IAEA Program on Tissue Banking RAS 7/008 (1985–2004) has promoted the use of gamma irradiation in the Asia-Pacific region, and that its corresponding program in Latin America (ARCAL) has promoted the use of irradiation in Latin American tissue banks.

Today, the benefits of gamma irradiation are well recognized. There is now a move in the USA to use gamma irradiation; no tissue bank in the

USA has ever used irradiation before. In Australia, the Therapeutic Goods Administration Act lists gamma irradiation as compulsory. A move is being made from the traditional 25 kiloGrays (kGy) used for gamma irradiation to 15 kGy — a step that is made possible by the use of clean processing room facilities to reduce the bioburden of the tissues being processed.

Because of the many incidences of disease transmission (especially in the USA, a country that does not use gamma irradiation) and because of the growing professional awareness of the many benefits of gamma irradiation (including the fact that radiation guarantees product sterility, something a surgical tissue bank can never do), radiation is now becoming a necessity in the processing of tissue grafts. As the standards for tissue banking by the American Association of Tissue Banks (AATB), European Association of Tissue Banks (EATB), Asia Pacific Association of Surgical Tissue Banks (APASTB), Australian Tissue Bank Forum (ATBF), and Latin American Association of Tissue Banks (ALABAT) are continually being renewed and upgraded, radiation is expected to constitute an integral part of the standards in all regions in the near future.

This book addresses the controversies surrounding gamma irradiation and its role in tissue banking. The dosage required to be delivered to the tissues is itself an enigma. Why is 25 kGy advocated? What is the evidence for such a dose? Why does Dr Dziedzic-Goclowska, an eminent radiation biologist at the Central Tissue Bank, Warsaw, Poland, advocate the use of 35 kGy? Australia — a country with the best regulations as well as compulsory auditing and licensing — is now seeking to implement a much lower dose of 15 kGy. How is this possible? With 15 kGy, could we not now also irradiate soft tissues? Until today, soft tissues have never been irradiated for fear that the dose of 25 kGy is too large and could weaken the collagen structure of tendons and ligaments. These and many more issues important to transplantation surgeons and tissue bankers alike will be discussed in detail in this book.

The book begins in Part I with a description of the many types of terminal sterilization that can be used for the processing of tissue grafts, and then sets the stage for why gamma irradiation is the preferred method.

Part II deals with some of the basic issues in tissue banking. These include the developmental history of tissue banking in the Asia-Pacific region; ethical, religious, legal, and cultural issues relating to tissue donors in Asia-Pacific countries; the requirements of setting up a tissue bank; and the training requirements needed for all tissue bank operators to provide good-quality control of tissue allografts for safe tissue transplantation practice.

Part III deals with the core issues of the basic science of radiation. How do tissues react to radiation, and what are the different types of radiation and irradiation facilities available? The radiation killing effects on bacteria and fungi are discussed. The effects of gamma irradiation on new emerging infectious diseases caused by viruses and prions, as well as on the biomechanical properties of bone and amnion, are also included.

Part IV deals with the processing and quality control of radiation. It covers dosimetry, requirements for process qualification, validation of the radiation dose delivered, and the importance of bioburden estimation. It discusses in great depth the various validation methods for the processing of freeze-dried bone grafts, amnion grafts, and femoral heads. It also includes dose setting and validation according to the IAEA Code of Practice (2004), as well as a quality system for the radiation sterilization of tissue grafts.

The clinical applications of irradiated bone grafts are described in Part V, and the applications of irradiated amnion grafts in Part VI.

This book includes three valuable sources of information in the Appendices: the Asia-Pacific Association of Surgical Tissue Banks (APASTB) Standards for Tissue Banking (January 2007), the IAEA Code of Practice for the Radiation Sterilization of Tissue Allografts (2004), and the IAEA Public Awareness Strategies for Tissue Banks (August 2002). The last appendix is particularly useful for tissue banks with a shortage of donors, as it provides a good guide on how to run public awareness campaigns.

This book is unique and very useful, as it provides a one-stop forum for tissue bankers who procure and process the grafts, radiation scientists who irradiate the grafts as the final processing step, and transplantation surgeons who use the irradiated products to learn about the latest developments in this multidisciplinary field of tissue banking and transplantation. The book is also a useful text for all tissue bankers, radiation scientists, and surgeons undergoing training in this field. This is especially so for participants of the National University of Singapore (NUS) distance learning Diploma Course in Tissue Banking, which is run by the IAEA/NUS International Training Centre in Singapore for the Asia-Pacific region, Latin America, Africa, and Europe; and also for participants of national training courses run by countries such as Korea.

Contents

LIST OF CONTRIBUTORS

Basril Abbas
BATAN Research Tissue Bank (BRTB)
Center for Research and Development
of Isotopes and Radiation Technology
BATAN, Jakarta 12070
Indonesia

Noriah Mod Ali
Secondary Standard Dosimetry Laboratory (SSDL)
Malaysian Nuclear Agency (NM)
Bangi, 43000 Kajang, Selangor
Malaysia

Febrida Anas
BATAN Research Tissue Bank (BRTB)
Center for Research and Development
of Isotopes and Radiation Technology
BATAN, Jakarta 12070
Indonesia

Zameer Aziz
NUH Tissue Bank
Department of Orthopaedic Surgery
Yong Loo Lin School of Medicine
National University of Singapore
Singapore

S. Bambang
Cicendo Eye Hospital, Faculty of Medicine
Padjajaran University, Bandung
Indonesia

Jocelyn L. L. Chew
NUH Tissue Bank
Department of Orthopaedic Surgery
Yong Loo Lin School of Medicine
National University of Singapore
Singapore

Aravazhi Ananda Dorai
Reconstructive Sciences Department
School of Medical Sciences, Health Campus
Universiti of Science Malaysia
16150 Kubang Kerian, Kelantan
Malaysia

Ferdiansyah
Biomaterial Center – "Dr Soetomo" Tissue Bank
Department of Orthopaedics and Traumatology
Dr Soetomo General Hospital
Airlangga University School of Medicine, Surabaya
Indonesia

Ahmad Sukari Halim
Reconstructive Sciences Department
School of Medical Sciences, Health Campus
Universiti of Science Malaysia
16150 Kubang Kerian, Kelantan
Malaysia

Asnah Hassan
Malaysian Nuclear Agency (NM)
Bangi, 43000 Kajang, Selangor
Malaysia

Susi Heryati
Cicendo Eye Hospital, Faculty of Medicine
Padjajaran University, Bandung
Indonesia

Nazly Hilmy
BATAN Research Tissue Bank (BRTB)
Center for Research and Development
of Isotopes and Radiation Technology
BATAN, Jakarta 12070
Indonesia

Getry Sukmawati Ibrahim
Department of Ophthalmology
Faculty of Medicine
Andalas University/M. Djamil Hospital
Padang
Indonesia

S. Indira
Cicendo Eye Hospital, Faculty of Medicine
Padjajaran University, Bandung
Indonesia

Kamarul Ariffin Khalid
Department of Orthopaedics, Traumatology and Rehabilitation
Kulliyah of Medicine
International Islamic University Malaysia
Malaysia

Chris C. W. Lee
NUH Tissue Bank
Department of Orthopaedic Surgery
Yong Loo Lin School of Medicine
National University of Singapore
Singapore

Aik-Ming Leow
Reconstructive Sciences Department
School of Medical Sciences, Health Campus
Universiti of Science Malaysia
16150 Kubang Kerian, Kelantan
Malaysia

Menkher Manjas
M. Djamil Hospital Tissue Bank
Department of Surgery, Faculty of Medicine
Andalas University, Padang
Indonesia

Hasim Mohamad
School of Medical Science
University of Science, Malaysia
Malaysia
and
Department of Surgery
Hospital Raja Perempuan Zainab II
Kota Bharu
Malaysia

Selamat S. Nadir
Malaysian Nuclear Agency (NM)
Bangi, 43000 Kajang, Selangor
Malaysia

Aziz Nather
NUH Tissue Bank
Department of Orthopaedic Surgery
Yong Loo Lin School of Medicine
National University of Singapore
Singapore

S.-H. Neo
NUH Tissue Bank
Department of Orthopaedic Surgery
Yong Loo Lin School of Medicine
National University of Singapore
Singapore

Paramita Pandansari
BATAN Research Tissue Bank (BRTB)
Center for Research and Development
of Isotopes and Radiation Technology
BATAN, Jakarta 12070
Indonesia

Eileen Sim
NUH Tissue Bank
Department of Orthopaedic Surgery
Yong Loo Lin School of Medicine
National University of Singapore
Singapore

Wan Azman Wan Sulaiman
Reconstructive Sciences Department
School of Medical Sciences, Health Campus
Universiti of Science Malaysia
16150 Kubang Kerian, Kelantan
Malaysia

Radiah Sunarti
Cicendo Eye Hospital, Faculty of Medicine
Padjajaran University, Bandung
Indonesia

Petrus Tarusaraya
Sitinala Leprosy Hospital
Tangerang
Indonesia

Norimah Yusof
Malaysian Nuclear Agency (NM)
Bangi, 43000 Kajang, Selangor
Malaysia

Ahmad Hafiz Zulkifly
Department of Orthopaedics, Traumatology and Rehabilitation
Kulliyah of Medicine
International Islamic University Malaysia
Malaysia

PART I.

TERMINAL STERILIZATION OF TISSUE GRAFTS

Chapter 1

Types of Terminal Sterilization of Tissue Grafts

Aziz Nather, Jocelyn L. L. Chew and Zameer Aziz

NUH Tissue Bank
Department of Orthopaedic Surgery
Yong Loo Lin School of Medicine
National University of Singapore
Singapore

Introduction

It is of crucial importance that surgeons use tissue grafts of high sterility in operations. In particular, they need to be vigilant about the presence of microorganisms, such as bacteria and viruses, as they have the potential to cause diseases and are also extremely small in size and invisible to the naked eye. Therefore, sterilization is important to inactivate or completely kill all types of microorganisms, thus preventing infection and the transmission of diseases.

Types of Sterilization

Sterilization can be classified into two main categories: physical and chemical methods. Physical sterilization includes thermal and nonthermal treatment. Examples of thermal treatment are steam and hot air, while non-thermal treatment includes radiation. Various types of radiation can and have been used in sterilization, such as cobalt-60 radiation (radioactive cobalt), high-voltage cathode irradiation, microwave sterilization, gamma radiation, and ionizing radiation. Chemical sterilization includes peracetic acid, ethylene oxide, hydrogen peroxide, beta-propiolactone, supercritical carbon dioxide, and glutaraldehyde.

Physical sterilization

Steam sterilization (Fig. 1) can be conducted in two ways, either by prevacuum method or by gravitational method. Both methods involve saturated steam at high temperature.

Prevacuum method

In the prevacuum method, air is removed from the chamber and steam is injected in. The graft under sterilization has to be exposed for 4 minutes at a temperature of 132°C and a pressure of 27 psi. The duration of one cycle is 45 minutes.

Gravitational method

The gravitational method involves the displacement of air as saturated steam enters the chamber. This occurs at 121°C at 15 psi. The graft exposure time is 15–30 minutes, and the whole cycle takes 1 hour. Steam sterilization will only occur if the steam and moisture come into contact with each surface

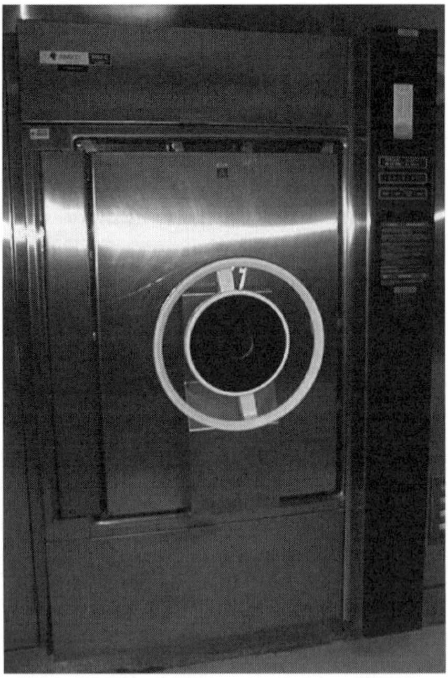

Fig. 1. Steam sterilizer.

area of the graft. For this to occur, all the air from the sterilizer chamber must be removed. In practice, it is impossible to remove all the air, but it is necessary to remove sufficient air so that the very small amount of air remaining will not impair the sterilization process.

Hot air sterilization

This method of sterilization involves hot air (Fig. 2), whereby the chamber is heated to 160°C for 2 hours.

Microwave irradiation

Microwave irradiation is a relatively new form of sterilization (Baqai and Hafiz 1992; Fitzpatrick *et al.* 1978). This method of bone allograft sterilization is a cheap and effective way to process contaminated bone (Ranft *et al.* 1995; Dunsmuir and Gallacher 2003). Dunsmuir and Gallacher (2003) found that no growth could be obtained in specimens subjected to microwave irradiation at 2450 MHz for 2 minutes or longer. Microwave irradiation has been shown to be effective in the destruction of bacteria, viruses, fungi, and parasites. To date, most studies have examined the use of microwaves in the

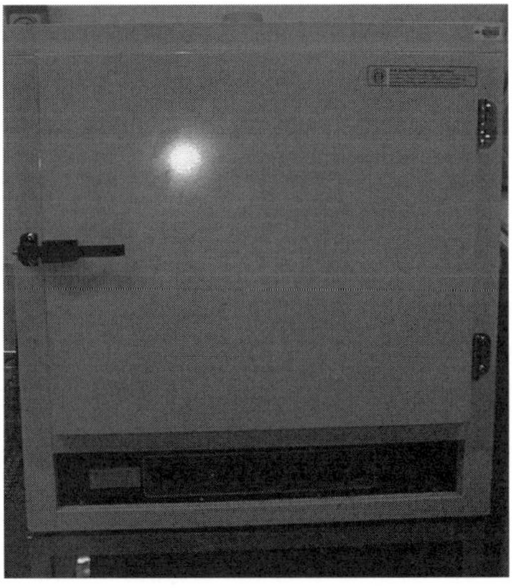

Fig. 2. Hot air sterilizer.

sterilization of contaminated laboratory equipment and surgical instruments (Latimer and Matsen 1977; Baysan *et al.* 1998).

Chemical sterilization

Chemical sterilization methods include peracetic acid (von Versen and Starke 1989; Pruss *et al.* 2003), ethylene oxide, hydrogen peroxide, beta-propiolactone (Hartman and Logrippo 1957; Melnikova *et al.* 1964; Savel'ev *et al.* 1965), supercritical carbon dioxide (Ishikawa *et al.* 1995), and glutaraldehyde.

Peracetic acid

Sterilization using 2% peracetic acid (Fig. 3) inactivates the critical microbial cell system, causing death. The liquid buffer is first drained into the chamber. The lid is closed and the chamber is filled with sterile water. The 35% peracetic acid is then aspirated into the chamber. All these take place at a low temperature of 50°C–55°C. The exposure time is 12 minutes, and the entire cycle takes less than 30 minutes.

Ethylene oxide

Sterilization by ethylene oxide (ETO) (Fig. 4) occurs at a temperature of 55°C–60°C under high pressure. Air is removed and ETO gas is channeled

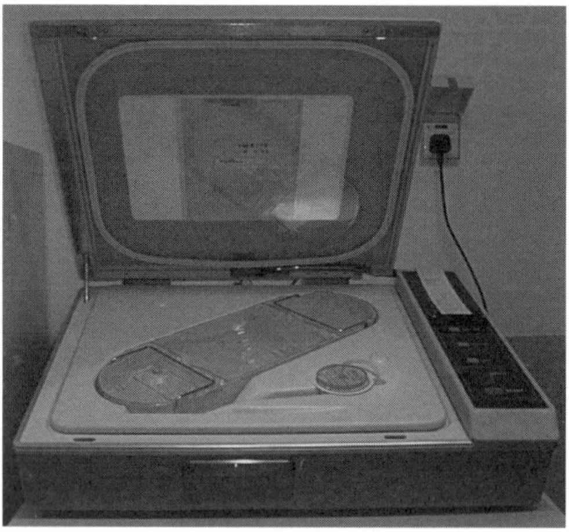

Fig. 3. Peracetic acid (STERIS).

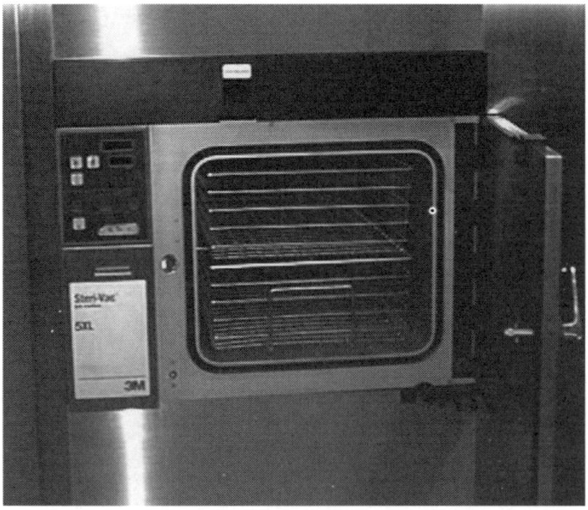

Fig. 4. Ethylene oxide sterilizer.

into the chamber. The ETO gas will diffuse into the items under sterilization. The exposure time is 2 hours, and the whole cycle takes 18–24 hours. A huge disadvantage of ETO is that it leaves toxic residues. The product has to be quarantined for approximately 2 hours before it can be used.

Hydrogen peroxide

Sterilization with hydrogen peroxide plasma (Fig. 5) disrupts the cell metabolism. Air is first removed and the H_2O_2 vial is punctured, upon which the H_2O_2 vaporizes and diffuses. Radiofrequency is then applied and the plasma is activated. This process occurs at 40°C. The exposure time is 16–20 minutes, and the entire cycle takes 75 minutes.

Beta-propiolactone

Beta-propiolactone is a type of gaseous chemosterilizer that is very penetrating. However, it is not recommended because of its toxic property.

Supercritical carbon dioxide

Another sterilization method is by using supercritical carbon dioxide, which can achieve a 12-log reduction in bioburden without compromising the structure and integrity of the transplanted skin, tendon, and bone. Supercritical CO_2 is also capable of achieving rapid inactivation of bacterial

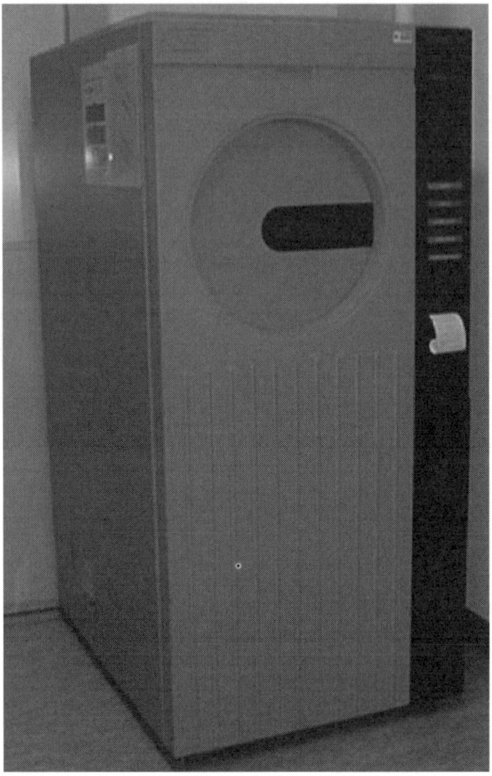

Fig. 5. Hydrogen peroxide (STERRAD).

endospores while in terminal packaging. NovaSterilis, Inc., a developer and provider of advanced medical sterilization technology, recently announced the commercial launch of its NOVA 2200™ Sterilization System — which employs supercritical CO_2 in a patented process to sterilize biomedical materials — to the tissue bank community. Ishikawa *et al.* (1995) found that microorganisms were effectively sterilized by the supercritical CO_2 treatment at 25 MPa and 35°C.

Glutaraldehyde

Sterilization with 2% glutaraldehyde (pH 8) (Fig. 6) requires an immersion time of at least 20 minutes. However, it is not often used, as it is toxic and can cause severe respiratory infection.

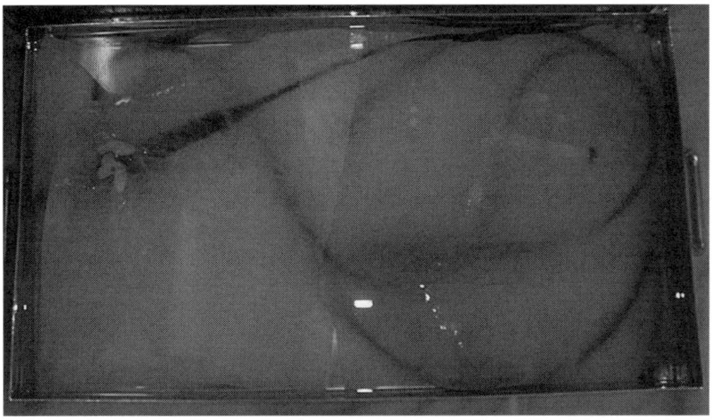

Fig. 6. Glutaraldehyde 2%.

References

Baqai R and Hafiz S (1992). Microwave oven in microbiology laboratory. *J Pak Med Assoc* **42**:2–3.

Baysan A, Whiley R, and Wright PS (1998). Use of microwave energy to disinfect a long-term soft lining material contaminated with Candida albicans or Staphylococcus aureus. *J Prosthet Dent* **79**:454–458.

Dunsmuir RA and Gallacher G (2003). Microwave sterilization of femoral head allograft. *J Clin Microbiol* **41**(10):4755–4757.

Fitzpatrick JA, Kwoa-Paul J, and Massey K (1978). Sterilization of bacteria by means of microwave heating. *J Clin Eng* **3**:44–47.

Hartman FW and Logrippo GA (1957). Betapropiolactone in sterilization of vaccines, tissue grafts, and plasma. *J Am Med Assoc* **164**(3):258–260.

Ishikawa H, Shimoda M, Shiratsuchi H, and Osajima Y (1995). Sterilization of microorganisms by the supercritical carbon dioxide micro-bubble method. *Biosci Biotechnol Biochem* **59**(10):1949–1950.

Latimer JM and Matsen JM (1977). Microwave oven irradiation as a method for bacteria decontamination in a clinical microbiology laboratory. *J Clin Microbiol* **6**:340–342.

Melnikova VM, Belikov GP, and Podkolzin VA (1964). Use of beta-propiolactone for the sterilization of some tissue grafts. *Ortop Travmatol Protez* **25**:33–36.

Pruss A, Gobel UB, Pauli G, Kao M, Seibold M, Monig HJ, Hansen A, and von Versen R (2003). Peracetic acid-ethanol treatment of allogenic avital bone tissue transplants — a reliable sterilization method. *Ann Transplant* **8**(2):34–42.

Ranft TW, Clahsen H, and Goertzen M (1995). Thermal disinfection of allogenic bone grafts by microwave. *J Bone Joint Surg Br* **77**(Suppl II):226.

Savel'ev VI, Danilova AB, Robiukova EN, and Degtiarev IP (1965). Beta-propiolactone sterilization of tissue grafts. *Vestn Khir Im I I Grek* **95**(7):108–110.

von Versen R and Starke R (1989). The peracetic acid/low pressure cold sterilization — a new method to sterilize corticocancellous bone and soft tissue. *Z Exp Chir Transplant Kunstliche Organe* **22**(1):18–21.

Chapter 2

Need for Radiation Sterilization of Tissue Grafts

Norimah Yusof

Malaysian Nuclear Agency (NM)
Bangi, 43000 Kajang, Selangor
Malaysia

Nazly Hilmy

BATAN Research Tissue Bank (BRTB)
Center for Research and Development of Isotopes and Radiation Technology, BATAN
Jakarta 12070, Indonesia

Introduction

Many tissue banks (including bone banks) have been established in many parts of the world. These banks supply a wide range of tissue grafts, both allografts and xenografts, to meet the growing demand for tissue transplantation.

Despite strict donor screening as well as good manufacturing and hygienic practices, there is always a risk of disease transmission caused by viruses, bacteria, or prions from donor to recipient; for instance, transmission of the hepatitis C virus from donor to recipient was reported in the USA from 2000 to 2002. During this time, 44 organs and tissues recovered from antibody-negative organ and tissue donors were transplanted into 40 recipients; among them, 6 received organs, 32 received tissues, and 2 received corneas. All of the tissues had been treated with surface chemicals or antimicrobials and the bone grafts ($n = 16$) had also undergone gamma irradiation, yet 8 cases of HCV genotype 1a were identified among the 40 recipients. Among the six organ recipients, posttransplantation serums were available for three, and definite cases occurred in all these three. Of the 32 tissue recipients, 5 probable cases occurred: one of the two recipients of saphenous vein, one of the three recipients of tendon, and all three recipients of tendon with bone. No cases occurred in recipients of skin ($n = 2$) or irradiated bone ($n = 16$) (CDC 2003).

A rare complication of musculoskeletal allografts was also reported by the Centers for Disease Control and Prevention (CDC) in 2002, whereby 26 cases of infection caused by *Clostridium sordellii* contamination were found, but no reports of disease transmission on demineralized bone products and radiation-sterilized products were made. Similarly, Conrad *et al.* (1995) observed that the hepatitis C virus can be transmitted by bone, ligament, and tendon, but found no cases with irradiated bone at 17 kGy.

Studies on the transmission of HIV from window period donations were conducted in the USA from 1999 to 2003. The window period allows donors with viral contamination to pass through the system undetected. The results stated that irradiation in sterilizing doses can significantly reduce the viral load and, in combination with appropriate donor screening and laboratory testing, significantly enhance and improve the safety of tissues being used for transplantation (Strong 2005).

New emerging diseases caused by viruses and prions — e.g. coronavirus (SARS), bird flu virus type H5N1, and West Nile virus — as well as several diseases caused by prions (proteinaceous infectious particles) — e.g. variant Creutzfeldt–Jakob disease (CJD) prion and mad cow disease (BSE) prion — have had an outbreak in several countries. For example, the West Nile virus has been transmitted through organ transplantations, blood transfusions, and needlesticks. The transmission of these new emerging diseases through contaminated allografts and xenografts obtained from unscreened donors increases the risk of grafts for transplantation (see chapter 10). Although the susceptibility of new emerging viruses to gamma irradiation or other sterilants is unknown, the routine use of terminal sterilization may provide some protection from transmission by tissue transplantation. More recently, several cases have been reported where the infecting organism was spore-forming bacteria or fungi rather than viruses; however, these microbes arose not from the donor, but from the environment during procurement and processing (Eastlund 2005). The fact that there is always some microbial contamination on processed tissues justifies the need for terminal sterilization.

The production of tissues has exceeded one million grafts worldwide annually, mainly by banks in the United States, Europe, Asia-Pacific, and Latin America. Standards are established at regional and international levels to ensure that only tissues procured from healthy living and dead donors are used (Loty 2005). Processing procedures recommended by any standard must first be validated by individual banks before using them on a routine basis. However, although each tissue is subjected to proper handling and even with ultimate attention, there is still some microbial growth on the processed tissue. Therefore, terminal sterilization not only inactivates microorganisms, but also attains a high level of sterility assurance for tissue products.

As is well known, microorganisms are a diverse group of life form. Some of their characteristics include the following:

- Extremely small and a nuisance
- Potential for causing disease
- Ubiquitous distribution
- Invisible to the naked eye

Tissue grafts, like other medical items, must be free from all forms of microorganisms.

Sources of Contamination

Sources of contamination in tissues can be described as follows:

- Screened donors may be contaminated by viruses during the window period or by viruses of new emerging diseases.
- Contamination by bacteria or fungi during procurement, processing, packaging, and storage is possible.

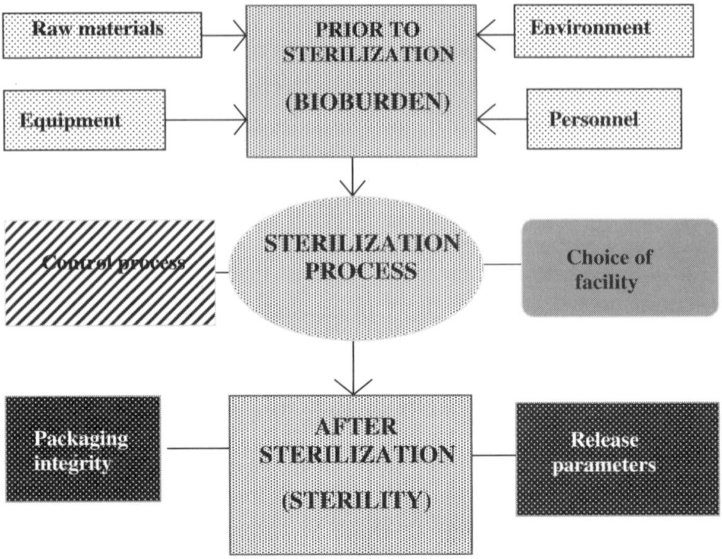

Fig. 1. Total sterility assurance program.

As depicted in Fig. 1, there are four main sources of contaminants during processing and handling prior to sterilization:

1. Raw materials, including procured tissues, chemicals or solutions used, and water
2. Equipment or machinery
3. Environment
4. Personnel/Manpower

The implementation of a total sterility assurance program prior to sterilization is therefore essential.

Raw materials

Tissues can only be procured after being subjected to a stringent donor screening process. Tissues are normally stored at $-10°C$ to $20°C$ while waiting for the microbiological and serological test results. Only tissues that pass the screening tests can be processed. Physical removal of extraneous tissue that was exposed during procurement is helpful in reducing contamination originating from the environment and handling. Additional handling during processing can cause additional contamination.

Guidelines for cleaning the processing room and practicing the aseptic technique used by the technicians involved should be implemented and followed (Winters and Nelson 2005). Chemicals and solutions for washings and treatments must comply with technical specifications in terms of consistent quality or grade. Tap water, if used, must be filtered. Distilled water, pure water, or deionized water must be sterile before use. Sterile procurement of tissues must be practiced (Nather 2001).

Equipment or machinery

All equipment and machineries are subjected to routine check-ups, frequent maintenance, and proper calibration. They must be kept clean at all times. Laminar airflow cabinets must be switched on at least 1 hour before being used. Autoclaves must function well to ensure adequate pressure and correct temperature for sterilization. Ovens must achieve the required temperature. Bandsaws must be cleaned after every use. No tissues are to be left unclean on any tool. Simple basic equipment such as balances, thermometers, pH meters, micropipettes, and even clocks must be calibrated.

Environment

The floor must be cleaned with detergent, and the surface wiped with proper disinfectant. Chemical disinfectants used in hospitals include alcohols, aldehydes, biguanides, halogens, phenolics, and quarternary ammonium compounds. The air-conditioning supply is preferably filtered. HEPA filters in clean rooms and clean cabinets must be replaced if they are damaged or not functioning, in addition to routine maintenance. The flow of air from room to room should be controlled; it should flow from a clean area to a less clean area. Periodic room monitoring, including particle count and microbial count, is encouraged. No living plants or pets are allowed near the processing room.

Personnel/Manpower

All personnel must be trained and retrained to use established procedures. They must be informed of any changes in the procedures, and must be educated about aseptic handling as well as how to do scrubbing and proper gowning before entering the processing room. They should always cover their hair (including beard) and wear a mask, and must not talk or cough during procurement and processing. They are not allowed into the processing area if they are not well, especially if they have caught a cold or flu. They are never to put on makeup or cosmetics, and must keep their fingernails tidy and short.

It is strongly advisable to do routine sampling for microbiological tests, specifically bioburden (i.e. colony-forming unit or microbial count for each batch of finished products), prior to sterilization. Bioburden tests should serve as a routine quality control measure, in addition to moisture content tests. Data on bioburden reveal not only the quality (cleanliness) of the graft produced, but also whether the environment in which the processing takes place is kept clean. Interestingly, one can also monitor if an operator has done the processing properly. Usually, new untrained operators produce tissue grafts with a high bioburden compared to those trained staff who can produce grafts with a reasonably consistent low bioburden.

Bioburden can still be found on the finished products, no matter how clean the environment is, how well-trained the operators are, or how strict the aseptic handling is practiced. Therefore, the products still need to undergo terminal sterilization.

Sterilization Process

Sterilization is the process in which all types of microorganisms are either inactivated (unable to reproduce) or completely killed. One should not be confused between sterilization and disinfection: disinfection is only meant to inactivate or remove pathogenic (disease-producing) microorganisms, with the exception of bacterial spores.

The aim of the sterilization process is to effectively kill all the microorganisms without causing any detrimental effects to the product. Tissue bankers can decide on the sterilization technique to be used, as long as the process allows the product to achieve a high sterility assurance level (SAL) for safe clinical application (Yusof 2000). This book only discusses radiation sterilization. Chapter 8 describes several types of irradiation facilities and the control process employed for the radiation sterilization process.

After Sterilization

Packaging integrity is the most important aspect to ensure that sterility is maintained. There is no such thing as an expiry date for sterility: the expiry date stated on the packaging is based on tissue product integrity, and sterility is maintained as long as the packaging is intact. Therefore, only those recommended packaging materials that are suitable for the chosen tissue sterilization process can be used. For instance, if radiation is decided as the method for sterilization, it is recommended that only radiation-compatible plastics (e.g. polyethylene) can be used. Chapter 14 describes various types of packaging materials.

Release parameters must be obtained from the facilities conducting sterilization, and the documents released must be kept as the product record. For radiation sterilization, release certificates must indicate the minimum and maximum absorbed doses as well as the type of dosimeter used to measure the absorbed doses.

Sterility tests must be carried out after the sterilization process (except for radiation sterilization, because the radiation dose is already selected based on product microbiological quality prior to sterilization). For products that are produced in limited numbers per each processing batch, such as tissue grafts, a small fraction of the tissues can be taken provided that this sample represents the overall tissues and undergoes processing along with the other tissues.

The products to be sterilized must be clean to a certain extent. One should never try to sterile "dirty" products, as it is unethical. Even though the microbes are killed, the sterilization process may not inactivate the endotoxin produced by the microbes. Thus, only products processed under good manufacturing practices, which result in low bioburden, can be easily sterilized.

Types of Sterilization Techniques

Basically, there are three main sterilization methods available to sterilize products in large quantities:

1. Thermal (dry or wet heat) — this method causes damage to the biological and physical properties of tissues. It cannot penetrate the product well.

2. Radiation — this method causes physical damage only at high doses. Gamma radiation can easily penetrate products, even in final packaging. It is a cold sterilization process.
3. Ethylene oxide (EtO) gas — this method leaves toxic residues and cannot easily penetrate tissues. It is also a cold sterilization process.

Of the three options, radiation is the best one. However, the lowest possible radiation dose must be identified so as to effectively kill microorganisms without causing significant damage to the tissues. Several tissue banks have conducted validation of a radiation sterilization dose of 25 kGy or lower for amnion and bone grafts; however, the radiation dose of 25 kGy is generally accepted.

Dose Response Curve

Different microorganisms in pure culture show different dose response curves to any sterilization process. Figure 2 shows three types of microorganisms with different radiation sensitivity results in distinctive response. The radiation dose is expressed as kilogray or kGy, with the following relationship between radiation dose and amount of calories:

$$1 \text{ gray (Gy)} = 100 \text{ rad} = 1 \text{ J/kg}$$
$$1 \text{ J} = 0.2389 \text{ cal}$$

The greater the slope or gradient, the more resistant the microorganism is to radiation. When the slope is steep, less radiation is required to lower the microbial count, and thus the microbe is more sensitive to radiation. The value of the slope or gradient, described as the reduction in growth per dose, can be calculated. The dose required to reduce one log cycle (by a factor of 10) of the microbial population is called the D_{10} value, which is sometimes referred to as the decimal reduction dose (Ley 1973). The linear plot of the graph can be mathematically expressed as

$$D_{10} = \frac{D}{\log_{10} N_0 - \log_{10} N} \text{kGy}$$

where N_0 is the initial number of viable microbes, and N is the number of microbes surviving after the dose D.

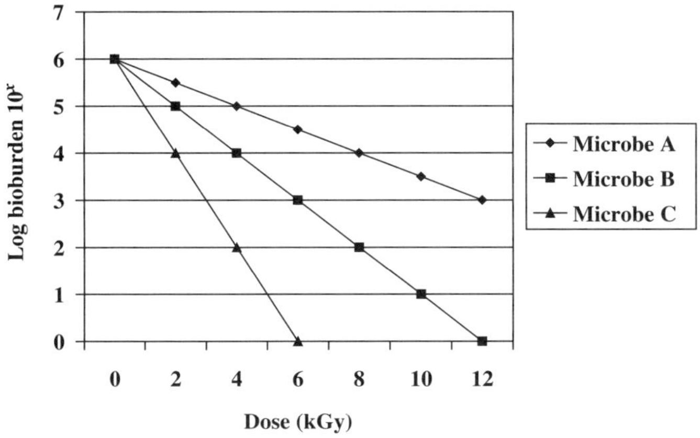

Fig. 2. Dose response curve for three microorganisms.

Therefore, the D_{10} value for the three microorganisms is calculated as follows:

1. Microbe A: 4 kGy
2. Microbe B: 2 kGy
3. Microbe C: 1 kGy

This means that microbe A is more radiation-resistant than microbe B, which is more radiation-resistant than microbe C. In other words, microbe C is more radiation-sensitive than microbe B, which in turn is more radiation-sensitive than microbe A. For example, if the D_{10} value for *Bacillus pumilus* is 2 kGy, this means that 2 kGy is required to reduce one log cycle of a population of the microbe. If the initial population (N_0) of the microbe is 10^6 colonies, then 12 kGy (D) is required to kill the population by sixfold to no population N, i.e. 6 log cycles $\times$ 2 kGy $=$ 12 kGy.

In the sterilization process, the microbe population is killed beyond level zero. Given that microbes are undetectable to the naked eye and ubiquitous in nature, only probabilities are dealt with. The sterilization process renders the tissues sterile to achieve a certain assurance level. Therefore, the sterility assurance level (SAL), the probability of obtaining a nonsterile among a population of products, is used. There are two levels of SAL:

1. SAL 10^{-3} — the possibility of obtaining not more than 1 nonsterile in 1000 product units. This SAL is used mainly for laboratory disposables, tools for external use, and packages.
2. SAL 10^{-6} — the possibility of obtaining not more than 1 nonsterile in 1 million product units. This SAL is used mainly for medical products and for items that are in contact with open tissues.

At present, only the SAL of 10^{-6} is used for medical devices and tissues. Generally, most tissue banks use gamma irradiation at 25 kGy for terminal sterilization, following recommendations by the International Atomic Energy Agency (IAEA) (2004). However, some American tissue banks use a lower dose of 15 kGy, while some in Poland use a higher dose of 35 kGy. In any case, the 25-kGy dose is no longer the magic dose for sterilization. Tissue bankers can actually decide to use either a lower or higher dose than 25 kGy, depending on the bioburden count and the types of contaminants commonly found on the products. Most importantly, the dose must be adequate enough to sterilize tissues in order to attain an SAL of 10^{-6} with minimal adverse effects on the physicochemical and biological properties of the tissues. Tissue bankers have to validate whatever dosage they have chosen. In principle, the following formula can be used to calculate the dose:

$$\text{Sterilization dose (SD)} = D_{10}(\log \text{bioburden} - \log \text{SAL})\ \text{kGy}$$

where D_{10} is the radiation dose required to reduce a microbial population by one log, and SAL is the sterility assurance level (normally at 10^{-6}).

The tissue banker, not the irradiation plant operator, is responsible for selecting the sterilization dose. The selected dose must be validated before being adopted, after which the irradiation plant delivers the required dose as accurately as possible. The IAEA Code of Practice (2004) (see Appendix 2) describes four methods to validate the sterilization dose. Chapters 16, 17, and 19 provide guidance on how to conduct the dose validation, and also discuss the applications and details of the Code.

Conclusion

Regardless of the processing method used or how clean the tissue-processing environment is, tissues still need to be sterilized in order to achieve a high SAL for safe clinical usage. Hygienic practices in procurement, processing, and packaging can minimize the types and number of viable microorganisms. Together with terminal sterilization treatment, a high SAL can thus be achieved. Radiation can offer terminal sterilization because the method is simple, it is widely used for medical devices, and — most importantly — its validation is possible.

References

Centers for Disease Control and Prevention (CDC) (2003). Hepatitis C virus transmission from antibody-negative organ and tissue donor. *MMWR Wkly* **52**(13):273–276.

Conrad EU, Gretch D, Obermeyer K, Moogk M, Sayers M, Wilson J, and Strong MD (1995). The transmission of hepatitis C virus by tissue transplantation. *J Bone Joint Surg* **77A**:214–224.

Eastlund T (2005). Viral infections transmitted through tissue transplantation. In: Kennedy JF, Phillips GO, and Williams PA (eds.), *Sterilisation of Tissues Using Ionising Radiations*, CRC Woodhead Publishing, England, pp. 255–278.

International Atomic Energy Agency (IAEA) (2004). Code of Practice for the Radiation Sterilization of Tissue Allografts: Requirements for Validation and Routine Control, Project No. INT/6/052, IAEA, Vienna.

Ley FJ (1973). The effect of ionizing radiation on bacteria. In: *Manual on Radiation Sterilization of Medical and Biological Materials*, IAEA Technical Report Series No. 149, IAEA, Vienna, pp. 37–63.

Loty B (2005). IAEA International Standards for Tissue Banks. In: Kennedy JF, Phillips GO, and Williams PA (eds.), *Sterilisation of Tissues Using Ionising Radiations,* CRC Woodhead Publishing, England, pp. 3–38.

Nather A (2001). Sterile procurement of bones and ligaments. In: Nather A (ed.), *Advances in Tissue Banking,* Vol. 5, World Scientific, Singapore, pp. 265–306.

Strong DM (2005). Effects of radiation on the integrity and functionality of soft tissue. In: Kennedy JF, Phillips GO, and Williams PA (ed.), *Sterilisation of Tissues Using Ionising Radiations*, CRC Woodhead Publishing, England, pp. 163–172.

Winters M and Nelson J (2005). Bacterial inactivation in tissues. In: Kennedy JF, Phillips GO, and Williams PA (eds.), *Sterilisation of Tissues Using Ionising Radiations*, CRC Woodhead Publishing, England, pp. 281–286.

Yusof N (2000). Gamma irradiation for sterilising tissue grafts and for viral inactivation. *Malays J Nucl Sci* **18**(1):23–35.

PART II.

TISSUE BANKING

Chapter 3

Tissue Banking in the Asia-Pacific Region — Past, Present, and Future

Aziz Nather*, Kamarul Ariffin Khalid† and Eileen Sim*

**NUH Tissue Bank*
Department of Orthopaedic Surgery
Yong Loo Lin School of Medicine
National University of Singapore
Singapore

†Department of Orthopaedics, Traumatology and Rehabilitation
Kulliyah of Medicine
International Islamic University Malaysia
Malaysia

Historical Development

The first tissue bank in the world was set up by Dr George Hyatt in 1949, and was named the US Naval Tissue Bank. At about the same time, in 1952, the Hradec Kralove Tissue Bank was set up at the Faculty Hospital, Czechoslovakia, by Dr Rudolf Klen; the Wakefield (later called the Yorkshire) Tissue Bank in the UK by Frank Dexter; the Poland Tissue Bank in Warsaw by Dr Janus Komender and Dr K. Ostrowski; and the Democritus Tissue Bank in Athens, Greece, by Dr N. Triantafyllou. Tissue banks gained recognition following the encouraging results of massive bone allograft transplantations reported by Dr Ottolenghi in 1966, Dr Parrish in 1973, and Dr Mankin in 1976.

In the USA, the development of tissue banks was pioneered by Professor Henry J. Mankin, who established the American Association of Tissue Banks (AATB) with about 30 tissue banks in 1990. At about the same time, Europe sprung into similar activity with an International Conference in Tissue Banking held in Berlin in 1991. The following year, in

June 1992, the European Association of Tissue Banks (EATB) was set up in Marseilles, France. In the Asia-Pacific region, tissue banking actually began in a few countries as early as the 1980s, e.g. Burma and Thailand in 1984. The Asia Pacific Association of Surgical Tissue Banks (APASTB) was established in October 1988 in Bangkok, Thailand, with Dr Vajaradul as its first president and secretary and Dr Nather as its first vice president.

There has been a resurgence of interest in tissue banking in the last decade, with the development of more new tissue banks in countries such as Korea, India, Malaysia, and Indonesia.

Allograft Transplantation

The bridging of large bone defects for tumor or trauma reconstruction poses a major challenge for orthopedic surgeons. Options include the following:

- Vascularized autologous cortical bone transplants
- Modular and custom-made prostheses
- Ceramics
- Cortical bone allografts

Vascularized bone transplants are not popular because the technique demands technical expertise as well as prolonged operating time and operating costs, and also mainly because the bone transferred (fibula) is too small to fill the volume of bone mass needed in the defect (usually a defect in the femur, tibia, or humerus). Modular prostheses are not favored because of the large cost factor, e.g. US$10 000–US$15 000 for a knee or shoulder prosthesis. Custom-made prostheses, although available in the USA, are not easily available in the Asia-Pacific region and have a bigger cost factor: the added cost of transportation and the time required before it becomes available. Ceramics are popularly used in Japan (A-W glass ceramics developed by Professor Yamamuro in Kyoto), but are not used elsewhere because of a similarly large cost factor and lack of availability as well as the time factor for transportation.

On the other hand, allografts provide a suitable alternative, provided they are issued by a tissue bank producing high-quality tissue allografts for safe tissue transplantation practice. Allografts provide enormous cost savings, e.g. a whole femur provided by a tissue bank costs around US$1000, which is 10 to 15 times cheaper than the cost of prostheses or ceramics. Also, the best solution for large bone defects is to replace bone with bone, i.e.

biological reconstruction. This does not incur the long-term complications of prostheses, such as loosening of components, metal disease (metallosis), and plastic disease (polyethylene disease).

Allografts therefore play an important role in massive bone defect reconstruction as any of the following:

- Allograft–autograft composite
- Allograft–prostheses composite
- Allograft–vascularized fibula composite (Cappana technique)
- Allograft–MSC composite, allograft–bone growth factor composite, or allograft–MSC–bone growth factor composite in the future

Issues in Tissue Banking

Before looking at the development of tissue banking in the individual countries in the Asia-Pacific region, the following key issues (Nather 2000a) must be examined:

- Ethical issues
- Legal issues
- Religious issues
- Cultural issues

Ethical issues

From an ethical point of view, tissue banking is good for Asia-Pacific countries because it helps to reduce health costs compared to its alternatives of prostheses or ceramics. For this reason, the governments of all Asia-Pacific countries support tissue banking activities. Bone allografts from commercial banks are also prohibitive in costs, e.g. a whole femur costs about US$4000 to US$5000.

Tissue donation must be viewed as an act of humanity to alleviate the suffering of fellow human beings. Therefore, it must not be allowed to promote any element of profit. It is hoped that tissue banks provide bone allografts on a noncommercial basis. Tissue banks should not be allowed to sell bone grafts. They are, however, allowed to charge "processing costs" — costs of procurement, processing, and distribution — if their countries have made a provision to allow for this in their laws. Processing costs are charged in countries such as Singapore, Malaysia, Japan, India, Sri Lanka, and Indonesia.

Legal issues

There is no universal law for tissue procurement and transplantation in the Asia-Pacific region. Where laws exist, in Singapore, Malaysia, India, Sri Lanka, Hong Kong, the Philippines, and Vietnam, they are based on similar Human Transplantation Acts in Europe and the USA. All the laws follow the "opting-in" framework, which requires consent from the donor or next of kin. However, some countries have no laws governing tissue banking, such as China, Thailand, and Myanmar.

Religious issues

According to the late Dr Hudson Silva, founder of the International Eye Bank in Sri Lanka, Buddhism is in perfect agreement with tissue donation because it is considered as an act of charity earning merit. Buddhism therefore favors tissue donation. Countries with a predominantly Buddhist population, such as Sri Lanka, Vietnam, and Thailand, have no shortage of donors.

Hinduism is parallel to Buddhism in many ways. Devotees of both religions practice cremation of the body — an act of destruction of the body. No resistance to tissue donation is expected, as seen in India.

The Islamic Koran does not forbid tissue donation *per se*. In fact, fatwas (religious rulings) promoting tissue donation have been issued in several Muslim countries, including Saudi Arabia, Pakistan, Bangladesh, Malaysia, and Indonesia. However, Muslims remain resistant to tissue donation because of cultural issues, and so these fatwas have failed.

Christianity also does not forbid organ and tissue donation. The late Pope John Paul II, in an audience with doctors and surgeons, expressed full support for organ and tissue donation when he quoted the Bible: " 'Give, and it will be given to you …' (Luke 6:38). We shall receive our supreme reward from God according to the genuine and effective love we have shown to our neighbour."

Cultural issues

Although religious issues generally do not disfavor tissue donation, the Asian cultural attitude is a big factor preventing many donors from coming forward. This Asian culture, which has become a strong part of the local mentality, is that God created us whole and so we prefer to return to Him whole so as not to displease him.

Muslim culture strongly disfavors tissue donation. Muslims bury almost everything that has been removed from their body, including amnion, foreskin of circumcised amnions, and amputated fingers and legs. This therefore explains the big shortage of donors in Muslim countries such as Pakistan, Bangladesh, and Indonesia.

In the Philippines, the population is predominantly Catholic. Whilst the religion favors tissue donation, this same Asian culture has caused a shortage of tissue donors in the country. In Korea, which has a 30% Catholic population, there is a shortage of deceased donors for the same reason.

More public awareness campaigns at the national level are required in these countries to change the cultural attitude of the people (Appendix 3).

IAEA Expert Missions

Under the Program for Tissue Banking by the International Atomic Energy Agency (IAEA), RAS 7/008 "Radiation Sterilization of Tissue Grafts", several experts were sent to countries in the Asia-Pacific region, including Dr Glyn Phillips, Dr Rudi von Versen, Dr Heinz Winkler, Dr Mike Strong, and Dr Aziz Nather. These missions were instrumental in helping set up tissue banks and developing tissue banking activities in several countries.

Dr Nather was contracted as a UN/IAEA expert to help set up tissue banks in 10 missions involving Malaysia (Kota Bahru and Kuala Lumpur), Vietnam (Ho Chi Minh City and Hanoi), Zambia, Myanmar, Argentina, Brazil, Cuba, Sri Lanka, and Korea. He was also invited to set up two tissue banks in Hong Kong by the Hong Kong Orthopaedic Association, namely at the Queen Mary Hospital and Prince of Wales Hospital in 1995; and to set up bone banks in Kobe, Japan, by Professor Maruo Souji in 1996. By conducting such missions, the author has gained good insight into the local situation of these countries.

Myanmar

Tissue banking began in the Asia-Pacific region in Burma in 1984, when Dr U. Pe Khin founded the Burma Tissue Bank in Rangoon, Burma. After his sudden death in 1987, Dr Myo Mint succeeded him in 1992 and reactivated the tissue bank project. However, his efforts were short-lived when he was transferred to Mandalay and succeeded by Dr Khin Maung Han in 1995.

There is no law for tissue donation in Myanmar, apart from the Eye Donation Law. Approximately 85% of the population are Buddhists, who favor tissue donation. There is a gamma irradiation facility, a gamma chamber belonging to the Department of Agriculture, that is available for their use.

Thailand

In light of the major setback suffered by Burma with the demise of its pioneer Dr U. Pe Khin, Thailand took over as the forerunner of the region. The Bangkok Biomaterial Center was set up by Dr Yongyudh Vajaradul at the Siriraj Hospital, Mahidol University, in December 1984.

Like Myanmar, there is no tissue donation law in Thailand. Thailand is predominantly a Buddhist country favoring tissue donation. The radiation sterilization of tissue grafts started in Thailand in 1986, when the bank acquired its own gamma chamber.

Singapore

The National University of Singapore (NUS) Bone Bank was set up in October 1988 as a research tissue bank for the Department of Orthopaedic Surgery by Dr Nather using an NUS Research Grant, RP 880334 "Bridging of Large Bone Defects by Allografts" (Nather and Wang 2002). However, the clinical demand for tissue allografts soon grew tremendously, and the bank was pushed into clinical activity fairly quickly.

In 1994, the Ministry of Education (Totalisator Board) awarded the bank a S$239 965 grant to upgrade its clinical facilities and functions, and to start the production of lyophilized gamma-irradiated morsellized bone allografts. It acquired two new freezers (in addition to its original two) and two sets of lyophilizer units (each lyophilizer unit included a band saw, a shaker bath, a lyophilizer, and a laminar flow cabinet). That same year, the NUS Bone Bank became the national bone bank supplying bone and soft tissue allografts to all nine hospitals in the country.

Tissue donation follows the Medical (Therapy, Education and Research) Act of 1972, whereby any person of sound mind and 18 years of age or above may give all or any part of his/her body for education or transplantation. The gift takes effect upon death. It is an "opting-in" law, requiring written consent from the donor or next of kin.

Tissue donation also follows the Ministry of Health's Multiorgan and Tissue Procurement System, a directive set up in 1992 by the Director of Medical Services, Dr Chen Ai Ju. With this centralized system, all donor solicitations are centrally coordinated and performed by a national team of transplant coordinators (mainly kidney and liver coordinators) for solid organs and tissues including kidney, liver, heart, cornea, skin, and musculoskeletal tissue. The bone team is activated only if the donors approached by the national team have consented to donate bones as well. Under this system, only about 10% of all kidney donors have also consented to donate bones and soft tissues. The situation could be improved if hospitals agreed to employ their own tissue transplant coordinators, who would then join the national team to better look after their own interests.

Singapore began irradiating deep-frozen long bones in September 1992 by sending the bones packed in Polylite containers with dry ice by air to the Malaysian Nuclear Agency (NM) in Bangi, Selangor. They are irradiated in a cobalt-60 plant (Sinagama) by Dr Norimah Yusof. Since 1994, with the production of lyophilized, gamma-irradiated morselized bones, these small grafts have been irradiated in a gamma chamber at the Department of Nuclear Medicine, Singapore General Hospital, by Dr Betty Xun Fei.

The National University Hospital (NUH) Tissue Bank was officially inaugurated in September 1995, and became a hospital cost facility in 1998. The bank has a wet processing laboratory, a dry processing laboratory, a documentation room, and a reception area with a space of 2000 square feet.

Japan

The Kitasato University Hospital Bone Bank was set up in April 1991 by Dr Moritoshi Itoman. It is illegal to procure tissues in Japan, except for cornea as stated in the Law for Transplantation of Kidneys and Corneas 1979. Radiation sterilization was introduced by Dr Itoman in 1994, with the cooperation of the Japan Atomic Energy Research Institute (JAERI).

Although legislation recognizing the concept of brain death was passed in 1997, few organs have been procured. In a landmark event on March 1, 1999, a liver, heart, and both kidneys were procured from a brain-dead donor in Kochi and airflown for transplantation to four recipients, each in a different city (Reuters). This event was thought to favor the environment of tissue donation in Japan; unfortunately, this did not happen.

There are at least 150 tissue banks present in Japan that deal only with femoral heads. They remain fairly inactive, waiting to spring into activity once tissue donation becomes more acceptable.

The Philippines

In Manila, the University of Philippines General Hospital Tissue Bank was set up by Dr Norberto Agcaoili in May 1990 at the Department of Orthopaedic Surgery, University of Philippines College of Medicine. Tissue donation follows the Republic Act 7170, 1991, an "opting-in" law whereby the legacy or donation of all or part of a human body after death for specified purposes must be authorized by the donor or next of kin. Whilst Filipinos are predominantly Catholic, their cultural attitudes do not support donation. All tissues are gamma-irradiated at the Philippines Nuclear Research Institute (PNRI) in Manila.

As a whole, tissue banking has yet to be active in the Philippines.

Malaysia

In Malaysia, two tissue banks were set up in 1991:

1. The Malaysian National Tissue Bank by Dr Hasim Mohamad at the Universiti of Science Malaysia, Kota Bahru, Kelantan
2. The Malaysian Institute for Nuclear Technology Research (MINT) Tissue Bank by Dr Norimah Yusof at MINT, Bangi, Selangor (later renamed the Malaysian Nuclear Agency or NM)

Like in other countries, tissue banking in Malaysia conforms to an "opting-in" law: the Laws of Malaysia, Act 130, 1974.

A Fatwa on Bone, Skin, and Amnion was passed by the Malaysia Islamic Centre in September 1995 — a religious ruling allowing Muslims to donate.

Despite this, there remains a shortage of Muslim donors due to cultural factors.

On November 5, 1994, the Malaysian National Tissue Bank was inaugurated by Dr Hasim Mohamad in Kota Bahru, Kelantan. A third tissue bank, the General Hospital Kuala Lumpur Bone Bank, was inaugurated by Dr Ruzlan in 1998 during the 7th Scientific Meeting of the APASTB held in Kuala Lumpur. In 2006, two more new tissue banks were set up: one at the University of Malaya Medical Centre, Kuala Lumpur; and one at the International Islamic University of Malaysia, Kuantan, in conjunction with a tissue engineering laboratory. All tissue allografts are sent to Dr Norimah Yusof at NM for gamma irradiation.

Under the leadership of Dr Hasim Mohamad and Dr Norimah Yusof, the development of tissue banking in Malaysia has expanded tremendously. The Malaysian Association for Cell and Tissue Banking was established in 2005. Moreover, on behalf of the APASTB, Malaysia will host the 5th World Congress of Surgical Tissue Banks — jointly organized by the APASTB, AATB, EATB, Australasia Tissue Bank Forum (ABTF), and Latin American Association of Tissue Banks (ALABAT) — in June 2008.

Indonesia

Dr Nazly Hilmy established Indonesia's first tissue bank, the BATAN Research Tissue Bank, at the Center for Application of Isotopes and Radiation (CAIR), National Atomic Energy Agency (BATAN), in Jakarta in 1990. Initially, due to the shortage of deceased donors, the bank processed both human and bovine bones for clinical application in addition to processing human amnion. The Indonesia 1992 Health Regulation is an "opting-in" law that allows retrieval of tissue from living donors only.

In 1986, Dr Nazly Hilmy managed to enact a Fatwa for Bone, Skin, and Amnion, thus permitting procurement from deceased donors as well. However, this religious breakthrough has not increased the attitude of donors due to cultural factors. Indonesia still faces a big shortage of deceased donors.

A second bone bank, the Dr M. Djamil Hospital Tissue Bank, has been set up in Padang, Sumatra, by Dr Menkher Manjas. In addition, the late Dr Abdurrahman inaugurated the Surabaya Bone Bank in Surabaya during the 8th Scientific Meeting of the APASTB in Bali in 2000.

Dr Abdurrahman also set up the Indonesian Association of Tissue Banks and became its first president. Unfortunately, his demise caused a major setback in the development of tissue banking in Surabaya. His leadership position at the Surabaya Bone Bank has since been succeeded by Dr Ferdiansyah.

China

The China Institute for Radiation Protection (CIRP) Tissue Bank was set up in 1988 in Taiyuan, Shanxi Province, by Dr Sun Shiquan and Dr Li Youchen. This was quickly expanded to become the first provincial tissue bank in China, the Shanxi Provincial Tissue Bank, in July 1993. In 1994, it secured approval from the government to distribute its tissue grafts to Beijing and other cities in China. There is no human transplantation act in China, but tissue banks in China follow the principle of obtaining written consent from donors before the procurement of tissues.

All tissue grafts are gamma-irradiated at the CIRP. In 2000, the Shanxi Provincial Tissue Bank was privatized by OsteoRad Biomaterial Co. Ltd. with modern up-to-date facilities. The CIRP has been conducting national training courses for tissue banking in China for several years.

It is still not known how many tissue banks exist in China or how big each facility is; indeed, China is a subcontinent in itself. Once the tissue banks in China become more known and active, they will have a major role to play in the development of tissue banking in the region.

Hong Kong

Two tissue banks have been set up at the two medical universities in Hong Kong. In 1990, Dr David Fang formalized a regional musculoskeletal tissue bank at the Queen Mary Hospital, University of Hong Kong. Dr T. L. Poon took over as the director in 1994; but with the resignation of Dr Poon, the bank has become rather inactive. In 1992, Dr Shekhar Kumta formalized another regional musculoskeletal tissue bank at the Sir Y. K. Pao Centre for Cancer, Prince of Wales Hospital, Chinese University of Hong Kong.

Both banks are supported by the Hong Kong Government. Tissue banking in Hong Kong follows the Human Organ Transplantation

Ordinance 1997, an "opting-in" law requiring consent from the donor or next of kin.

Vietnam

Dr Tran Bac Hai was instrumental in developing the Biomaterial Research Laboratory University Training Centre for Health Care Professionals in Ho Chi Minh City in January 1993. The bank procures amnion and lyophilized morselized chip grafts. All of the grafts are sent to Dalat for irradiation. At around the same time, the Hanoi Tissue Bank — a skin bank — was set up at the Laboratory of Biomaterial Preparation (Vinatom) by Dr. Pham Quang Ngoc. The bank processes skin and amnion grafts. All of the tissues are sent to the Hanoi Irradiation Centre for irradiation.

With both Dr Tran and Dr Pham now retired, no good successors have come forward. As a result, tissue banking has become rather inactive in Vietnam.

Sri Lanka

The Sri Lanka Model Human Tissue Bank was set up by the late Dr Hudson Silva and his wife. Dr Silva is renowned for having procured more than 40 000 corneas to be distributed to several countries in the world on humanitarian grounds. In 1993, an agreement was signed between the IAEA and the Ministry of Health in Sri Lanka, upon which the Government gave a big piece of land for the development of the tissue bank. The bank was inaugurated on May 8, 1996, by the Prime Minister of Sri Lanka.

This project was defined as a model project because there were many donors in this predominantly Buddhist country, and it was thought that they could supply the much-needed grafts to other countries in the region with a great shortage of donors. Unfortunately, this plan was poorly conceived and could not happen, as the laws between countries do not allow tissues to cross borders easily.

Sri Lanka follows an "opting-in" law, the Human Tissue Transplantation Act No. 48 of 1987, requiring consent from the donor or next of kin. The bank has its own gamma irradiation facility — a Gamma Cell 200 — on its own premises.

Sri Lanka suffers a big problem in the utilization of the tissue grafts it produces by surgeons in the country. More professional education is needed in Sri Lanka to address this problem.

Australia

Four tissue banks in Australia incorporate radiation processing for the terminal treatment of grafts by the Australian Nuclear Science and Technology Organisation (ANSTO). These include the following:

1. Queensland Bone Bank (led by Dr David Morgan)
2. Donor Tissue Bank of Victoria (led by Dr Lyn Ireland)
3. Perth Bone and Tissue Bank (led by Professor David Wood)
4. South Australia Tissue Bank

Tissue banks in Australia have to comply with the Australian Code of Good Manufacturing Practice for Therapeutic Goods – Human Tissues, September 1995. This Code adopts and applies basic quality system principles from the ISO 9000 series of standards to tissue banking.

The strength of tissue banking in Australia lies in the high standards that these tissue banks are required to comply with, according to the Therapeutic Goods Administration (TGA) Act, in order to obtain yearly licensing. The banks are audited yearly. In contrast, in the USA, the AATB has set very high standards, but accreditation is not compulsory. In Europe, the European Council will issue European Council Standards that must be complied with by all tissue banks in Europe; however, it will take some years before common standards for the whole of Europe can be implemented. Singapore follows the Australian system of compulsory auditing and licensing; indeed, Singaporean auditors are trained by TGA authorities in Australia.

A private tissue bank with two clean rooms has recently been developed in New South Wales at a cost of about A$1 million. It is not in operation yet. A large institutional tissue bank costing A$12 million has also been set up in Brisbane by the Government of Queensland, with six clean rooms and state-of-the-art facilities. Both of these banks will play a role in influencing tissue banking not only in Australia, but perhaps also in the Asia-Pacific region.

India

The Tata Memorial Hospital Tissue Bank was set up in 1988 by the late Dr N. M. Kavarana at the Tata Memorial Hospital, Mumbai, in collaboration with the IAEA. Tissue banking follows the Bombay Anatomy Act 1949, which covers the use of unclaimed or donated bodies for therapeutic purposes, medical education, or research; and the more recent Transplantation of Human Organs Act 1994, in which consent is required from the donor or next of kin. The irradiation of tissue grafts is performed in a Gamma Chamber 900 donated by the Atomic Energy Commission, Government of India. The current director of this tissue bank is Dr Astrid Lobo Gajiwala.

In 2006, there was great interest in the resurgence of activities to set up tissue banks in many parts of India, such as Chennai (Dr Mayil Natarajan), Coimbatore, Kerala, New Delhi, Mumbai, Kolkata, etc. Like China, India is a subcontinent that has recently sprung into activity. The development of such new tissue banks in India will play a major role not only in influencing tissue banking in India, but also in the rest of the region.

Korea

The Korea Biomaterial Research Institute was established in 1990 by Dr Chang Joon Yim at the College of Dentistry, Dankook University, in Cheonan, Korea. The tissue grafts are irradiated by the Korea Atomic Energy Research Institute (KAERI) in Taejon, Korea.

Brain death was legally recognized in Korea in February 2000. Since then, there has been tremendous activity in setting up new tissue banks in Korea, notably at the Catholic University Hospital in Seoul, Korea, by Professor Yong Koo Kang (St. Vincent's Hospital). More than 20 new tissue banks have already been established.

Plans are underway to set up one or two regional tissue banks in Korea. Two private tissue banks have also been set up with government approval: Bioland and Hans Biomed.

Tissue Banking in the Asia-Pacific Region

Two major driving forces have been responsible for the development of tissue banking in the Asia-Pacific region:

- IAEA Program on Tissue Banking in the Asia-Pacific region from 1985 to 2004
- Asia Pacific Association of Surgical Tissue Banks, which was established in October 1988 (Nather *et al.* 2005a)

"Golden Age" of Tissue Banking in the Asia-Pacific Region

The tissue banking program run by the IAEA was indeed responsible for the "golden age" of tissue banking in the Asia-Pacific region.

The Regional Cooperative Agreement (RCA) was an agreement among 16 member states in the Asia-Pacific region, namely Australia, Bangladesh, China, India, Indonesia, Japan, Korea, Malaysia, Mongolia, Myanmar, Pakistan, the Philippines, Singapore, Sri Lanka, Thailand, and Vietnam. The RCA Project RAS 7/008: Radiation Sterilization of Tissue Grafts (1985–2004) was responsible for setting up and developing 15 tissue banks in 12 member states, i.e. Bangladesh, China, India, Indonesia, Korea, Malaysia, Myanmar, Pakistan, the Philippines, Sri Lanka, Thailand, and Vietnam. These banks were provided with equipment, and experts were sent to these countries. Scientific visits and fellowships were also given to the tissue banks in these countries.

RAS 7/008 was refined to a Thematic Model Project under the capable leadership of Professor Glyn Phillips, technical advisor to the Deputy Director-General, Department of Technical Cooperation, IAEA (Mr Qian Jihui). The objective was to raise the quality standards of tissue banking to an international level. Efforts were directed to harmonize the quality standards of tissue banks in the region, thus facilitating the exchange of grafts from one country to another in the long term.

A curriculum on tissue banking was assembled for the first time in Suzhou in 1994, with each country contributing assigned chapters. This IAEA draft curriculum was piloted in a regional training workshop in Singapore in September 1995, involving 21 trainers and 35 trainees. It was during this workshop that the NUH Tissue Bank was inaugurated as a hospital tissue bank. This bank became a cost center in 1998.

The decision was made to develop a Regional Training Centre (RTC) in the Asia-Pacific region that would run a 1-year distance learning course leading to university diploma certification. The author is extremely grateful to Professor Phillips for choosing Singapore to be this RTC. With a S$225 500 grant from the National Science and Technology Board, the RTC was built on level 2 of NUH with a purpose-built wet processing laboratory, dry processing laboratory, documentation room, and reception bay. About S$100 000 of this grant was used to convert the IAEA draft curriculum into

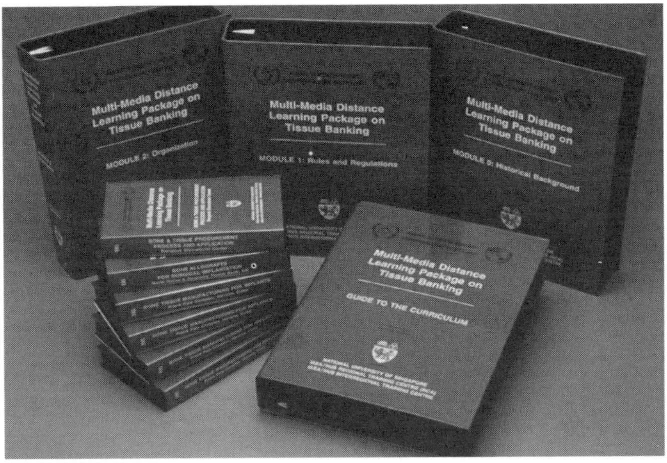

Fig. 1. Multi-Media Curriculum.

the IAEA/NUS Multi-Media Curriculum (collectively owned by the region) with booklet modules, case studies, videotapes, and box containers (Fig. 1).

The IAEA/NUS Regional Training Centre was launched on November 3, 1997, by the Deputy Vice Chancellor of NUS, Professor Chong Chi Tat. The IAEA was represented by Mr Thomas Tisue, special advisor to the Deputy Director-General (Mr Qian Jihui). The first IAEA/NUS diploma course in tissue banking was simultaneously launched with 17 participants (Nather 2000b).

The conversion to the Multi-Media Curriculum was completed in April 1998, and a regional training workshop called "Training the Trainers" was held that same month. Directors of tissue banks from all countries in the region who would act as trainers for students in their own countries were each given one set of the curriculum, and were taught how to use it and how to conduct student supervision. The first convocation was held in October 1998, with 12 candidates convocating (Fig. 2).

Along with centralized training, the IAEA started sending experts to audit tissue banks in the region in November 1998. All banks must now conform to a standardized procedure manual and quality control manual with standards acceptable by the IAEA.

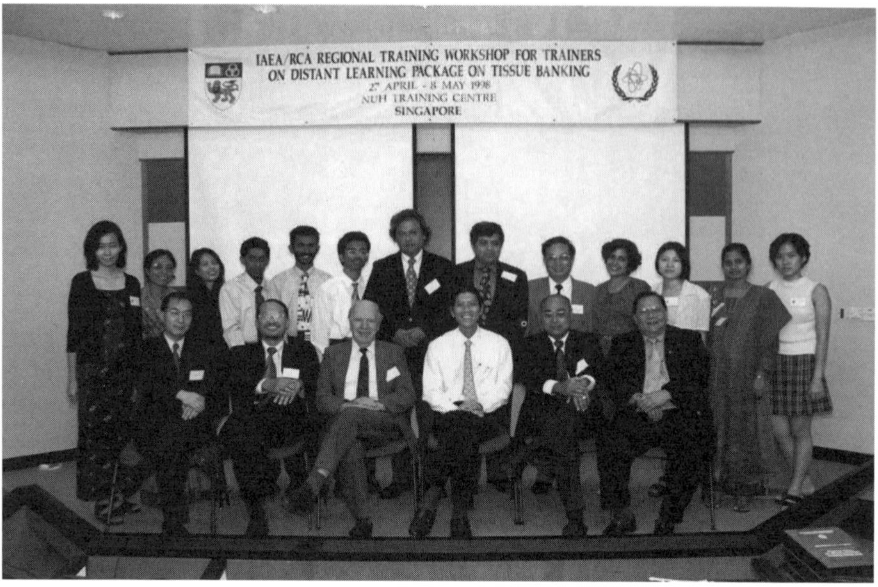

Fig. 2. Convocation ceremony of first diploma course in October 1998.

Technology transfer to Latin America

With the success of the RCA Program on Tissue Banking in the Asia-Pacific region, the IAEA decided that Latin America could also benefit by technology transfer from the RCA to the Regional Cooperative Agreement for the Advancement of Nuclear Science and Technology in Latin America and the Carribean (ARCAL). An interregional trainers workshop was held in October 1998 with delegates from ARCAL member states, namely Argentina, Brazil, Chile, Mexico, and Peru. Each delegate was presented with one set of the Multi-Media Curriculum. This curriculum (in English) was translated into Spanish for use in Latin America, and Argentina was trained by Singapore to function as the RTC for Latin America. This interregional project was successful. Buenos Aires began functioning as the RTC for Latin America in 2002.

Curriculum update

In 2000, the seven videotapes of the Multi-Media Curriculum were converted into two VCDs and a companion book — *Radiation and Tissue*

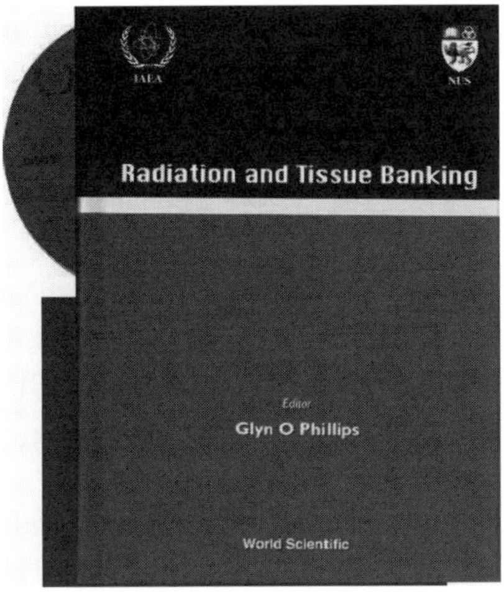

Fig. 3. Curriculum update.

Banking (Phillips 2000) — was introduced as an update to the Multi-Media Curriculum (Fig. 3). In 2002, *The Scientific Basis of Tissue Transplantation* (Nather 2001) was introduced as a text for the basic sciences component of the course.

Workshop/Training courses held by the IAEA

During the "golden age", the IAEA hosted one to two workshops/training courses yearly on key issues for tissue banking, including quality control, public awareness, radiation, sterilization of tissues, etc. The IAEA made participation by all member countries of the APASTB possible by scheduling such workshops and training courses to coincide with the following APASTB Meetings:

4th APASTB Meeting	1991	Manila, Philippines
5th APASTB Meeting	1994	Suzhou, China
6th APASTB Meeting	1996	Gold Coast, Australia
7th APASTB Meeting	1998	Kuala Lumpur, Malaysia
8th APASTB Meeting	2000	Bali, Indonesia
9th APASTB Meeting	2002	Seoul, Korea

Since the IAEA Program ended in 2004, participation of IAEA Meetings has only been from Australia, India, Indonesia, Korea, Japan,

Malaysia, Singapore, and Hong Kong. Participation from Bangladesh, China, Myanmar, Pakistan, Sri Lanka, and Vietnam has stopped since the last IAEA workshop cum 9th APASTB Meeting in Seoul in 2002.

Development of internet diploma course in tissue banking

It was decided that the text booklet and CD-based curriculum should be converted into internet form for online delivery as an internet course. It was felt that this could save the enormous costs of bringing students and lecturers to the 2-week foundation course held in Singapore at the start of each batch (Nather 2001).

Singapore was appointed as the Interregional Training Centre in 2002. A server was installed at the NUS by the IAEA. The curriculum was to be served to participants online in three packages quarterly. This internet course had to be completed via a face-to-face terminal examination at the NUS at the end of the 1-year distance learning course in order to validate the students enrolling for the course.

A memorandum of understanding was signed between the Government of Singapore (Dean, Faculty of Medicine, NUS) and the IAEA (Deputy Director General, Department of Technical Cooperation, IAEA) on July 4, 2002, making Singapore the International Coordinating Centre (ICC) (Fig. 4).

The role of the ICC includes the following:

- Assisting the IAEA in the development of the internet curriculum
- Acting as a depository of the IAEA/NUS Curriculum
- Coordinating and implementing training via internet using the IAEA/NUS Curriculum
- Assisting other RTCs, e.g. in case the server in Argentina crashes
- Assisting national training centers (e.g. Korea) with their own national training courses using the English internet curriculum

The development of the Internet Centre was deemed to be extremely important because it was the first internet diploma course ever to be developed by the NUS, as well as the first one with university accreditation on tissue banking in the world.

The online curriculum conversion was completed in January 2004. The ICC launched its first internet course in February 2004 with its sixth batch.

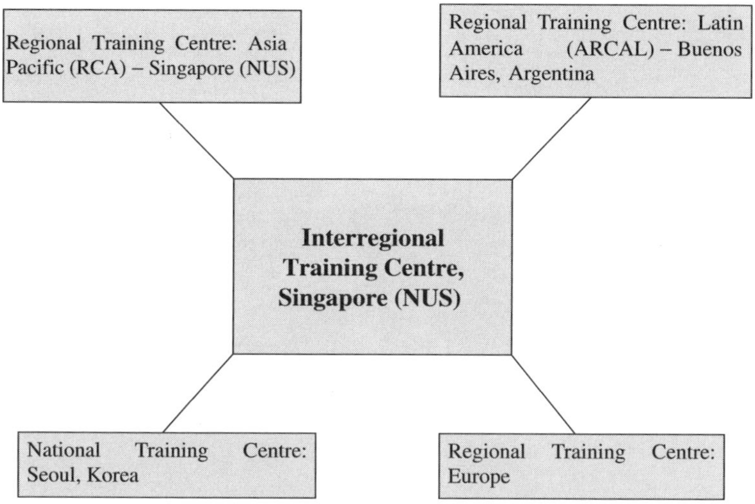

Fig. 4. Role of Singapore as the International Coordinating Centre.

The curriculum was served online in three packages quarterly, with three assignments served online for each package (Fig. 5).

Courses held

As of 2007, eight courses have been held. A total of 160 tissue bank operators have registered with the NUS diploma in tissue banking. Of these, 133 are from the Asia-Pacific region (15 countries), 6 from Latin America (Brazil, Chile, Cuba, Peru, Uruguay), 9 from Europe (Greece, Slovakia, Poland, Ukraine), 12 from Africa (Zambia, Libya, Egypt, Algeria), and 2 from Australia (Table 1) (Nather *et al.* 2005b).

As of 2006, seven convocations have been held. A total of 102 tissue bank operators have convocated with an NUS diploma in tissue banking, namely orthopedic surgeons, pathologists, microbiologists, radiation scientists, and technologists. Of these, 20 have graduated with distinction, 45 with credit, and 37 with pass only (Table 2) (Nather *et al.* 2005b).

Post-IAEA ERA: Gloom for Asia-Pacific Region

The region faced much difficulty when the IAEA suddenly ended the program without any warning or communication. US$100 000 had been spent

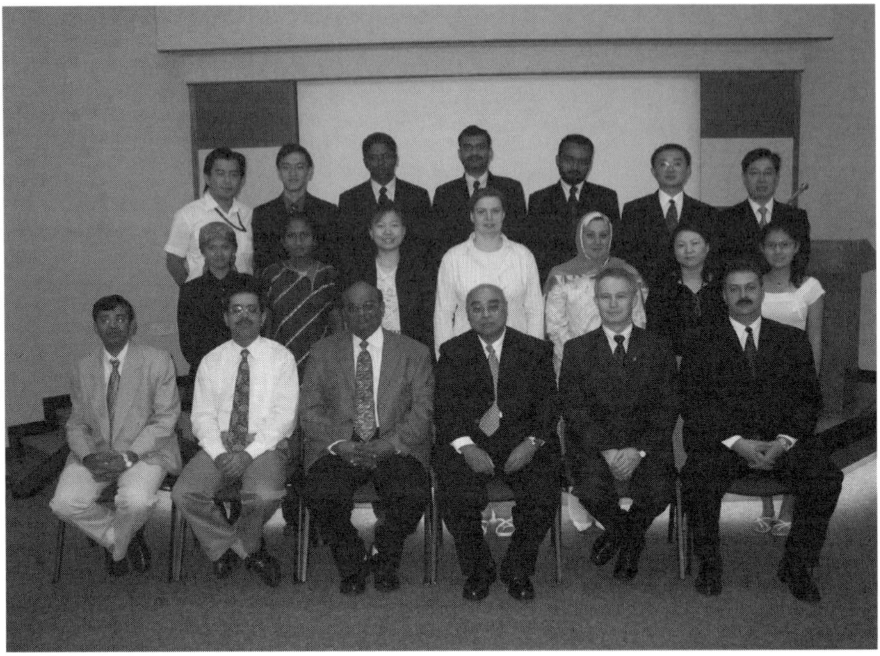

Fig. 5. Convocation of first internet course in 2005 (sixth batch).

on building the online curriculum, and another US$100 000 on setting up hardware at the ICC; yet after only running one internet course, the IAEA disappeared from the scene. As a result, the ICC and the regions (Asia-Pacific, Latin America, and Korea) were left to fend for themselves. The less developed countries like Bangladesh, Pakistan, Myanmar, Sri Lanka, and Vietnam stopped sending students to the ICC; in fact, they disappeared from tissue banking activities altogether and stopped attending APASTB Meetings as well.

Korean national training course

In the midst of this gloomy post-IAEA era, the hustle and bustle of activities stirring in Korea was a comfort to the region, the ICC, and the APASTB.

Korea had initially translated the Multi-Media Curriculum into Korean in 2003. In November 2003, the first Korean national training course (KNTC) was held. It was hosted by the course director, Professor Yong Koo Kang;

Table 1. Regional distribution of tissue bank operators registered (1997–2006).

Batch no.	No. of students registered				
	Asia-Pacific	Latin America	Africa	Europe	Australia
First batch (Nov 1997–Oct 1998)	18	0	0	0	
Second batch (Apr 1999–Mar 2000)	16	0	0	1 (Slovakia)	
Third batch (Apr 2000–Mar 2001)	19	2 (1 Brazil) (1 Chile)	0	0	
Fourth batch (Apr 2001–Mar 2002)	19	0	3 (2 Zambia) (1 Algeria)	2 (1 Greece) (1 Slovakia)	
Fifth batch (Apr 2002–Aug 2003)	14	3 (1 Cuba) (1 Peru) (1 Uruguay)	3 (1 Egypt) (1 Libya) (1 Zambia)	1 (Poland)	
Sixth batch (Feb 2004–Feb 2005)	12	1 (USA)	2 (1 Libya) (1 Algeria)	5 (3 Slovakia) (1 Ukraine) (1 Poland)	
Seventh batch (Mar 2005–Mar 2006)	17				
Eighth batch (Apr 2006–Apr 2007)	18		2 (South Africa)		2
Total	133	6	12	9	2

Table 2. Results of the IAEA/NUS diploma courses conducted (1997–2006).

Batch no.	No. of students registered	No. of students convocated	Results			
			Distinction	Credit	Pass	Fail
First batch (Nov 1997–Oct 1998)	18	12	4	5	3	6
Second batch (Apr 1999–Mar 2000)	17	15	2	5	8	2
Third batch (Apr 2000–Mar 2001)	21	17	1	5	11	4
Fourth batch (Apr 2001–Mar 2002)	24	19	1	11	7	5
Fifth batch (Apr 2002–Aug 2003)	21	14	3	8	3	7
Sixth batch (Feb 2004–Feb 2005)	19	12	4	5	3	7
Seventh batch (Mar 2005–Mar 2006)	18	13	5	6	2	5
Eighth batch (Apr 2006–Apr 2007)	22					
Total	160	102	20	45	37	36

and was jointly run by the Korean Association of Tissue Banks (KATB), of which Professor Kang is the president, and the Korean Musculoskeletal Transplantation Society (KMTS), of which Professor Kang is the chairman of the Education Subcommittee. The first convocation ceremony was held in December 2004, with 11 out of 12 students convocating (Fig. 6).

The second KNTC was held in December 2004 with 12 students, of which 10 students convocated in December 2005 (Fig. 7). The third KNTC was conducted in December 2005 with 22 students, with 18 students convocating in December 2006 (Fig. 8). The fourth batch was launched in December 2006 with 25 students. After a 3-year term, Dr Il-Young Park was appointed as the new course director for the KNTC (2006–2009), replacing Dr Yong Koo Kang.

Korea has clearly set an example for other countries to follow. The IAEA and NUS have developed an "expressway" with the ICC and the IAEA/NUS internet curriculum. It is up to individual countries to build roads linking this expressway to their own countries and to run their own national

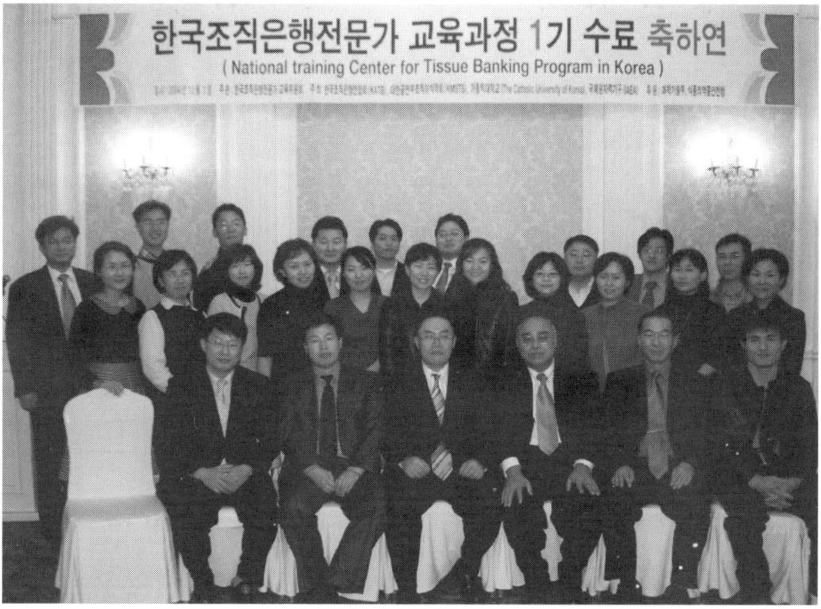

Fig. 6. Convocation ceremony of 1st KNTC in 2004.

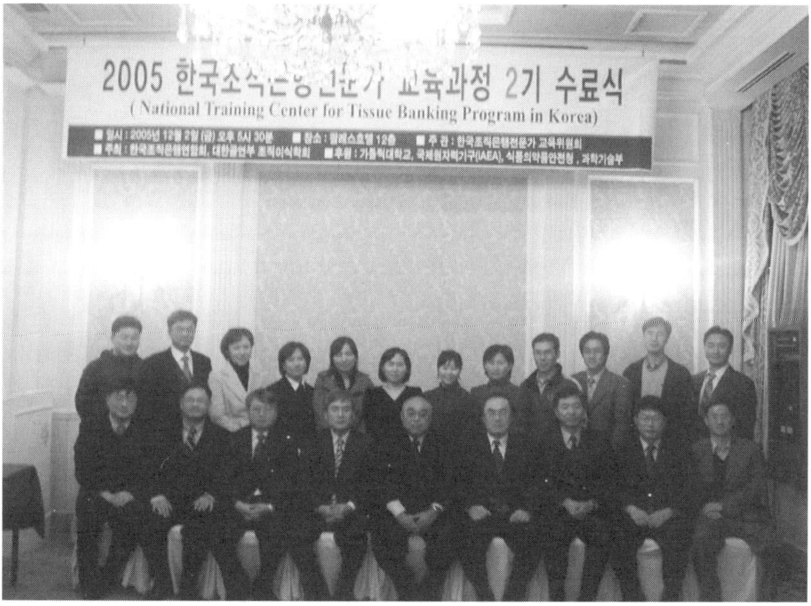

Fig. 7. Convocation ceremony of 2nd KNTC in 2005.

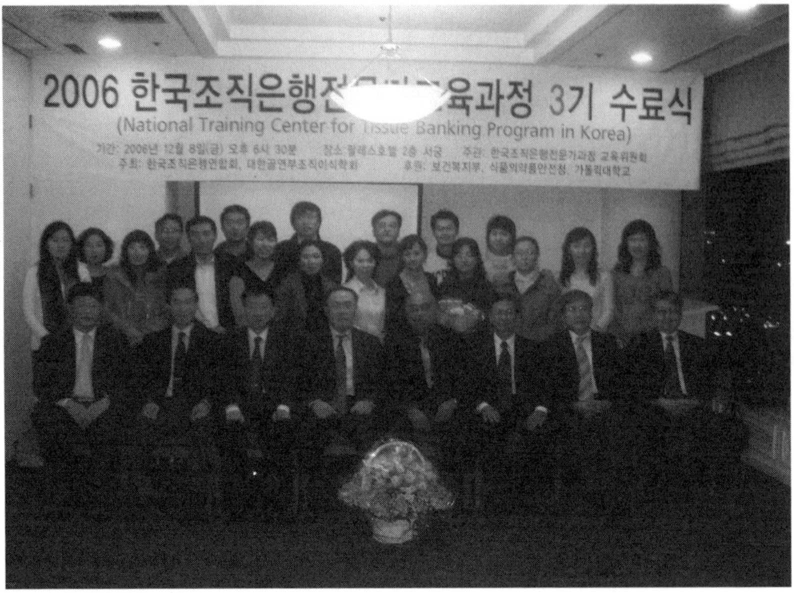

Fig. 8. Convocation ceremony of 3rd KNTC in 2006.

training centers. Potential countries to do this include India, Malaysia, and Indonesia.

Asia Pacific Association of Surgical Tissue Banks (APASTB)

The APASTB was set up in October 1988 with its secretariat initially in Bangkok, and with Dr Vajadul as its first president and Dr Nather as its first vice president (Nather *et al.* 2005a).

Presidents of the APASTB

Dr Yongyudh Vajadul	Thailand	1988–1990
Dr Aziz Nather	Singapore	1990–1992
Dr Moritoshi Itoman	Japan	1992–1994
Dr Norberto Agcaoili	Philippines	1994–1996
Dr Sun Shiquan	China	1996–1998
Dr David Morgan	Australia	1998–2000

Dr Hasim Mohamad	Malaysia	2000–2002
Dr Abdurrahman	Indonesia	2002–2004
Dr Chang Joon Yim	Korea	2004–2006
Dr Shekhar Kumta	Hong Kong	2006–2008

Scientific meetings of the APASTB

Inaugural	Thailand	1989	Dr Y. Vajaradul
Second	Singapore	1990	Dr A. Nather
Third	Japan	1991	Dr M. Itoman
Fourth	Philippines	1992	Dr N. Agcaoili
Fifth	China	1994	Dr Tang Zhongyi
Sixth	Australia	1996	Dr D. Morgan
Seventh	Malaysia	1998	Dr H. Mohamad
Eighth	Indonesia	2000	Dr Abdurrahman
Ninth	Korea	2002	Dr J. Y. Chang
Tenth	Hong Kong	2004	Dr S. Kumta
Eleventh (Fig.9)	India	2006	Dr A. L. Gajiwala
Twelfth	Malaysia	2008	Dr H. Mohamad
Thirteenth	Singapore	2010	Dr A. Nather

Current office bearers of the APASTB, 2006–2008

Immediate Past President	Chang Joon Yim	Korea
President	Shekhar Kumta	Hong Kong
First Vice President	Astrid Lobo Gajiwala	India
Second Vice President	Norimah Yusof	Malaysia
Third Vice President	Yong Koo Kang	Korea
Secretary-General	Menkher Manjas	Indonesia
Assistant Secretary-General	Il-Young Park	Korea
Treasurer	Abdul Halim Sukari	Malaysia
Auditors	Moritoshi Itoman	Japan
	Hasim Mohamad	Malaysia
Editors	Aziz Nather	Singapore
	Norimah Yusof	Malaysia

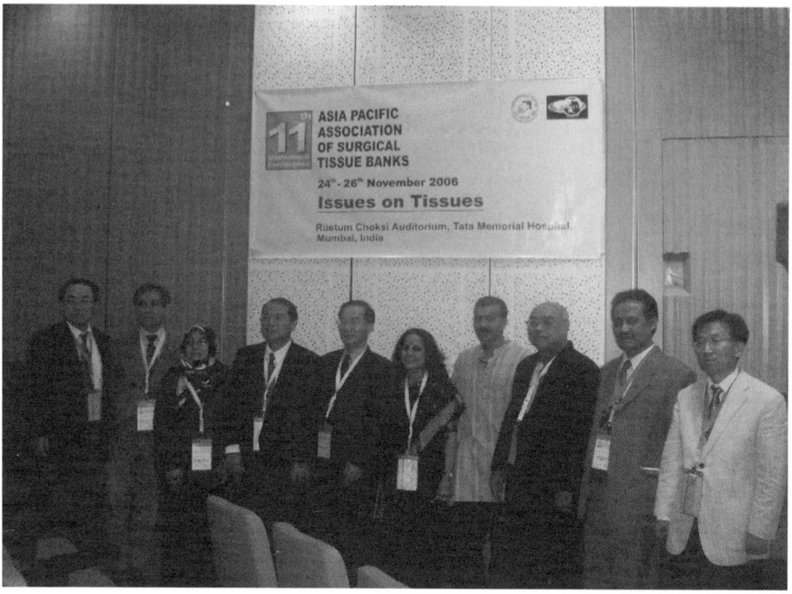

Fig. 9. 11th APASTB Meeting in Mumbai, India, on November 26–28, 2006.

Current status of the APASTB

There are now up to 200 members in the APASTB. The APASTB produces a yearly newsletter. It has just completed its first edition of "Standards for Tissue Banking", which was printed in January 2007 for distribution to all members (Fig. 10) (Appendix 1).

World congresses on tissue banking

- The 1st World Congress on Tissue Banking — involving the APASTB, EATB, and AATB — was hosted by the APASTB in October 1996 at the Gold Coast, Australia. Chairman: Dr David Morgan.
- The 2nd World Congress on Tissue Banking and the 8th International Conference of the EATB were held in Warsaw, Poland, on October 7–10, 1999. Chairman: Dr Janus Komender.
- The 3rd World Congress on Tissue Banking was held in Boston, USA, in 2002. Chairman: Dr Samuel Doppelt.
- The 4th World Congress on Tissue Banking was held in Brazil, Latin America, in May 2005. Chairperson: Dr Marisa Herson.

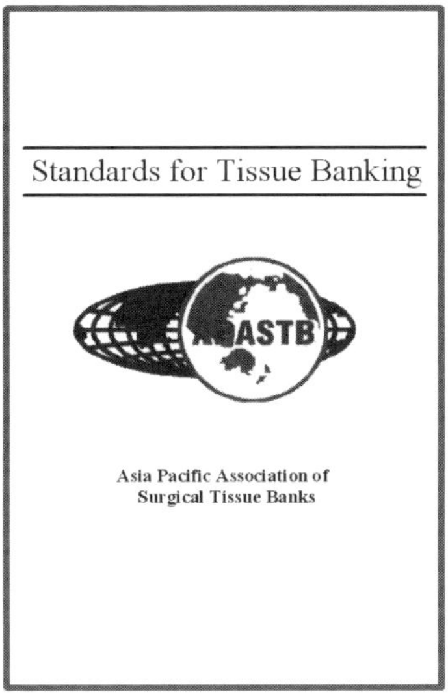

Fig. 10. APASTB Standards for Tissue Banking.

- The 5th World Congress on Tissue Banking — in conjunction with the 12th International Conference of the APASTB — will be hosted by the APASTB in June 2008 in Kuala Lumpur, Malaysia. Chairman: Dr Hasim Mohamad; Secretary: Dr Norimah Yusof.

Future of Tissue Banking in the Asia-Pacific Region

Threat of tissue engineering

Despite the advances in tissue engineering, tissue banks continue to thrive. The failure to produce scaffolds capable of fulfilling both the biological and biomechanical functions of the tissues replaced has been a big failure for tissue engineering.

Existing artificial scaffolds for bone — tricalcium phosphate, hydroxyapatite, and polycaprolactone — are only of cancellous strength (about 30 megapascals), but scaffolds of cortical strength (about 200 megapascals) are needed. In the absence of the latter, bone allografts (natural scaffolds) currently present as the best scaffolds for tissue engineering. Until technology improves further, natural scaffolds will still remain the best scaffolds. The situation with scaffolds for ligaments is even worse, as poly(L-lactide) and polyglycolic acid are only of suture strength. Again, ligament allografts (natural scaffolds) are the best scaffolds at present.

The way forward is to combine the use of bone and ligament allografts with mesenchymal stem cells (MSCs) and growth factors. Dr Nather has shown that the addition of MSCs to cortical bone allografts in adult rabbits enhanced union at the host–graft junction and improved the biological incorporation of the allograft in terms of increased resorption index, cortical new bone formation index, and osteocyte index. He also showed that the addition of autologous platelet-rich plasma (PRP) enhanced union in an identical model of the host–graft junctions; increased resorption activity greatly; and increased the new bone formation index and osteocyte index slightly, but not to the same degree as seen with MSCs. More research is needed on the value of PRP. Research is also needed to see if MSCs added with PRP in combination to allografts produce similar or better results than when MSCs and PRP are added to bone allografts in isolation. In the near future, it is anticipated that the use of MSCs and growth factors using Good Manufacturing Practice (GMP) facilities in combination with bone and ligament allograft transplantation in patients will give better results.

Factors influencing the development of tissue banking in the Asia-Pacific region

These include the following:

- China factor — There must be 100 or more tissue banks in China. They run large national training centres, but have remained quiet so far. Once China modernizes, it will have a large influence on the region.
- India factor — India is another subcontinent that has just awakened. Chennai, Coimbatore, Kerala, Kolkata, Mumbai, and New Delhi are setting up new tissue banks and no longer using formalin-preserved allografts, which posed a major obstacle to the progress of tissue banking in India to follow internationally accepted standards for nearly two decades. 2006 proved to be a good year. Six centers have approached Dr Nather to set up new tissue banks that meet international standards. Dr Nather is confident that India will set up not only new tissue banks, but also its own national training program (possibly in Chennai) with Dr Mayil Natarajan (current

president of the Indian Orthopaedic Association) leading the way. Once developed, India is also expected to exert a large influence on the region.

- Australia factor — The development of a private tissue bank in New South Wales by Australian Biotechnologies (a for-profit organization) and a mega-institutional bone bank in Brisbane is expected to have a possible influence on tissue banking in the region.
- Privatization factor — Privatization is growing in the region. There are already two private tissue banks in Korea (Bioland and Hans Biomed) and one in Australia. This will have a large influence on the balance of tissue banking in the region. On the whole, most countries in the Asia-Pacific region are against for-profit organizations, but may not be averse to nonprofit organizations.

Role of the World Health Organization

The World Health Organization (WHO) has taken an active lead in the global field of tissue banking now that the IAEA has relinquished its role. The WHO intends to set up the ICC in Singapore as a WHO center within 1 or 2 years. The whole world is now looking towards the WHO to play an active role in regulating and promoting tissue banking activities in the wake of the large vacuum left behind by the IAEA.

References

Nather A (2000a). Tissue banking in Asia Pacific region — ethical, legal, religious, cultural and other regulatory aspects. *ASEAN Orthop Assoc* **13**(1):60–63.

Nather A (2000b). Diploma training for technologists in tissue banking. *Cell Tissue Bank* **1**(1):41–44.

Nather A (ed.) (2001). *The Scientific Basis of Tissue Transplantation*. World Scientific, Singapore.

Nather A, Ong HJC, Feng MCB, and Aziz Z (2005a). Asia-Pacific Association of Surgical Tissue Banking — past, present and future. *ASEAN Orthop Assoc* **17**(1):17–19.

Nather A, Teo WY, and Wang LH (2005b). Diploma course training of tissue bank operators: 7 years of experience. In: Nather A (ed.), *Bone Grafts and Bone Substitutions: Basic Science and Clinical Applications*, World Scientific, Singapore, pp. 213–226.

Nather A and Wang LH (2002). Bone banking in Singapore — fourteen years of experience. *ASEAN Orthop Assoc* **15**(1):20–29.

Phillips GO (ed.) (2000). *Radiation and Tissue Banking*. World Scientific, Singapore.

Reuters AFP (1999). Media frenzy shocks heart-donors family. Breaking of taboo. *The Straits Times*, Tuesday, March.

Chapter 4

Ethical, Religious, Legal, and Cultural Issues in Tissue Banking

Aziz Nather*, Ahmad Hafiz Zulkifly† and Eileen Sim*

**NUH Tissue Bank*
Department of Orthopaedic Surgery
Yong Loo Lin School of Medicine
National University of Singapore
Singapore

†Department of Orthopaedics, Traumatology and Rehabilitation
Kulliyah of Medicine
International Islamic University Malaysia
Malaysia

Introduction

Every country has its own set of ethical, religious, legal, and cultural factors that affects the development and success of local tissue banks. This chapter discusses the common issues encountered in tissue banking in the Asia-Pacific region.

Ethical Issues

Tissue donation is an act of humanity, as it enables one to alleviate the sufferings of fellow human beings. Ideally, tissue banks should not sell tissues, but rather provide tissue grafts on a noncommercial basis without any profit motive. As costs are incurred during procurement, processing, and distribution, tissue banks may charge "processing costs", provided the law (if any) of the country makes provisions to allow for the retrieval of such costs. A common acceptable practice in institution banks is to work out the total costs of such procurement and processing — including manpower costs, equipment maintenance costs, cost of consumables, electricity and water consumption costs, etc. — and then charge the recipients using these tissues to pay for such costs (Nather 2000). Some tissue banks in the Asia-Pacific region charge processing costs, e.g. Japan, Singapore, Malaysia, Sri Lanka, and India.

In the Asia-Pacific region, commercial tissue banks do not operate in most countries. Only Korea has two or three commercial tissue banks; in the remaining countries, commercial banks are generally not favored. The view held by most countries in terms of developing commercial or private banks is to favor not-for-profit institutions, and most of them are against for-profit institutions if commercialization is to take place at all.

In Europe, tissue banks are obliged to comply with the Ethical Code of the European Association of Tissue Banks (EATB). Likewise, in the United States, the American Association of Tissue Banks (AATB) publishes standards to help ensure that the conduct of tissue banking meets acceptable norms of technical and ethical performance. No similar formal ethical code has been produced for the Asia-Pacific region, however. Nevertheless, tissue banks in this region also comply with all of the principles enunciated in the Ethical Code of the EATB. The guiding principle followed by all tissue bank operators is based on moral principles, human duty, and proper conduct, as enshrined in the Hippocratic Oath (which requires doctors and health workers to *non nocere* or "not injure").

Tissue banking helps to reduce a country's healthcare costs (Hachiya *et al.* 1999). Allogeneic bone grafts are less expensive than custom-made prostheses or ceramics, which can be costly. Commercially produced bone allografts are also prohibitive in costs. However, bone allografts produced by noncommercial or institution tissue banks are often either provided free of charge or at nominal costs ("processing costs only"), thus reducing the patient's medical costs.

Religious Issues

Tissue donation is a sensitive issue that invokes important concerns regarding the dignity of the living and the dead, the concept of brain death, and the concept that tissue donation is the greatest gift one can bestow upon fellow human beings after one's death. The answers to these questions are inextricably tied to the dominant religious and cultural mindsets within each country. In this regard, the culture of an ethnic group is often inseparable from the religion followed by that group. Hence, religion plays a major role in promoting or retarding the development of tissue banking in each country. The major religions in the Asia-Pacific region are Buddhism, Islam, Christianity, and Hinduism.

Buddhism

The attitude of Buddhism is in perfect agreement with tissue donation (Nather 2000). In Buddhist scriptures, there are stories where the donation of tissues has been referred to as acts of charity that earn merit. Buddhists are expected to meditate about the impermanence of life. The body will decay, just as a beautiful fragrant flower withers and decays. The concept of tissue donation is encouraged not only after death; even while living, tissue donation is considered to be a meritorious act.

In countries where Buddhism is the predominant religion, there is no shortage of tissue donors. These countries include Sri Lanka, Thailand, Vietnam, and Myanmar. The most successful public awareness programs on tissue donation have been achieved in Thailand, Sri Lanka, and Vietnam. The decision to set up the Model Human Tissue Bank in Sri Lanka by the International Atomic Energy Agency was greatly influenced by the world-renowned success of the Eye Donation Society — which, led by Dr Hudson Silva, achieved its target of procuring 40 000 eyes by May 1999 — coupled with the abundance of tissue donors in this predominantly Buddhist country (more than 90% are Buddhists).

Buddhism is also one of the major religions, although not the predominant one, in Korea (about 30%) and Singapore (about 30%). The success of the National University Hospital Tissue Bank in Singapore is largely due to the fact that the Buddhist community in Singapore strongly supports the tissue transplantation program. All tissue donors in Singapore are Buddhists.

Islam

Muslims are by far the most vocal group against tissue donation. The Islamic states in the Asia-Pacific region include Pakistan, Bangladesh, Malaysia, and Brunei. In addition, Islam is the predominant religion in

Indonesia, a secular country that follows the five principles of *Pancasila*. There are about 200 million Muslims in China, another secular country. Islam is also an important religion in other secular countries, such as Singapore (about 20%) and India (about 40%) (Nather 2000).

The Koran respects life and values the needs of the living over those of the dead. This means that organ donation and transplantation can be considered in circumstances when it would save a person's life. No mention is made about allowing transplantation to improve the quality of life of a recipient. As a result, Muslims are more likely to allow kidney donation and less likely to allow tissue donation, as the latter is perceived as merely improving the quality of (rather than saving) life. Nevertheless, while interpretations of the Koran vary according to different religious leaders, e.g. between the ustazs and the ulamas, tissue donation is not explicitly forbidden in the Koran (Nather 2000).

Countries with a significant Muslim presence have their own muftis. A mufti is a religious official who is appointed by the government to deal with all Islamic matters in the country, including the issue of organ and tissue donation. Fatwas are religious rulings made by a fatwa committee as an official stand by the government on certain issues, e.g. the tissue donation and transplantation issue. The fatwa committee — chaired by the mufti — may include prominent religious leaders, lawyers, doctors, and members of the public.

A common misconception among Muslims is that organ and tissue donation is not permitted by the Islamic Law. However, fatwas concerning organ donation have been declared in several countries in the Asia-Pacific region, including Malaysia, Brunei, and Singapore. A fatwa was passed in Saudi Arabia in 1985 sanctioning both the live and cadaveric donation of organs. Likewise, in 1998, a fatwa was passed in the United Arab Emirates that sanctioned live and cadaveric organ donation as well as organ donation from Muslims to non-Muslims, and that accepted the concept of brain death (El-Shahat 1999).

A milestone event for fatwas specific to tissue donation occurred on September 4, 1995, when the first fatwa on bone, skin, and amnion was introduced by the Malaysian Islamic Centre. This was followed on June 29, 1997, by a fatwa on bone, skin, and amnion in Indonesia, sanctioning tissue procurement from deceased donors. This was a great leap forward for

Indonesia, as the previous law — the Indonesia 1992 Health Regulation — allowed tissue procurement only from living donors. Unfortunately, efforts by Dr Nather since 1995 to seek a similar fatwa for Muslims in Singapore from the *Majlis Ugama Islam Singapura* (Religious Council of Islamic Singapore) have not succeeded so far, although a fatwa for cornea was passed in 1999 — the first fatwa for tissues in Singapore.

However, fatwas are not legally binding, and so the decision to donate remains very much the prerogative of the individual and his/her family. Hence, the introduction of favorable fatwas is only the first step in promoting public acceptance of tissue donation among Muslims.

Another important consideration for Muslims is that they must bury the body as soon as possible after death. Therefore, procedures like tissue procurement, which may delay the burial, are not taken very kindly.

Culturally, Muslims accept that God created them whole and they prefer to return to Him whole. It is a common practice among many Muslims to bury amputated limbs, foreskins from circumcision, and amnions from delivery. This is a cultural practice, not a religious requirement. Not all Muslims follow this practice.

In addition, there is the less obvious *halal* and *haram* concept. Muslims cannot consume certain food items such as pork (which is considered *haram* or "forbidden") and alcohol. Food allowed for consumption are called *halal*. However, it is permissible for medical purposes to use porcine heart valves and medicines containing alcohol. Nevertheless, strict Muslims may choose to avoid all *haram* items altogether and seek other options instead. As a result, many Muslims tend to reject organs and tissue from non-Muslims, who consume pork and do not observe the *halal* and *haram* concept. The concept of a *halal* tissue from a Muslim donor for transplantation to a Muslim recipient is very attractive to them. Indeed, *halal* hospitals have proven to be very popular in Malaysia. However, in countries where Muslims form a minority, e.g. in Singapore (where only 20% of the population are Muslims and nearly all of the donors are Buddhists), such practices are not feasible.

Therefore, it does not come as a surprise that there is a big shortage of bone donors in countries where Islam is the predominant religion, including Pakistan, Bangladesh, Malaysia, and Indonesia. The lack of donors also slows down the development of tissue banking in these countries. They have been successful in procuring amnion, but not bones and ligaments, from deceased donors.

In Islam, the *waris* issue is also important. When a person dies, the *waris* or "next of kin" plays a key role as to what happens to the body of the deceased. Even if the donor has consented, the next of kin must also consent if tissue donation is to be allowed. For Muslims, therefore, consent is required not only from the patient, but also from his/her next of kin or *waris*.

Nevertheless, the demand for tissues in these countries is great and steadily increasing. Indonesia and Malaysia have resorted to the production of bovine bone xenografts for bone transplantation until such time that public awareness programs can produce better results (Nather 2000). Specific fatwas for bone have been passed in both countries, but they have not produced significant changes in the Muslim population's attitude towards tissue donation. More public education is needed to change entrenched cultural practices and beliefs, along with the passing of fatwas, before more Muslims will come forward and pledge to be tissue donors.

Christianity

Christianity is the predominant religion in the Philippines and Australia. Nather (2000) showed that it is also one of the major religions, though not the predominant one, in Korea (about 30%) and Singapore (about 30%).

Tissue donation is considered to be consistent with the ecclesiastical Christian dogma of loving one's neighbor as oneself, as it is thought to be an act of genuine altruism — of giving something up at little or no cost to the donor to save the lives of others. This was reiterated by the late Pope John Paul II while attending the Congress of the Society for Organ Sharing on June 20, 1991, when he quoted from the Bible: "'Give, and it will be given to you; good measure, passed down, shaken together, running over, will be put into your lap' (Luke 6:38). We shall receive our supreme reward from God according to the genuine and effective love we have shown to our neighbor." These words are in full support of organ and tissue donation and transplantation. Christian communities in Europe and the USA support tissue transplantation. For instance, on the weekend of November 13–15, 1998, churches and synagogues across the US encouraged their faithful to sign donor cards (*Japan Times* 1998).

Despite the strong Christian presence in the Philippines and Korea, however, other factors (including cultural factors) have led to a shortage of donors in these countries. The cultural concept is again that God created them whole and they would like to return to Him whole, not physically altered by the act of tissue donation.

Hinduism

Hinduism is the predominant religion of India, a secular country. It is also an important religion in Sri Lanka (about 10%), Singapore (about 10%), and Malaysia (10%).

Hinduism is parallel to Buddhism in many ways, and it has no objection to tissue donation and transplantation. Devotees of both religions practice cremation of the body, which is in fact an act of destruction of the body, in front of and with full knowledge of the relatives. Therefore, resistance to the concept of tissue donation is not expected (Nather 2000).

Legal Issues

There is no universal law governing tissue procurement and tissue transplantation for the various countries in the Asia-Pacific region. If regulatory laws are present in some of these countries, they are based on similar human transplantation acts practiced in Europe and the USA. These acts cover a wide range of issues, including the definition of brain death, the definition of tissues and organs, the issue of consent for organ donation (either by the donor or next of kin), and the prohibition of trade in human organs.

Two different legal frameworks are seen to be operating in the Asia-Pacific region: the "opting-in" system based on informed consent, and the "opting-out" system based on presumed consent. For instance, while Malaysia follows the opting-in system for kidneys and corneas, Singapore follows the opting-out system under the 1987 Human Organ Transplant Act for kidneys only; in 2004, this opting-out act was extended to include corneas. It should be noted that in almost all countries, these laws are specifically designed for organ transplantation. Tissue procurement can be carried out only by following such laws for organs.

Singapore

Tissue procurement in Singapore follows the Medical (Therapy, Education and Research) Act of 1972, whereby "any person of sound mind and eighteen years of age or above may give all or any part of his body for education … transplantation. . . . The gift takes effect upon death" (Nather 2000).

More recently, the Human Organ Transplant Act was passed in 1987. It is based on presumed consent, and "makes provision for the removal of kidneys from the bodies of persons who are citizens or permanent residents, who have died from accidents, for transplantation purposes only. Muslims and persons over 60 years old are exempted from provisions of this Act." The seven criteria for brain death are also described in this Act. An amendment to the Act in 2004 extended the list of tissues procured to include the liver, heart, and cornea, and extended the donor pool to nonaccidental causes of death, among other changes.

Australia

The donation of human tissue in Australia is regulated by the legislation in each of the eight states and territories under substantially uniform acts (known as the Human Tissue Act in some states, and as the Transplantation and Anatomy Act in others), which were passed in the late 1970s and early 1980s. Most provisions require consent from the donors or from the families of brain-dead heart-beating donors, with the exception of tissues removed at autopsies that can be used for transplant, therapeutic, educational, and research purposes without further reference to the next of kin. Nonetheless, the tissue banking sector in Australia has, for the most part, sought to include consultation with next of kins in their protocol for practical and ethical purposes (Ireland and McKelvie 2003).

India

The procurement of tissues for transplantation in India is governed by the Transplantation of Human Organs Act, which was enacted in 1994. However, as healthcare comes under the purview of state governments, this Act is applicable only when a state adopts it. Fourteen states have yet to approve of it (Gajiwala 2003).

A human organ as defined by this Act is any part of the human body consisting of a structured arrangement of tissues that cannot be replicated by the body if wholly removed. There is no specific mention of particular organs. Under the Act, therapeutic purposes are defined as the systemic treatment of any disease or the measures to improve health according to any particular method or modality. The Act recognizes brain stem death, which needs to be certified by four qualified medical practitioners approved by the state. The removal of organs is subject to prior written consent from the deceased or from the person who is lawfully in possession of the dead body, with the exception of the removal of organs from bodies sent for postmortem examination. In the latter case, the Act authorizes the removal of organs for therapeutic purposes, provided there were no known objections from the deceased person.

While regulations specific to tissue banking have yet to be developed, the Transplantation of Human Organ Rules was issued by the Government of India in 1995 to combat the illegal trading of human organs. It has since been adopted by the state of Maharashtra (Gajiwala 2003).

Malaysia

The transplantation of cadaveric tissues in Malaysia is governed by the Human Tissues Act 1974, which enables the removal of tissues from cadavers for therapeutic, medical education, and research purposes under two conditions: at the express request of the donor, which may be given at any time either in writing or orally stated during the deceased's last illness in the presence of two witnesses; or in the absence of objection from the deceased and with the consent of the next of kin (Kassim 2005).

The word "tissue" is not defined in this Act. Likewise, "the person lawfully in possession of the body" is not defined, nor is there an articulation of a hierarchy of relatives deemed to be the next of kin. More significantly, the current Act does not provide an exact definition of death. Presently, the Act only requires two fully registered medical practitioners to confirm (upon personal examination of the body) that life is extinct. There is no inclusion of brain death in this Act as a method of determining death, although brain-dead donors are a source of organs in cadaveric organ transplantation. With regard to fatwas specific for tissue donation, the first fatwa on bone, skin, and amnion was introduced by the Malaysian Islamic Centre on September 4, 1995 (Nather 2000).

Sri Lanka

Sri Lanka follows The Human Tissue Transplantation Act No. 48 of 1987, which requires consent from the donor or next of kin.

Philippines

In the Philippines, tissue donation follows The Republic Act 7170, 1991, which authorizes the legacy or donation of all or part of the human body after death for specified purposes (Nather 2000).

Vietnam

Tissue procurement in Vietnam is provided for by the Civil Code, Article 32, Chapter 2, where consent is needed from the donor or next of kin; and by The People's Health Protection Code, Chapter 4, which provides for tissue transplantation (Nather 2000).

Indonesia

Indonesia is unique in the region in that its legislation for tissue procurement is incomplete. The Indonesian 1992 Health Regulation provides for the procurement of tissues from living donors, but not from deceased donors. A fatwa for bone, skin, and amnion was introduced by the Religious Council on June 29, 1997, permitting tissue procurement from cadaveric donors (Nather 2000).

Japan

Japan has the Law Concerning Human Organ Transplants, which was passed in 1997. According to this Law, organs can be removed only if the donor has expressed his/her intention with respect to the definition of death and organ donation in a written document beforehand, and if the family has already signed the donor card and also agreed with organ removal (the family has the authority to veto an individual's organ donation by refusing to sign the donor card). Brain death is defined under this Law as "an irreversible cessation of all functions of the entire brain including brain stem." Under the Law, individuals are able to choose a definition of death, either brain death or traditional cardiac death, according to their own personal views on human death.

As of December 2005, only 33 brain-dead cases have been used for organ transplantation (Bagheri 2005). The first of these cases was performed on February 28, 1999, when a liver, a heart, and two kidneys were legally procured from a brain-dead donor in Kochi and air-flown for transplantation to four recipients in four other Japanese cities (Reuters/AFP 1999). It was hoped that this landmark event would change the legal environment to favor tissue transplantation in Japan (Nather 2000). Unfortunately, this has not happened.

Korea

The Organ Transplantation Law was passed in Korea in 2000. Under the Law, brain death is defined as the irreversible cessation of the whole brain function, and has to be diagnosed by two specialist doctors and the patients' physician as well as approved by a brain-death determination committee. Donor consent is required for organ removal, but the family has strong veto power towards organ transplantation. The Korean Network for Organ Sharing is a centralized authority for organ procurement. Since the Law was enacted, the number of brain death diagnoses and donations has decreased. Before the Law was enforced, 162 cases were diagnosed as brain dead; as of 2003, only 43 cases were diagnosed (Bagheri 2005).

Bangladesh

The Tissue Donation and Transplantation Act was passed in Bangladesh in April 1999, permitting donation from live and cadaveric donors (Nather 2000).

Countries with no law

In contrast, several countries in the Asia-Pacific region do not have any law concerning tissue procurement and transplantation. Such countries include Thailand, China, and Myanmar.

In Myanmar, no law for tissue donation exists, apart from the Eye Donation Law. In China, although there is no human transplantation act, transplantation is nevertheless practiced in accordance with the principle of written consent for donation prior to the patient's death or from the next of kin.

Cultural Issues

Culturally, certain issues have to be resolved before organ donation and transplantation can take off in any country. These issues include the concept that organ harvesting is a form of disrespect towards the dead because the body is no longer as intact as before, and the dangers of commodifying body parts.

Culturally, Muslims accept that God created them whole and they prefer to return to Him whole. Islam does not explicitly forbid donation. However, the cultural practice among many Muslims is to bury amputated limbs, and even foreskin from circumcision and amnion from delivery. There is thus a big shortage of bone donors in Muslim countries. Likewise, Christianity promotes organ and tissue donation. However, there is a shortage of donors in Christian-dominant countries like the Philippines, due to the cultural attitudes of the people who also prefer to return to God whole.

To overcome cultural barriers, there is a need for more public awareness programs on the need for and benefits of tissue donation and tissue transplantation in the community. This is needed to address the cultural and religious issues that may hinder tissue donation. In addition, there is also a need for professional awareness among doctors to encourage surgeons to carry out more tissue transplantations.

References

Bagheri A (2005). Organ transplantation laws in Asian countries: a comparative study. *Transplant Proc* **37**:4159–4162.

El-Shahat YIM (1999). Islamic viewpoint of organ transplantation. *Transplant Proc* **31**:3271–3274.

Gajiwala AL (2003). Setting up a tissue bank in India: the Tata Memorial Hospital experience. *Cell Tissue Bank* **4**:193–201.

Hachiya Y, Sakai T, Narita Y, Izawa H, and Yoshizawa K (1999). Status of bone banks in Japan. *Transplant Proc* **31**:2032–2035.

Ireland L and McKelvie H (2003). Tissue banking in Australia. *Cell Tissue Bank* **4**:151–156.

Japan Times (1998). November 15.

Kassim PN (2005). Organ transplantation in Malaysia: a need for a comprehensive legal regime. *Med Law* **24**:173–189.

Laws of Malaysia (1974). Act 130: Human Tissues Act, 1974. Ketua Pengarah Percetakan.

Nather A (2000). Tissue banking in Asia Pacific region — ethical, legal, religious, cultural and other regulatory aspects. *J ASEAN Orthop Assoc* **13**:60–63.

Reuters/AFP (1999). Media frenzy shocks heart-donors family. Breaking of taboo. *The Straits Times*, March.

Chapter 5

Setting Up a Tissue Bank

Aziz Nather and Chris C. W. Lee

NUH Tissue Bank
Department of Orthopaedic Surgery
Yong Loo Lin School of Medicine
National University of Singapore
Singapore

Introduction

Dr Nather has been contracted by the International Atomic Energy Agency as an IAEA expert to set up tissue banks in several countries. Between the years 1994 to 2000, he helped to set up tissue banks in several countries, including 1 in Japan, 3 in Malaysia, 2 in Vietnam, 1 in Sri Lanka, 1 in Myanmar, 2 in Hong Kong, 1 in Zambia, 1 in Argentina, 1 in Brazil, and 1 in Cuba. More recently, he has set up 1 tissue bank in Korea, 1 in Indonesia, 2 more in Malaysia, and 1 in India.

In setting up a tissue bank, one must consider the following factors in detail:

- Religious and cultural issues of the population in the country
- Legal status of organ or tissue procurement and transplantation in the country
- Level and extent of support provided by the government
- Demand for tissue allograft transplantation in the country
- Commitment of the professionals setting up the tissue bank

Religious and cultural issues

These issues play a crucial role in deciding whether a bank will succeed or not. In countries where the population is predominantly Buddhist, tissue banking is likely to prosper. This is because the philosophy of Buddhism is in perfect harmony with favoring organ and tissue donation (Nather 2000a). In Sri Lanka, Thailand, and Vietnam, countries where Buddhism is the predominant religion, there is no shortage of donors. In contrast, organ and tissue donors are not forthcoming in countries where the religion is predominantly Islam, e.g. Bangladesh, Pakistan, Malaysia, and Indonesia. To be sure, Islam does not explicitly forbid tissue donation. However, culturally the Muslims prefer to return to God whole. They bury everything alongside a deceased's body, including amputated limbs, foreskin from circumcision, and even amnion from delivery (Nather 2000a).

Legal issues

The presence of the Tissue Transplantation Act has been a significant factor in promoting the development of tissue banks in several countries, such as Singapore, Hong Kong, and India (Nather 2000a). In Japan, although the concept of brain death was introduced into law in 1997, tissue donation has not progressed. In contrast, with the introduction of the brain death concept into law in Korea in 2000, tissue banking has prospered and many new banks have been set up. On the other hand, the absence of any law for tissue procurement has not hampered the progress of tissue banking in several countries, including China and Thailand.

Potential government support

In countries where the government — specifically the Ministry of Health — is keen to back the tissue banking program (usually in alignment with kidney, liver, and cornea transplantation programs), the program is likely to succeed. Strong government support has been responsible for the success of tissue banking in Singapore, Hong Kong, and Malaysia (Nather 2000a). In contrast, in countries where the government priority is on other aspects of health, the development of tissue banking is fraught with difficulty.

Demand for tissue transplantation

Before any tissue bank can grow, there must be a big market for tissue grafts. The failure of the Model Human Tissue Bank in Sri Lanka to grow, despite the large number of available donors, was due to the small number of grafts used by surgeons in the country (Nather 2000a). Several campaigns had been carried out to increase professional awareness of tissue banking and transplantation in the country, but they proved to be unsuccessful.

Commitment of professionals setting up the tissue bank

The single most important factor for the development of a tissue bank is the vision, mission, and commitment of the director and his/her team who have been tasked to set up and run the tissue bank. Setting up a tissue bank is a complex venture. Dynamism and commitment are required to face the many obstacles that need to be overcome — from the institution, from the government, etc. Without dedicated team members who are prepared to persevere and overcome these obstacles, the mission is unlikely to succeed.

Planning Required for Setting Up a Tissue Bank

In setting up a tissue bank, careful planning must be required to address the following key elements:

- Building design of the tissue bank
- Manpower organization of the tissue bank
- Facilities required
- Equipment required
- Manpower
- Budget requirements for running costs

Building design

Unless a portion of the space in the department of an institution has been apportioned for the development of a tissue bank, nothing further can be done. One is indeed limited by the size of the space apportioned.

The main limiting factor in almost any country is space. Space is limited. Indeed, space is precious everywhere. Because of such a constraint, the minimum space requirement must provide for the following:

- Two separate rooms for the processing of tissues

  1. A wet processing room or an isolation room for the reception of donor tissues. Wet processing includes dissection, cutting, washing, and pasteurization (Nather 2000b).
  2. A dry processing room or a clean room. Dry processing includes lyophilization, packing, and labeling. Dry processing rooms should ideally be laminar flow rooms, but this is not the case in almost all countries in the Asia-Pacific region. However, clean processing is usually done under laminar flow conditions, with a laminar flow cabinet rather than a laminar flow room. The cost of constructing a room with laminar flow is between S$500 000 to S$1 000 000, a cost that almost all tissue banks in the Asia-Pacific region cannot afford. Besides, with the recommended practice of using end-sterilization of all tissue graft products by gamma irradiation at 25 kGy, there is no need for such a laminar flow room.

- A documentation room for allowing the proper filing of all documentation records whilst maintaining strict confidentiality (Nather 2000b).

If sufficient space is available in the construction of a building, then the design should be constructed to allow for the following ideal flow chart for tissue processing (Fig. 1).

Although it is advantageous to have a separate distribution area, distribution work and documentation can also be performed in the reception/documentation/distribution area in cases where space is limited. In this situation, the building is constructed to allow for a modified flow chart for tissue processing (Fig. 2).

Renovation costs are always required to convert the space given into the various laboratories as per the adopted or chosen flow chart for tissue processing.

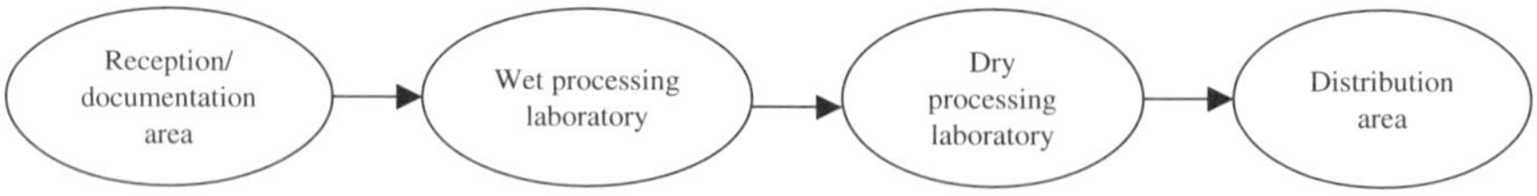

Fig. 1. The ideal flow chart for tissue processing.

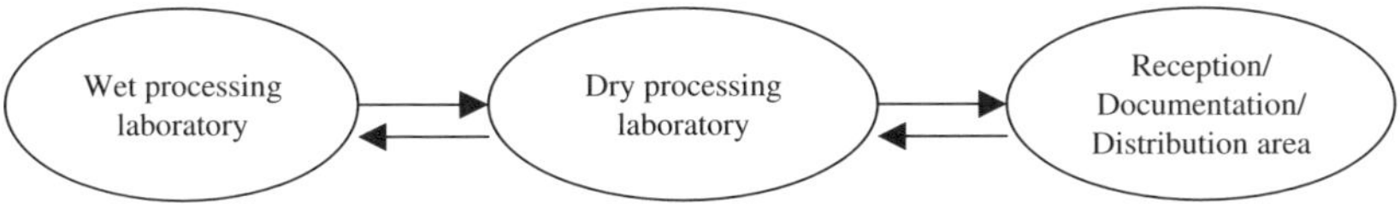

Fig. 2. A modified flow chart for tissue processing.

Figure 3 shows the building design of the National University Hospital (NUH) Tissue Bank in Singapore, which essentially has a separate wet processing laboratory, a separate dry processing laboratory, and a central bay for reception/documentation/distribution. Before entering each laboratory, the technician must first go through a changing area and change his/her attire and shoes.

Manpower organization structure

Before a tissue bank is planned, its manpower organization structure must first be clearly thought through for the tissue bank to function efficiently and successfully. From the onset, it must be decided which organization or institution will be responsible for supporting and financing the tissue bank. Approval must first be sought from the relevant organization or institution to accept this responsibility before any plan to set up a tissue bank can proceed. Approval must first be obtained from all key personnel for their involvement with the tissue bank.

In the Asia-Pacific region, tissue banks have been developed by three different institutions or organizations: universities, hospitals, and radiation institutions. In Singapore, Dr Nather has established the National University Hospital (NUH) Tissue Bank as a hospital venture (although the department is part of the National University of Singapore) because the tissue bank is financially viable as a cost center of the National University Hospital (Nather and Wang 2002).

It is important to establish the following manpower organization sub-structures (Nather 2000b): the Advisory Board, the Tissue Bank Committee, and the Management Committee. The manpower organization structure of the NUH Tissue Bank is shown in Fig. 4.

Advisory board

The Advisory Board or Administration Board must include the key personnel in the institution, e.g. the chairman of the medical board, deputy

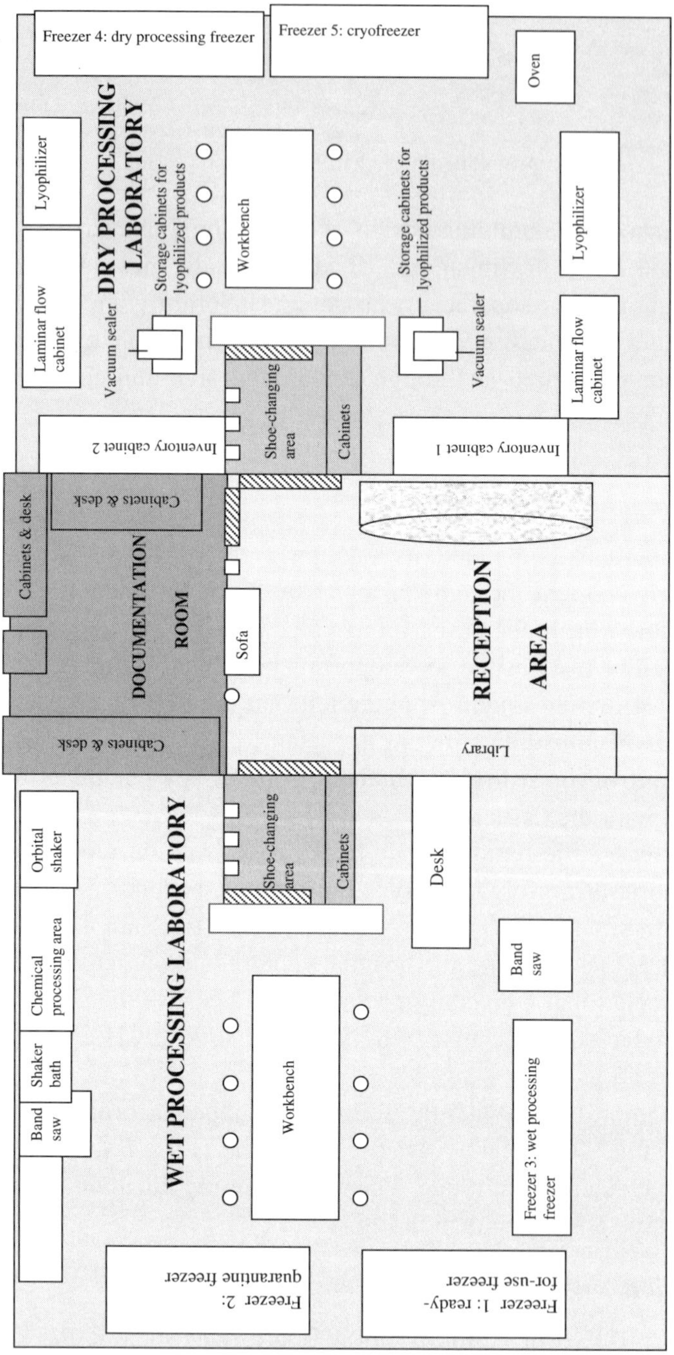

Fig. 3. The building design of the NUH Tissue Bank.

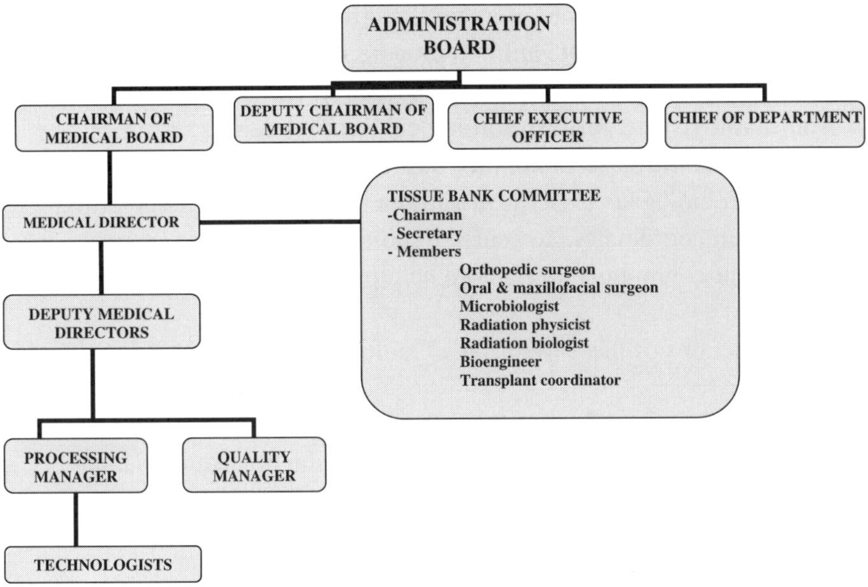

Fig. 4. The manpower organization structure of the NUH Tissue Bank.

chairman of the medical board, chief executive officer of the hospital, director-general of the radiation facility, deputy director-general, etc. The functions of the Advisory Board include the following:

- Monitor the functions and progress of the tissue bank
- Evaluate reports by the tissue bank
- Review all recommendations made by the Tissue Bank Committee
- Endorse all guidelines in the procedure and quality manual produced by the Tissue Bank Committee
- Endorse new amendments made by the Tissue Bank Committee

Tissue bank committee

It is important to set up this Committee, which is to be chaired by the director of the tissue bank, in order to promote tissue-banking activities. Important persons that should be included in this committee should include the following:

- Orthopedic surgeons to promote the procurement and transplantation of bones and soft tissues

- Maxillofacial surgeons to promote the utilization of bones
- Obstetricians to promote amnion procurement
- Plastic surgeons to promote the utilization of amnion
- Microbiologists to perform serological tests for donors
- Pathologists to source donors for tissue procurement
- Radiation biologists to perform gamma sterilization of tissue grafts
- Transplant coordinators to source donors for tissue procurement
- Prominent community workers to help promote public awareness

The functions of the Tissue Bank Committee include the following:

- Formulate procedural guidelines for the procurement, processing, and distribution of tissue grafts to be adopted in the procedure manual
- Formulate quality assurance policies to be adopted in the quality manual
- Monitor the functions and progress of the tissue bank
- Promote public awareness of tissue banking
- Promote professional awareness of tissue banking and tissue transplantation
- Report to the Advisory Board regarding all of the activities of the tissue bank

Management committee

This committee, also to be chaired by the director of the tissue bank, is responsible for the day-to-day running of the tissue bank. Members of the committee should include the director, deputy director, and technologists. The committee should meet at least weekly to discuss the following issues:

- Number of tissues procured
- Number of tissues transplanted
- Complications or problems encountered
- Administrative matters
- Personnel matters
- Other matters

An effective management committee is needed if the tissue bank is to function efficiently and successfully.

Facilities required

Electricity supply to tissue bank

Electrical freezers in the tissue bank should be supplied with red sockets (emergency electrical supply), if possible, so that emergency power is automatically restored to the red sockets in the event of electrical failure. This is possible in hospitals with emergency backup generators. For example, in the NUH Tissue Bank, all five electrical freezers are provided with red sockets (Nather 2000b).

Where red sockets are not provided, electrical freezers must be equipped with battery-operated liquid CO_2 backup systems. When electrical failure occurs, the cabinet temperature of the freezer will rise. When the temperature reaches above $-65°C$, liquid CO_2 from the cylinder will be infused into the freezer to stop the temperature from rising any higher.

Biohazard disposal facilities

Facilities must be available for the speedy and safe disposal of biohazard wastes. In a hospital facility, this is easily provided, as biohazard wastes are sent to the mortuary for disposal by incineration.

Equipment required

Wet processing laboratory

- $-80°C$ electrical freezer installed with a thermograph and liquid CO_2 backup system (Fig. 5)
- Stainless steel band saw (Fig. 6)
- Shaker bath (Fig. 7)
- Orbital-wrist shaker (Fig. 8)

Dry processing laboratory

- Lyophilizer (Fig. 9)
- Laminar airflow cabinet (Fig. 10)
- Vacuum sealer (Fig. 11)
- Electronic balance (Fig. 12)

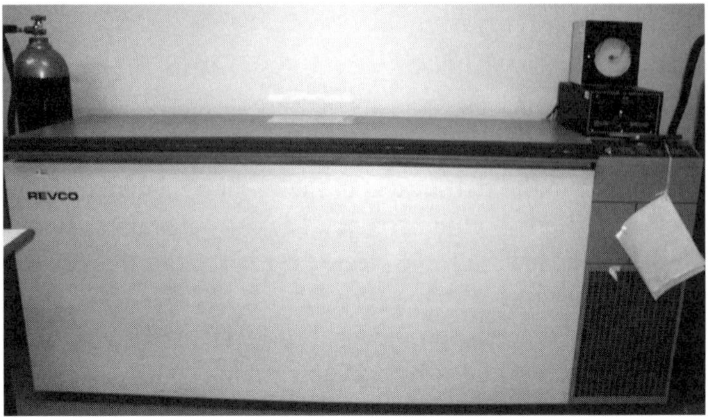

Fig. 5. A −80°C electrical freezer.

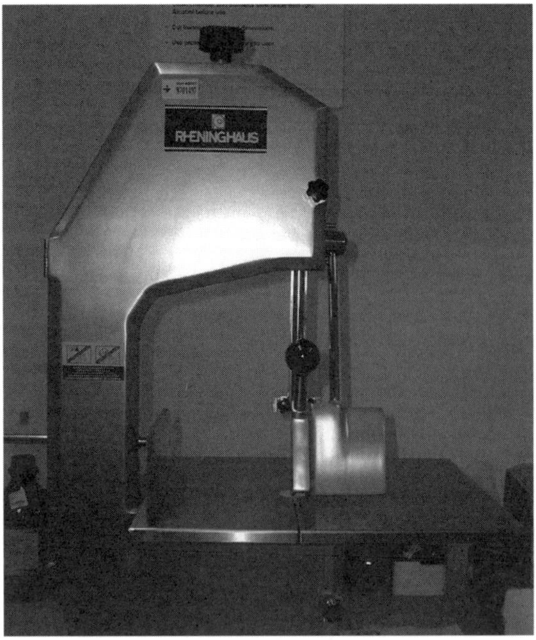

Fig. 6. A stainless steel band saw.

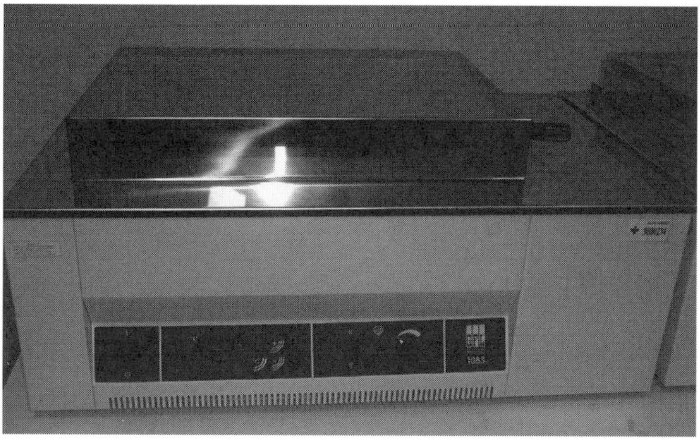

Fig. 7. A shaker bath.

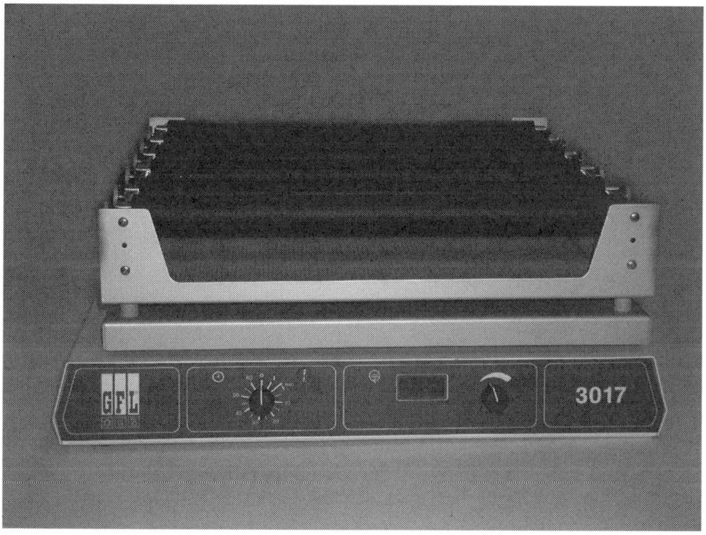

Fig. 8. An orbital-wrist shaker.

Equipment costs

A guide as to the estimated costs for the abovementioned minimum equipment that must be acquired to set up a tissue bank is shown in Table 1. As indicated in the table, a fund of about S$100 000 is needed to purchase the minimum equipment required.

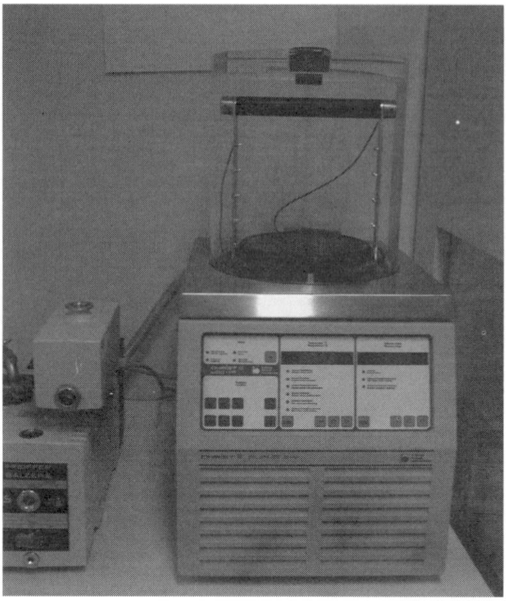

Fig. 9. A lyophilizer.

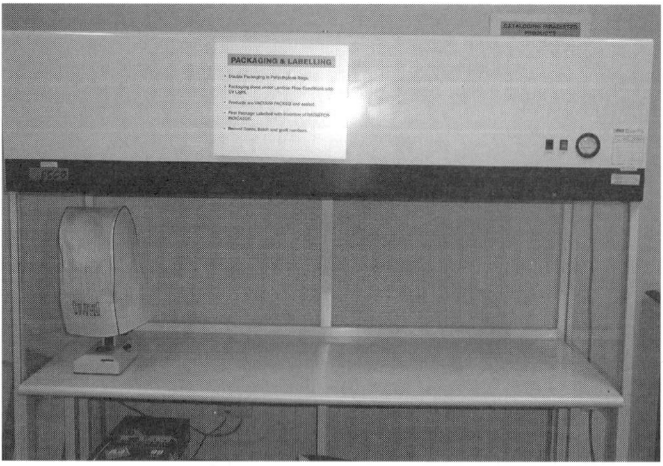

Fig. 10. A laminar airflow cabinet.

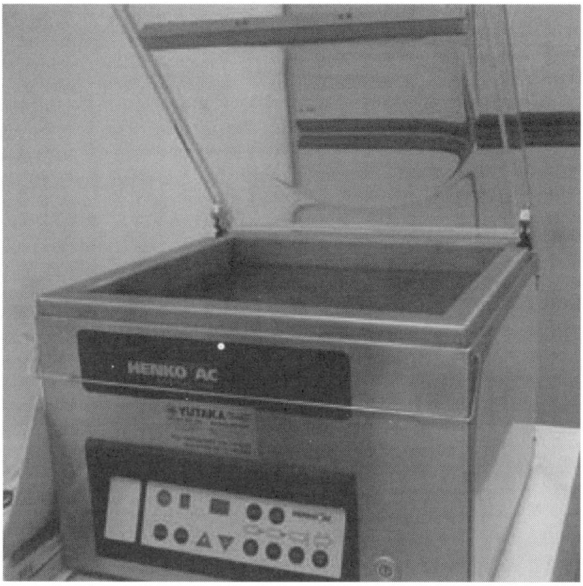

Fig. 11. A vacuum sealer.

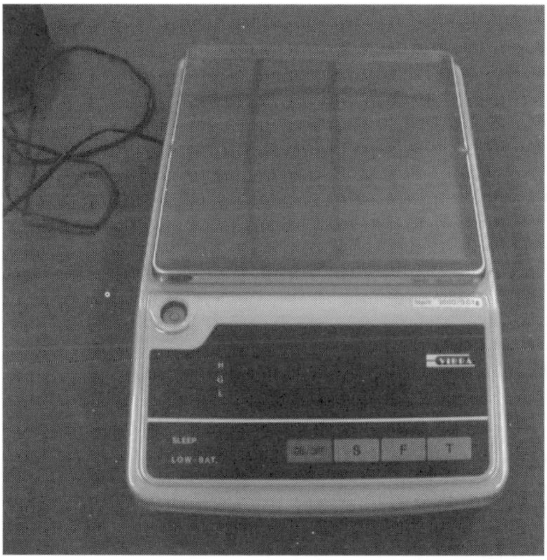

Fig. 12. An electronic balance.

Table 1. Equipment costs.

	SGD	USD*	RM*
−80°C electrical freezer with thermograph, liquid CO_2 backup	$30 000	$18 934	$69 861
Stainless steel band saw	$7000	$4418	$16 301
Shaker bath	$3000	$1893	$6986
Orbital-wrist shaker	$2000	$1262	$4657
Lyophilizer	$30 000	$18 934	$69 861
Laminar airflow cabinet	$10 000	$6311	$23 287
Vacuum sealer	$6000	$3787	$13 872
Oven	$3000	$1893	$6986
Electronic balance	$2000	$1262	$4657
Total	**$93 000**	**$58 697**	**$216 569**

*Rates as of Oct 2006.

Manpower requirements

The bank must be run by two full-time laboratory technicians. They must be proficient in (and receive training in) all aspects of tissue banking, including the donor selection criteria, methods of procurement, processing techniques, documentation, and distribution of tissue grafts. In the case of the NUH Tissue Bank, all staff should have at least a diploma in tissue banking from the National University of Singapore (NUS) (Nather 2000c).

In Singapore, manpower costs are expensive. Each laboratory technologist is paid a salary of about S$30 000 a year. Therefore, the annual manpower cost for running the tissue bank is at least S$60 000 per year.

Yearly budget for running costs

A yearly budget (such as the one in Table 2) must be submitted and the necessary funds provided to meet the yearly running costs incurred by the tissue bank. This annual expenditure must be approved by the funding institution.

Financial Considerations

Running a tissue bank is a business venture requiring capital expenditure, maintenance costs, manpower costs, etc. On average, giving allowance to a

Table 2. Planning a budget.

	SGD	USD*	RM*
Manpower costs (salary for 2 technicians)	±$60 000	±$37 869	±$133 972
Equipment maintenance costs	±$10 000	±$6312	±$23 287
Electricity	±$3000	±$1893	±$6986
Water consumption	±$1500	±$947	±$3493
Consumables	±$10 000	±$6312	±$23 287
	±$85 000	**±$53 648**	**±$197 940**

*Rates as of Oct 2006.

one-off capital expenditure of about S$100 000 (which should be provided by a grant from the hospital or relevant institution), the yearly running cost is approximately S$85 000. No organization is willing to fund such a large amount indefinitely. Instead, the supporting institution usually funds the running costs for at least 2 to 5 years, after which the tissue bank is expected to become self-sustaining.

To achieve this, tissue processing costs may be charged to recipients using the tissue grafts provided by the tissue bank, on the condition that the law of the country allows for the recovery of such tissue processing costs. To arrive at the real costs to be charged for tissue processing, the tissue bank must do a detailed analysis of all the running costs in one year versus the number of tissue grafts processed annually, and then calculate the production costs for each type of graft produced. The recommended tissue processing cost charged is 20% higher than the cost of production in order to allow for cost recovery.

Conclusion

Setting up a tissue bank is indeed a serious business requiring detailed planning and approval from various levels, including the department, the institution, and the government. It must be approached in a systematic and comprehensive manner. First, space allocation must be secured from an institution. Next, approval must be obtained from the institution to fund this venture. Once this approval is obtained, it is also necessary to obtain approval from key personnel in the institution to be part of the manpower organization structure that has to be established. Only then can one begin to plan the building design for the bank. Technologists to run the tissue bank must be recruited. With the availability of the required funds, which often must be procured from a research grant, the purchase of the necessary equipment then begins in stages.

In today's context, it is now more cost-effective to set up a "three-in-one" establishment: a tissue bank, a tissue engineering laboratory, and a tumor bank. Such a center saves space and costs, and avoids the duplication of equipment and facilities. It is recommended that new institutions be set up in such an enterprising three-in-one venture.

References

Nather A (2000a). Tissue banking in Asia Pacific region — ethical, legal, religious, cultural and other regulatory aspects. *J ASEAN Orthop Assoc* **13**:60–63.

Nather A (2000b). Organization systems. In: Phillips GO (ed.), *Radiation and Tissue Banking*, World Scientific, Singapore, p. 237.

Nather A (2000c). Diploma training for technologists in tissue banking. *Cell Tissue Bank* **1**:41–44.

Nather A and Wang LH (2002). Bone banking in Singapore — fourteen years of experience. *J ASEAN Orthop Assoc* **15**:20–29.

Chapter 6

A Comprehensive Training System for Tissue Bank Operators — 10 Years of Experience

Aziz Nather, Shu-Hui Neo and Chris C.W. Lee

NUH Tissue Bank
Department of Orthopaedic Surgery
Yong Loo Lin School of Medicine
National University of Singapore
Singapore

Introduction

The daily activities of a tissue bank are performed by technologists. It is therefore essential that they are well trained to perform all of the duties required of them. These include the following:

- Screening of potential donors (both living and deceased)
- Performing serological investigations
- Procurement of tissues
- Processing of tissues
- Documentation
- Distribution of tissues
- Promotion of public awareness of tissue banking and transplantation
- Promotion of professional awareness of tissue banking and transplantation

Thus, there is a great need for the formal training of technologists in tissue banks not only in the Asia-Pacific region, but also in other regions such as Latin America, Africa, and Eastern Europe, where the directors of tissue banks are mostly part-time volunteers (Nather 2000; Nather *et al.* 2003). The only full-time staff employed to run the tissue banks are the technologists. This is in contrast to large banks in the USA and Europe, many of which are run by large corporations as business ventures.

For a long time, the only available training programs were the short 2-week courses conducted by the American Association of Tissue Banks. There was therefore great demand for a structured year-long training program with a comprehensive curriculum leading to diploma certification by an internationally recognized university.

IAEA/RCA Program on Radiation Sterilization of Tissue Grafts (RAS 7/008)

In 1985, the International Atomic Energy Agency (IAEA) — under the Regional Cooperative Agreement (RCA) for member states in the Asia-Pacific region — began running a program on the "Radiation Sterilization of Tissue Grafts" (RAS 7/008) involving tissue banks in 13 countries, namely Bangladesh, China, India, Indonesia, Korea, Malaysia, Myanmar, Pakistan, the Philippines, Singapore, Sri Lanka, Thailand, and Vietnam (Nather 1999; Nather 2000; Nather *et al.* 2003). The IAEA provided capital expenditure for the purchase of equipment needed to set up one tissue bank in each of 12 member states (Singapore was not a recipient country under this program, but rather has participated as a contributing country providing available expertise where necessary). National coordinators from each member state spent several years developing and writing an IAEA/RCA draft curriculum on tissue banking, with Professor Phillips as the coordinating editor. The first draft curriculum was successfully assembled during the RCA Workshop in Suzhou, China, in 1994, and was the first of its kind in the world.

The curriculum was piloted in Singapore during the IAEA/RCA Regional Workshop on the "Dissemination of Information on Procedures for Production and Radiation Sterilization of Tissue Allografts" in September 1995. Twenty-one trainers used the curriculum to teach 35 trainees. This was the largest workshop ever held for curriculum training and it was deemed to be successful, as the curriculum was found to be effective and very suitable for training tissue bank operators. The NUH Tissue Bank was inaugurated as a hospital tissue bank during the opening ceremony of this workshop (Nather 2000).

Development of the Regional Training Centre (RTC) for the Asia-Pacific Region in Singapore

In September 1996, the NUH Tissue Bank was appointed by the IAEA to become the IAEA /NUS Regional Training Centre (RTC) for training tissue bank operators in the Asia-Pacific region (Nather 1999; Nather 2000). The Government of Singapore (represented by the Ministry of Environment), with the National Science and Technology Board (NSTB) as the funding agency, awarded a S$225 500 grant to build a new purpose-built tissue bank cum regional training center. The National University Hospital provided a space of 2000 square feet for this purpose. The center was designed with separate wet and dry processing laboratories, a documentation/distribution room, and a reception area.

The RTC was inaugurated during the IAEA/RCA regional training course for the "Delivery of Curriculum to Tissue Bank Operators" in November 1997. At the same time, the first ever NUS diploma course in tissue banking for tissue bank operators was launched — another first in the world.

NUS Diploma Course in Tissue Banking

The NUS tissue banking course is a 1-year distance learning diploma course. The minimum criteria for admission are at least five passes in the GCE O-Level Examination (or its equivalent), experience in working in a tissue bank or association with a tissue bank for at least 1 year, and proficiency in English. The course fee is only US$100.

The curriculum for the NUS diploma course includes the following:

- The conversion of the IAEA draft curriculum on tissue banking into the Multi-Media Curriculum, which consists of 8 modules, accompanying sets of slides, 7 video demonstrations, and 1 audio cassette (Fig. 1). The components of each module are contained in specially designed box containers (Nather 2000; Nather *et al.* 2003). The production costs of this curriculum (about S$100 000) are borne by the NSTB. The eight modules comprise the following:

  Module 0: Historical Background
  Module 1: Rules and Regulations

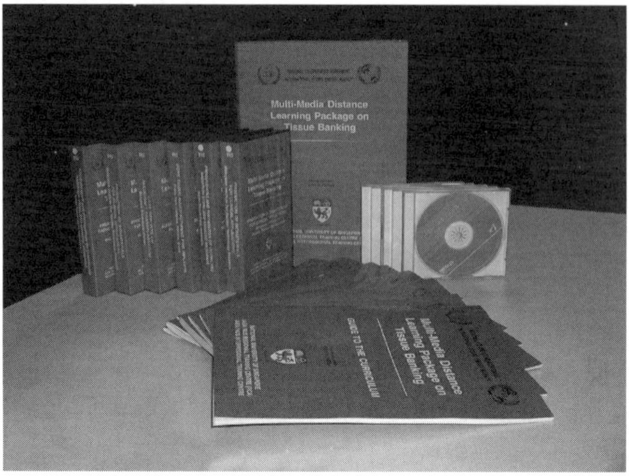

Fig. 1. The IAEA/NUS Multi-Media Curriculum produced by Singapore.

Module 2: Organization
Module 3: Quality Assurance
Module 4: Procurement
Module 5: Processing
Module 6: Distribution and Utilization
Module 7: Future Developments in Tissue Banking
plus Module: Guide to Curriculum

- Lectures on basic sciences. The basic science subjects include basic anatomy, basic microbiology, introduction to transmissible diseases, basic immunology, principles of sterile technique, basic radiation science, biology of healing of tissue transplantation, and biomechanics of tissue transplantation.
- Recommended textbook: *The Scientific Basis of Tissue Transplantation, Advances in Tissue Banking*, Vol. 5 (Nather A, ed., World Scientific, Singapore, 2002).

The course structure consists of three components:

- A 2-week foundation course at the RTC, Singapore, with lectures and practical demonstrations, ending with a theory and practical (OSPE) examination (phase I)

- Three assignments given at quarterly intervals, the last assignment being a practical assignment
- A terminal examination conducted by the NUS over 1 week at the RTC (phase II)

The mark allocation scheme for the diploma course is as follows:

• Foundation course exam (theory, practical)	20%
• Assignments	40%
• Terminal NUS exam (theory, practical, viva)	40%

The NUS diploma in tissue banking is awarded in three categories:

• Distinction	>80 marks
• Credit	70–79 marks
• Pass	50–69 marks

Unsuccessful candidates are allowed to resit for the examination up to a maximum of three attempts during the main or supplementary examinations.

IAEA/NUS diploma courses held

The first diploma course was launched on November 3, 1997, with 17 candidates; and the first NUS diploma examination was held in October 1998. Overall, 12 candidates graduated; of these, 4 passed with distinction, 5 with credit, and 3 with pass only (Nather 2000; Nather *et al.* 2003).

Between 1997 and 2006, eight courses were conducted by the RTC with a total of 160 tissue bank operators. Of these, 133 were from the Asia-Pacific region (13 countries) including 2 from Iran, 12 were from Africa (Zambia, Libya, Egypt, Algeria), 6 from Latin America (Brazil, Chile, Cuba, Peru, Uruguay), 9 from Europe (Greece, Slovakia, Poland, Ukraine), 2 from Australia, and 2 from South Africa. The last (eighth) batch involved 22 students who registered in April 2006 and are due to sit for the terminal examination in April 2007. Currently, seven batches have completed diploma training. A total of 102 tissue bank operators have convocated with an NUS diploma in tissue banking; of these, 20 have completed the course with distinction, 45 with credit, and 37 with pass only (Table 1). Thirty-six students did not complete the diploma course. Increased participation from regions outside the Asia-Pacific has been seen from the fourth batch onwards (Table 2).

Table 1. The results of the IAEA/NUS diploma courses conducted (1997–2006).

Batch no.	No. of students registered	No. of students convocated	Results			
			Distinction	Credit	Pass	Fail
First batch (Nov 1997–Oct 1998)	18	12	4	5	3	6
Second batch (Apr 1999–Mar 2000)	17	15	2	5	8	2
Third batch (Apr 2000–Mar 2001)	21	17	1	5	11	4
Fourth batch (Apr 2001–Mar 2002)	24	19	1	11	7	5
Fifth batch (Apr 2002–Aug 2003)	21	14	3	8	3	7
Sixth batch (Feb 2004–Feb 2005)	19	12	4	5	3	7
Seventh batch (Mar 2005–Mar 2006)	18	13	5	6	2	5
Eighth batch (Apr 2006–Apr 2007)	22					
Total	160	102	20	45	37	36

Technology transfer to Latin America

In October 1998, an IAEA interregional trainers workshop on the "Distant Learning Use of the Curriculum Package on Tissue Banking" was conducted by Professor Phillips and Professor Nather in Singapore with participant trainers from Argentina, Brazil, Chile, Cuba, Mexico, and Peru (Nather 2000). One copy of the Multi-Media Curriculum (English version) was presented to each trainer from Latin America with the compliments of the Singapore Government. The curriculum was subsequently translated into Spanish for use by Latin American countries, with Argentina established as the RTC for Latin America.

Technology transfer to Africa

Similar technology transfer was attempted in Africa. Professor Phillips and Professor Nather conducted an IAEA regional training course on tissue

Table 2. The regional distribution of tissue bank operators registered (1997–2006).

Batch no.	No. of students registered				
	Asia-Pacific	Latin America	Africa	Europe	Australia
First batch (Nov 1997–Oct 1998)	18	0	0	0	
Second batch (Apr 1999–Mar 2000)	16	0	0	1 (Slovakia)	
Third batch (Apr 2000–Mar 2001)	19	2 (1 Brazil) (1 Chile)	0	0	
Fourth batch (Apr 2001–Mar 2002)	19	0	3 (2 Zambia) (1 Algeria)	2 (1 Greece) (1 Slovakia)	
Fifth batch (Apr 2002–Aug 2003)	14	3 (1 Cuba) (1 Peru) (1 Uruguay)	3 (1 Egypt) (1 Libya) (1 Zambia)	1 (Poland)	
Sixth batch (Feb 2004–Feb 2005)	12		2 (1 Libya) (1 Algeria)	5 (3 Slovakia) (1 Ukraine) (1 Poland)	
Seventh batch (Mar 2005–Mar 2006)	17	1 (USA)			
Eighth batch (Apr 2006–Apr 2007)	18		2 (South Africa)		2
Total	133	6	12	9	2

banking in June 1999 in Algiers, Algeria. Six countries — Algeria, Egypt, Ghana, Libya, Nigeria, and Zambia — participated in this course (Nather 2000).

Curriculum update

The curriculum has been updated in three phases (Nather *et al.* 2001):

- Phase 1 — seven video tape demonstrations on the procurement, processing, and transplantation of tissues were converted into two compact discs in March 2000 (Fig. 1).
- Phase 2 — text booklets for modules 0 to 7 were updated as a companion book, *Radiation and Tissue Banking* (Phillips GO, ed., World Scientific, Singapore, 2000), in July 2000 (Fig. 2).

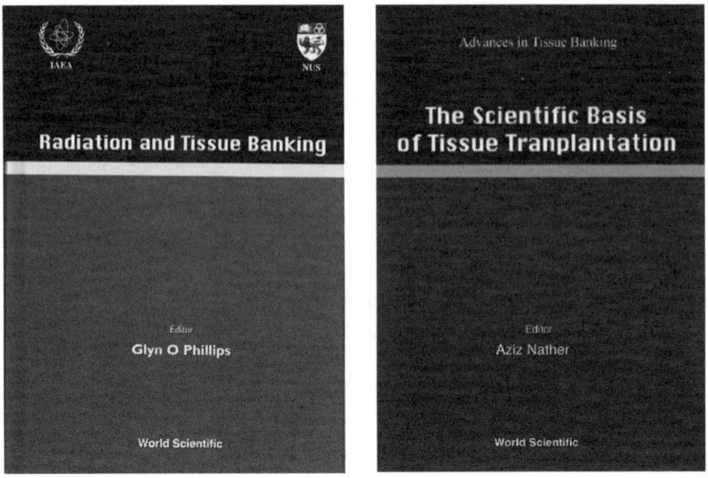

Fig. 2. The curriculum updates, *Radiation and Tissue Banking* (left) and *The Scientific Basis of Tissue Transplantation* (right).

- Phase 3 — a text on basic sciences was produced for the first time as a textbook, *The Scientific Basis of Tissue Transplantation*, in January 2002 (Fig. 2).

Development of the NUS Internet Diploma Course

The demand for training has increased exponentially over the years not only for technologists in the Asia-Pacific region, but also for tissue bank operators in other regions like Africa and parts of Eastern Europe (Nather *et al.* 2001; Nather *et al.* 2003). The financial costs borne by the IAEA were very large. For each foundation course (phase I), the cost incurred for sponsoring 6 overseas lecturers and 20 students from 13 member states (Asia-Pacific region) was about US$100 000. In addition, the cost incurred for holding the phase II 1-week terminal examination at the end of the year (including sponsoring the same students plus three overseas examiners) was about US$40 000. From 1997 to 2003, the total cost incurred for five batches was approximately US$700 000, a staggering amount.

If the IAEA was to continue sponsoring similar courses in the future, these costs had to be substantially reduced. Also, it was not possible for the IAEA to continue sponsoring such courses indefinitely. Thus, plans had to be made by the RTC in Singapore to continue running such courses on its own, without the financial support of the IAEA. In other words, the RTC had to become self-sufficient. Likewise, member states had to start paying for the training costs of their own tissue bank operators.

An effective solution was to convert the diploma course into an internet course. In October 2000, the IAEA approached Singapore to consider such a conversion (Nather *et al.* 2001; Nather *et al.* 2003) and it was largely responsible for funding the cost of this development, which began in 2001. With the introduction of this internet course, the need for a foundation course could be eliminated. However, for the NUS to confer a diploma, the terminal examination still had to be held in the RTC, Singapore; instead of 1 week and three examiners, it could be held for just 3 days and involve only one external examiner. The estimated cost for the exam would then be only about US$15 000. Had the training course been designed as a distance learning internet course from the start, the cost incurred by the IAEA for the first five batches (1997–2003) would have been only US$75 000 plus the cost of registration fees (US$500 × 101 = US$50 500) — i.e. a total of US$125 000 instead of US$700 000, a fivefold decrease in the expenditure that has been spent.

Instruction materials for internet delivery

The instruction materials for internet delivery include the following:

- IAEA/NUS Multi-Media Curriculum — eight modules (text booklets), two compact discs, and accompanying sets of slides
- Companion book — *Radiation and Tissue Banking*

Requirements for internet course

- National training centers in participating countries. Only countries that have recognized tissue banks with recognized trainers are allowed to participate in the internet course. Without the foundation course, good and close supervision of each trainee by a qualified and recognized trainer in the students' own country is mandatory.
- IT facilities in national training centers. National training centers must have the following IT facilities (Nather *et al.* 2001): a 486 (or equivalent)

processor, 16 MB (or greater) of RAM, a 2-GB (or greater) hard drive, a 56-Kbps modem, a CD-ROM drive, a printer, and Version 3 (or similar) of Netscape Navigator/Internet Explorer.

- IT facilities for the Internet Training Centre, Singapore. A web server was provided by the IAEA in March 2003. In addition, a senior systems analyst — cofunded by the IAEA and NUS (80% and 20% shared costs, respectively) — was employed for a period of 1 year to develop the online course and to function as the webmaster.

Internet project team

An NUS Internet Project Team (Nather *et al.* 2001) was assembled, including Associate Professor Aziz Nather (principal investigator), Ms Chang Hseuh Fun (systems analyst, Dean's Office), and Ms Lim May Ying (analyst programmer, Center for Instructional Technology Accessibility).

MOU for the development of the Interregional Training Centre (ITC) in Singapore

In October 2000, the NUS approved the development of the NUS internet diploma course in tissue banking (Nather *et al.* 2001). A memorandum of understanding (MOU) was signed between the NUS (represented by the dean, Faculty of Medicine) and the IAEA (represented by the deputy director-general) on July 4, 2002 (Nather *et al.* 2003). With this memorandum, Singapore was appointed as the IAEA/NUS Interregional Training Centre (ITC) for four regions: the Asia-Pacific, Latin America, Africa, and Europe (Fig. 3). All of the local costs for the development of the ITC were borne by a local grant obtained from the Lee Foundation (S$85 000) in Singapore.

Current status of the internet diploma course in tissue banking

The internet course was piloted with the fourth batch of diploma students in April 2001, and with the fifth and sixth batches in 2002 and 2003, respectively. The first internet course was launched on February 9, 2004, with 16 students sponsored by the IAEA. The IAEA funded the costs of the new registration fees (US$500 $\times$ 16 = US$8000). In addition, there were three other self-sponsored students. The terminal examination for this first internet course was held in February 2005.

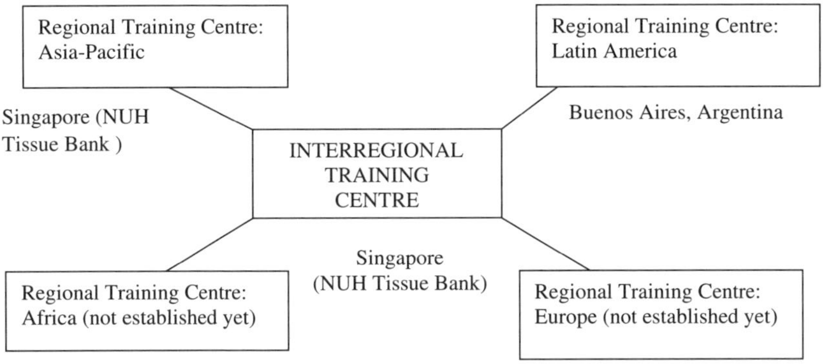

Fig. 3. The network of the IAEA training program, with Singapore as the Interregional Training Centre for the Asia-Pacific, Latin America, Africa, and Europe.

Delivery packages of the online course

The curriculum is delivered in three packages:

- Package 1
  - Online delivery of modules 0 to 2
  - Basic sciences: anatomy, matrix biology, physiology of tissues, and immunology (recommended textbook: *The Scientific Basis of Tissue Transplantation*)
  - Online delivery of assignment I
- Package 2
  - Online delivery of modules 3 to 5
  - Basic sciences: radiation sciences
  - Online release of CD demonstrations for module 4 (procurement) and module 5 (processing)
  - Online delivery of assignment II
- Package 3
  - Online delivery of modules 6 and 7
  - Basic sciences: biology of healing of allografts, biomechanics of healing of allografts
  - Online release of CD demonstrations for module 6 (distribution and utilization)
  - Online delivery of assignment III

The mark allocation scheme for the internet diploma course is as follows:

— Assignments I, II, III 60%
— Terminal examination (theory, practical, viva) 40%

Post-IAEA Era

The IAEA stopped sponsoring the program in 2005. The Training Centre in Singapore has continued to run the internet diploma course, with students in the seventh batch paying for their own enrollment. The response has been encouraging. In 2005, 17 students (who were recruited without IAEA involvement) participated in the seventh batch, and 22 students registered the following year in the eighth batch. Clearly, there is a need for more training.

National Training Programs

The Korean National Training Center has been set up in St Vincent's Hospital, Catholic Medical University, Seoul, Korea, with Professor Yong Koo Kang as the director. This center is jointly run by the Korean Association of Tissue Banks (KATB) and the Korean Musculoskeletal Transplantation Society (KMTS). The center uses the IAEA Multi-Media Curriculum translated into the Korean language with funds from the IAEA, largely due to the efforts of Dr Chang Joon Kim, Dr Glyn Phillips, and Mr J. Morales. The first Korean national training course (KNTC) was launched in 2003 with IAEA support. Eleven students participated using the Multi-Media Curriculum printed in Korean.

The structure of the course (also a 1-year distance learning program) is similar to the IAEA/NUS diploma course run in Singapore, and consists of the following:

- A 1-week foundation course (optional)
- Three assignments
- Three weekend courses (with lectures, assignments, and practical demonstrations)
- A terminal face-to-face examination

The KNTC is run in collaboration with the IAEA/NUS Training Centre in Singapore, which serves all Korean students with the internet curriculum in English.

The first examination was held at St. Vincent's Hospital in November 2004, with Dr Nather as the IAEA consultant and external examiner. All 11 students passed. The second KNTC commenced in November 2004 with 12 participants. The examination was held in November 2005, again with Dr Nather as the external examiner with IAEA support. Ten students passed. At the same time, 22 students enrolled in the third KNTC without IAEA involvement. The examination was conducted in December 2006, with Dr Nather as the external examiner.

Conclusion

Singapore has played a key role in the global training of tissue bank operators over the last 10 years, providing training not only to the Asia-Pacific region, but also to Latin America, Africa, and Europe. Its Regional Training Centre has grown and, as of February 2004, now functions as an Interregional Training Centre. It is grateful to the IAEA for making the NUH Tissue Bank part of a very meaningful and successful venture.

As the IAEA program came to an end in 2005, the center aims to continue the training courses on its own. In order to succeed, it has forged partnerships with key countries in the Asia-Pacific region, namely Korea, Malaysia, and Indonesia. These countries have indicated their interest to run national training programs in collaboration with Singapore. So far, only Korea has started its own national training course in the Korean language, supported by resources from the ITC in Singapore. Malaysia and Indonesia are planning to run similar national training courses in English, with Singapore providing the internet curriculum.

Acknowledgments

The author is grateful to Professor Glyn O. Phillips for all his advice and supervision since the inception of the RTC in conducting all the diploma courses. He is also grateful to Professor Phillips, Mr J. Morales, and Ms E. Dosekova for contributing to the development of the internet diploma course and the ITC in Singapore; and to Ms J. Baharim for all the secretarial assistance provided in typing this manuscript.

References

Nather A (1999). Tissue banking in the Asia Pacific region — the Asia Pacific Association of Surgical Tissue Banking. In: Phillips GO, Strong DM, von Versen R, and Nather A (eds.), *Advances in Tissue Banking*, Vol. 3, World Scientific, Singapore, pp. 419–425.

Nather A (2000). Diploma training for the technologists in tissue banking. *Cell Tissue Bank* **1**:41–44.

Nather A, Phillip GO, Cheong HF, and Ling MY (2001). Development of IAEA/NUS internet diploma course in tissue banking. *J ASEAN Orthop Assoc* **14**:5–7.

Nather A, Phillips GO, and Morales J (2003). IAEA/NUS distance learning diploma training course for tissue bank operators — past, present and future. *Cell Tissue Bank* **4**:77–84.

PART III.

BASIC SCIENCE OF RADIATION

Chapter 7

Interaction of Radiation with Tissues

Norimah Yusof

Malaysian Nuclear Agency (NM)
Bangi, 43000 Kajang, Selangor
Malaysia

Introduction

Tissue allografts are being widely used with a growing demand worldwide. In 2002 alone, more than 800 000 grafts were used in the US, and more than 160 000 grafts were applied in the Asia-Pacific region. The need to sterilize tissue grafts is becoming an increasingly important consideration, following a few cases of disease transmission after tissue transplants. Radiation has been widely used to terminally sterilize tissues, especially in the Asia-Pacific region following the successful International Atomic Energy Agency (IAEA) regional program promoting radiation sterilization.

This chapter describes the basic physical processes through which ionizing radiation interacts with processed tissue components, explaining the practical implications for radiation sterilization. Even though processed tissue is considered as a nonliving cell, the interaction process provides a useful background for understanding the mechanism that leads to changes in the tissue physicochemical properties. As this chapter only deals with the effects of radiation on processed tissues, details of the mechanism through which ionizing radiation inactivates or kills microorganisms are given in chapter 9.

Similar to thermal or chemical processes, changes by radiation are caused by the deposition of energy. The binding energy of molecular bonds is generally below 12 eV. Ionizing radiation energy is imparted to the system mainly in quanta of 10 eV or more, with the result that practically any chemical bond may be broken and any potential chemical reaction may take place.

Ionizing Radiation

Ionizing radiation refers to radiation that has high enough energy to dislodge electrons from atoms or molecules and convert them to electrically charged particles called ions. These ions then interact with water molecules to form radicals. The formation of ions and radicals in the system that leads to a series of chemical changes is called the ionization process. Ionizing radiation includes many types of incoming particles: those that are directly ionizing, e.g. heavy and light charged particles; and those that are indirectly ionizing or uncharged particles, e.g. neutrons and X- and gamma-ray photons.

Radiation Unit

The absorbed dose (gray, Gy) is the amount of energy absorbed per unit mass of irradiated product. The relation between Gy and the old unit rad is as follows:

$$1\,\text{Gy} = 1\,\text{J/kg} = 100\,\text{rad}$$
$$1\,\text{kGy} = 1 \times 10^3\,\text{J/kg} = 238.9\,\text{cal/kg}$$
$$(\text{at} \sim 0.24°\text{C})$$

The absorbed dose rate is the absorbed dose per unit time (e.g. Gy/s, kGy/min, kGy/h).

Interaction of Ionizing Radiation with Aqueous System

Biological tissues contain more than 80% water; even when processed and dried (either air- or freeze-dried), tissues still contain some water at less than 10%. About 40% of the damage is caused by direct ionization, while the remaining 60% is caused by indirect damage. The direct effect of radiation involves the simple interaction between ionizing radiation and critical biological molecules, causing the excitation, lesion, and scission of biopolymeric structure (Yusof 2000). The indirect effect involves the formation of ionized products of water molecules or radiolysis of water, as illustrated below.

Radiolysis of water

1. Ionization
   (a) Direct ionization — electrons are ejected from water molecules:

$$H_2O \rightarrow H_2O^+ + e^-$$

   (b) Indirect ionization — water molecules further decompose into hydrogen and hydroxyl radicals:

$$e^- + H_2O \rightarrow H_2O^-$$
$$H_2O^+ \rightarrow H^+ + OH^*$$
$$H_2O^- \rightarrow H^* + OH^-$$

2. Recombination

$$e^- + H_2O^+ \rightarrow H_2O^*$$
$$H^* + OH^* \rightarrow H_2O$$
$$H^+ + OH^- \rightarrow H_2O$$

3. Decomposition

$$H_2O \rightarrow H^* + OH^*$$

Therefore, the radiolysis of water molecules releases aqueous electrons and free radicals, summarized as follows:

$$H_2O \rightarrow e^-aq + OH^* + H^*$$

These products in irradiated water will last for only $\sim 10^{-9}$ seconds after high-energy radiation passes through. As described further in chapter 9, the amount of radiolytic products produced per 100 eV radiation energy is influenced by many environmental factors (e.g. water content, temperature, oxygen levels, presence of radical scavengers) and radiation quality (i.e. dose rate and radiation type). These free radicals interact further as shown below.

1. Interaction among free radicals (H^*, OH^*)

$$H^* + H^* \rightarrow H_2$$
$$OH^* + OH^* \rightarrow H_2O_2 \text{ (hydrogen peroxide)}$$
$$H^* + OH^* \rightarrow H_2O$$

2. Interaction with water molecules or reaction products

$$H_2O + H^* \rightarrow H_2 + OH^*$$
$$H_2O_2 + OH^* \rightarrow H_2O + HO_2^*$$

3. Interaction with biologically important molecules in tissues/cells
   (a) With organic molecules (RH):

$$RH + OH^* \rightarrow R^* + H_2O$$
$$RH + H^* \rightarrow R^* + H_2$$
$$RH \rightarrow R^* + H^*$$
$$RH + HO_2^* \rightarrow R^* + H_2O_2$$

   (b) With oxygen:

$$H^* + O_2 \rightarrow HO_2^* \text{ (hydroperoxy radicals)}$$
$$R^* + O_2 \rightarrow RO_2^* \text{ (organic peroxy radicals)}$$

   (c) With tissue constituents

These free radicals R^* react with biologically important molecules in tissues, such as the following:

1. Organic molecules: collagen, fibers, protein, enzyme
2. Inorganic molecules: salts, minerals, hydroxyapatite
3. Water molecules

These chain reactions of indirect effect are generally held responsible for major radiation damages in tissue components. Tissue is a complex matter, which can give rise to various effects. For example, bone is an organic matrix containing mainly collagen impregnated with calcium salts (generally calcium phosphate) in the form of crystalline hydroxyapatite. Sometimes, changes may not be due at tissue constituents, but rather at secondary structures (Yusof 2000).

Interaction with tissues

The practical uses of irradiated biological tissues in clinical applications have increased tremendously in the past 10 years, following the great achievements of the IAEA regional program on the radiation sterilization of tissues in the Asia-Pacific and Latin America. A great deal is known about the effects of radiation on various types of tissues that determine their end use. It is important that the irradiated tissues are capable of their intended function in the body after transplantation. Bone, used as a scaffold for instance, should be invaded and ultimately incorporated by living tissue from the host.

The availability of sterile tissue graft materials is of great importance, and the radiation dose selected to sterilize tissues must be sufficient to inactivate/kill all micoorganisms on the tissue with no detrimental effects on the tissue. However, radiation while sterilizing tissues has other effects on their physical properties. Therefore, the conditions for the radiation sterilization of tissues need to be specified and well controlled. By understanding the radiation effects, we can sterilize tissues while minimizing the deleterious effects, maintaining the native structure as well as the biochemical and biomechanical properties of tissues — hence, maintaining the functional characteristics.

Effects on Tissue Constituents

Collagen

Generally, changes in the physical properties of collagen are relatively small with respect to changes in chemical compositions (Yusof 2000). Instead, the changes are mainly in terms of a disorganized secondary structure. The tensile strength of hydrated collagen has been shown to reduce to one third of its original tensile strength only after a very high dose of 460 kGy.

Radiation at 10–50 kGy induced minor cleavage of alpha chains of the collagen triple helix molecule (Tomford 2005). Intramolecular and intermolecular hydrogen bonds were broken at 10 kGy, mainly due to scission and structure breakdown. Cross-link at 50–100 kGy was suppressed below 0°C, as the movement of reactive free radicals was limited in the frozen state. The amino acid composition in collagen did not alter, even at high doses of 50–1000 kGy (Yusof 2000).

Fibril structure

The fibril structure only changed at doses higher than 100 kGy (Yusof 2000).

Tendon

The tensile strength of irradiated tendons reduced by two thirds when irradiated at 180 kGy (Yusof 2000). Irradiation at 25 kGy and freeze-drying did not change the histological pattern, comparable to fresh at 6 months after implantation; while irradiation at 20 and 40 kGy showed no effect on biomechanical properties 6 months after surgery.

Therefore, most effects of radiation on tissue constituents are observed at very high doses more than 25 kGy (Yusof 2000).

Effects on Tissues

The effects of radiation on nonviable tissues are not the summation of effects on all tissue constituents. Desirable effects of radiation may include decrease in immunogenicity and increase in resorbability, while undesirable effects include reduction in biomechanical properties and decrease in osteoinductive capacity. These effects are influenced by the type of tissue, the type of radiation source, and the conditions during irradiation.

Radiation is not used solely, but apparently is applied after tissues have been subjected to washing and preservation (including freezing, drying, and freeze-drying/lyophilization for prolonging storage). Therefore, the resulting effects are the effects of the combined treatment of radiation with other physical and chemical processes carried out prior to sterilization.

Soft tissues

Both gamma and electron have been used with doses ranging from 17 to 80 kGy to evaluate the effects of radiation on various soft tissues including cartilage, heart valves, dura mater, skin, fascia, sclera, amnion, meniscus, and tendons (Strong 2005). Damage generally occurs with increasing doses of irradiation. At lower doses (17–20 kGy), the effects on strength and modulus are not consistently significant; but at doses higher than 25 kGy, biochemical, biophysical, mechanical, and material properties are more significantly altered. Only tissue grafts that are not required to maintain structural integrity, but rather are used as coverings (such as amnion) or in non–weight-bearing reconstruction (such as cartilage) have more clinical success.

Work carried out by Dziedzic-Goclawska in 1976 indicated that radiation at 35 kGy in the dry-frozen state increased the solubility of dried collagen–derived membrane used for wound dressing by 50%, due to the direct effect of scission of polypeptide chains — hence, decreased tensile strength (Yusof 2000). When irradiated in the presence of water, the solubility decreased due to random reactions of free radicals on collagen structure.

Even though freeze-drying is used to reduce the water content of tissues in order to minimize the indirect effect of radiation, the process itself has been shown to have detrimental effects on tissue structure (Yusof 2000). The physical properties of air-dried amnion were better than those of freeze-dried amnion, and were not affected even after 5 years of storage and irradiation at 17–25 kGy. Skin, both freeze-dried and irradiated, reduced the tensile strength by 25%. Frozen heart valve irradiated at 29 and 32 kGy maintained the biomechanical strength of the aortic wall; but when freeze-dried, the heart valve irradiated at 25 and 33 kGy decreased in tensile strength, cracked, and became brittle due to damage in structure. Freeze-dried dura mater irradiated at more than 25 kGy changed in biomechanical properties and decreased in permeability. Freeze-dried fascia lata irradiated at 25 kGy decreased in permeability and needed a longer time to reach a steady state.

Bone and musculoskeletal tissues

Radiation sterilization of musculoskeletal tissue grafts was initiated more than 50 years ago, from the use of cathode rays in 1955 to the current use of gamma irradiation. The progress is in parallel to the popularity of bone transplantation (Tomford 2005). Long bone and osteoarticular grafts, by virtue of their massive size, are easily sterilized by high penetration of gamma radiation. The effects of radiation on bone are not only on the collagen that sustains the biomechanical properties of bone, but also on the osteoinductive factors (i.e. bone growth factors).

Radiation at 25–30 kGy has a minimal adverse effect on bone biomechanical properties and healing; however, effects on osteoinductivity need further research. Doses greater than 30 kGy produce irreparable damage to the collagen; therefore, tissues can only be sterilized between 20 and 25 kGy, preferably in a frozen state where free radicals are inactive, to prevent an extensive inflammatory response to the irradiated collagen.

Although the combined treatment of radiation and freezing has no effect on the elastic and strength properties of collagen, the treatment significantly decreases the capacity to absorb load. Frozen massive allografts irradiated at 25 kGy using gamma gave encouraging clinical results with no infection after 3 years. Kang *et al.* (2005) confirmed that when both deep-frozen and freeze-dried allografts irradiated at 15 to 25 kGy were used in reconstruction for malignant bone tumors, the clinical results were as good as those for nonirradiated allografts. However, rapid thawing may be the major cause of cellular damage and delayed rupture in cryopreserved arterial allografts; thus, slow thawing is recommended.

Freeze-drying (lyophilization) causes deterioration to biomechanical characteristics, and the effect is exaggerated after irradiation (Yusof 2000). The freeze-drying and lipid extraction of femoral heads reduced compressive strength by 20%; and when irradiated at 25 kGy, it further reduced to 42.5% (Tomford 2005). Deep-freezing when combined with 25 kGy neither changed the scanning electron microscope (SEM) structure nor reduced the elasticity of bone, but freeze-drying with radiation caused microcracks and reduced elasticity (Yusof 2000).

Conclusion

Radiation sterilization is used to increase the safety of tissue grafts in order to prevent the transmission of diseases from donor to recipient. However, the radiation doses used must not cause structural changes to the tissue. Tissues irradiated in the frozen state sustain much less degradation than tissues irradiated at room temperature. Freeze-drying enhances radiation damage. Doses less than 25 kGy with no damaging effects on tissue and its constituents can be selected to sterilize tissues that have been properly processed under good hygienic practices. In addition, tissue bankers must be able to choose the proper processing method for a particular type of tissue, depending on the functional roles of the tissue. For instance, the combination of radiation and freeze-drying is not recommended for weight-bearing large bones, but is still the best procedure for freeze-dried bone chips and morselized bones, as they are easily transported and stored at room temperature. Despite its detrimental effects, gamma radiation is still an effective method to sterilize tissues.

References

Dziedzic-Goclawska A (1976). Personal communication.

Kang YK, Jeong JY, Chung YG, Babk WJ, and Rhee SK (2005). Complications of structural allografts for malignant bone tumours. In: Kennedy JF, Phillips GO, and Williams PA (eds.), *Sterilisation of Tissues Using Ionising Radiations*, CRC Woodhead Publishing, England, pp. 157–162.

Strong DM (2005). Effects of radiation on the integrity and functionality of soft tissue. In: Kennedy JF, Phillips GO, and Williams PA (eds.), *Sterilisation of Tissues Using Ionising Radiations*, CRC Woodhead Publishing, England, pp. 163–172.

Tomford WW (2005). Effects of gamma irradiation on bone — clinical experience. In: Kennedy JF, Phillips GO, and Williams PA (eds.), *Sterilisation of Tissues Using Ionising Radiations*, CRC Woodhead Publishing, England, pp. 133–140.

Yusof N (2000). Gamma irradiation for sterilising tissue grafts for viral inactivation. *Malays J Nucl Sci* **18**(1):23–35.

Chapter 8

Types of Radiation and Irradiation Facilities for Sterilization of Tissue Grafts

Norimah Yusof*, Noriah Mod Ali* and Nazly Hilmy†

**Malaysian Nuclear Agency (NM)*
Bangi, 43000 Kajang, Selangor
Malaysia

†BATAN Research Tissue Bank (BRTB)
Center for Research and Development of Isotopes and Radiation Technology, BATAN
Jakarta 12070, Indonesia

Introduction

Tissue allografts comprise a wide range of tissues. Those that are currently radiation sterilized include bone, cartilage, fascia, dura mater, skin, and amnion. Tissue allografts are not medical products of commercial production processes involving large numbers of samples; therefore, the levels of microbial contamination are not consistently low, and extra attention and handling are required during sterilization (IAEA 2004). Prior to using radiation sterilization for tissues, the effects of radiation on the tissues and their components must be considered. The interaction of radiation with tissues is discussed in chapter 7.

Types of Radiation

Radiation is a form of energy emitted from a source, and travels through tissue material either as particles or waves. They lose their energy mainly through ionizations and excitations. Chapter 9 describes direct and indirect actions of ionizing radiation. Two radiation types that are commonly used in commercial and large-scale sterilization processes, having primary energies ranging from 10 keV to 10 MeV, are the following:

1. High-energy charged particles (i.e. electron beams)
2. Electromagnetic radiation (i.e. X-rays and gamma rays)

High-energy charged particles

Electron beams are usually generated by machines such as ion accelerators (cyclotrons) and electron accelerators. An electron beam machine is similar to a television set (25 keV), but the former has a higher voltage (3000 keV) and electrons are accelerated through a vacuum tube. Basic properties of electron beams include the following:

- Limited penetration, thus needing to increase penetration by increasing the voltage
- High current that results in an increased number of charged particles, thus increasing the dose rate
- Chemical effects that are similar to electromagnetic radiation (upon contact with the material, electrons alter various chemical and molecular bonds, including those of the reproductive cells of microorganisms).

Electromagnetic radiation

Photon fields are produced either as X-rays resulting from intense electron beams striking a high atomic number of metallic targets, or as gamma rays from powerful radionuclide sources such as cobalt-60 (half-life, 5.26 years; energy, 1.17 MeV and 1.33 MeV) and caesium-137 (half-life, 30 years; energy, 0.66 MeV). Generally, gamma rays have a higher energy than X-rays (NM 2004).

Cobalt-60 is naturally unstable and decays back to stable, nonradioactive nickel-60 at a rate of approximately 1% per month. Both gamma rays (energy, 1.17 MeV and 1.33 MeV) have excellent penetrating power that enables the treatment of products in their final hermetically sealed packaging, ensuring sterility until the product is removed from its package and put into use. It does not make the product radioactive. Cobalt-60 has a half-life of 5.26 years, and each source is typically in use at an irradiator site for at least 20 years. Agreements are in place whereby the suppliers of cobalt-60 sources accept the return of these low-activity sources back for re-encapsulation, recycling, or disposal at the end of their useful life. The security of cobalt-60 transportation to minimize theft, loss of control, or misuse of product has received particular attention from international and national regulators around the world in addressing terrorist threats. Over 800 million curies (approximately 80 000 sources) of cobalt-60 have been safely and securely shipped to irradiators worldwide. There has never been an accident.

Both X-rays and gamma rays have short wavelengths and high energies to cause ionizations (note: ultraviolet and infrared rays may initiate chemical changes, but not via ionization; therefore, they are not ionizing radiation), as shown in Table 1. Figure 1 shows the energy spectrum of electromagnetic radiation (X-rays, cosmic rays, and gamma rays) as well as the penetration of α, β, and γ rays. X-rays and gamma rays have the same properties and effects on materials, even though they come from different origins: X-rays are generated by man-made machines; whilst gamma rays are emitted by radionuclides, cobalt-60, or caesium-137, depending on the source strength.

Source strength

- Non-SI unit: 1 curie (Ci) $= 3.7 \times 10^{10}$ disintegration/disintegration per second
- SI unit: 1 becquerel (Bq) $= 2.7 \times 10^{-11}$ Ci

Table 1. Wavelengths of ionizing and nonionizing radiation.

Radiation	Wavelength (meters)
Radiowaves	10^{8}–10^{-3}
Microwaves	10^{-1}–10^{-6}
Visible light rays	10^{-2}–10^{-7}
Ultraviolet rays	10^{-7}–10^{-11}
X-rays	**10^{-8}–10^{-12}**
Gamma rays	**10^{-10}–10^{-14}**
Synchrotron	10^{-12}–10^{-14}

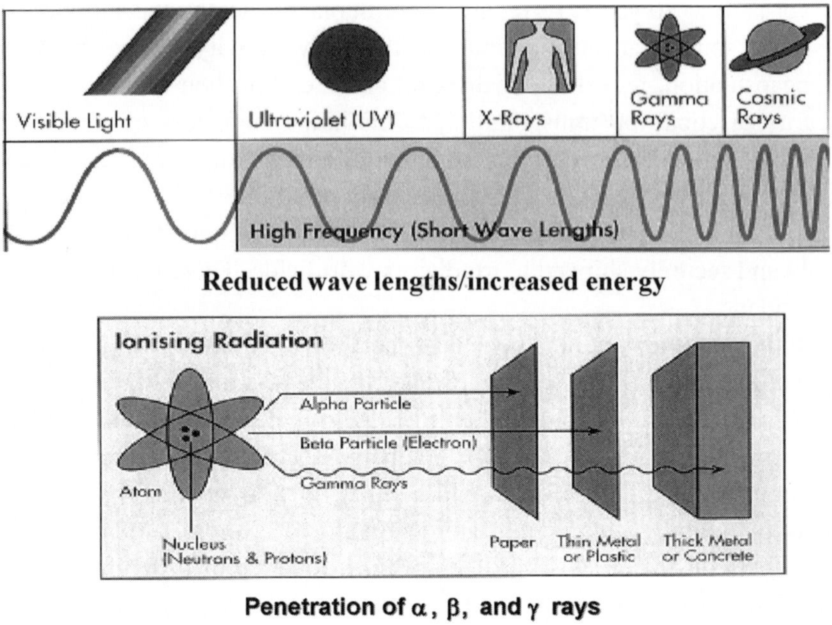

Fig. 1. Energy spectrum of electromagnetic waves and penetration mode of α, β, and γ rays.

Industrial Irradiators

Commercial irradiators have either gamma rays emitted by cobalt-60 or electrons generated by an electron accelerator. Table 2 summarizes the different characteristics between the two.

Table 2. Comparison between gamma and electron irradiators.

Characteristic	Gamma	Electron
Energy	1.17 and 1.33 MeV	0.2–10 MeV
Power	1.48 kW/100 kCi	4–400 kW/unit
Dose rate	Low (kGy/h)	High (kGy/s)
Maintenance	Replenishment of cobalt-60, decay 1%/month	Replacement of electronic parts
Penetration	High (43 cm in water)	Low (0.35 cm/MeV)
Energy utilization efficiency	Low (~40%)	High (90%)
Product thickness (assume product density 0.5 gcm^{-3})	80–100 cm	8–10 cm (double-sided irradiation)

In choosing radiation as the sterilization process, several factors have to be considered:

1. Type of radiation: Gamma rays are preferred due to their deep penetration that allows tissues to be irradiated after final packaging in a box. Electron beams with a high dose rate can irradiate in a shorter time, but have limited penetration; only an accelerator with a high energy level (5–10 MeV) can have better penetration. The uniformity of radiation dose distribution must be close to 1.
2. Radiation dosage: A 25-kGy or 2.5-Mrad dose is the most commonly used radiation dose for sterilization, but tissue bankers can decide the dosage used to sterilize their tissues. The dose can be selected depending on the bioburden or microbial count on the tissue prior to sterilization, and on the types of microbes (more specifically, the most commonly found and radioresistant microbes). Dose setting for the radiation sterilization of tissue, as described in chapter 19, requires a radiation facility that can deliver very accurate doses for validation work (i.e. verification dose $\pm 10\%$).
3. Temperature and condition during irradiation: For air- and freeze-dried tissues, irradiation is conducted at room temperature, while chilled and frozen tissues must be irradiated at the appropriate temperature. It is a great challenge to irradiate frozen tissues, as the frozen temperature needs to be maintained before, during, and after irradiation.
4. Product integrity: Product density and configuration in a box help to improve the radiation dose distribution in the box. It is advisable not to mix different types of products with a wide range of density in a box. The packaging material used must be compatible with radiation, and must stay intact after irradiation and throughout storage.

Components for Irradiation Facilities

An irradiation plant looks like any other warehousing facility. It requires a special site license from the appropriate national licensing authority, and is regulated by radiation safety authorities. The irradiation facility consists of four main components:

1. The irradiation cell — a source room with a concrete biological shield.

2. Radiation source — a gamma source, unlike an electron beam machine, cannot be switched off and emits rays even when the plant is not in operation. The radioactive source, sealed in stainless steel tubes, is lowered into a pool of water 6–9 m deep to shield the environment from gamma radiation.
3. An automatic product conveyor/carrier system — the system carries the product from the unprocessed product area to the irradiation room, and then brings it to the processed product area after treatment.
4. A control, safety, and auxiliary system — product scheduling, tracking, treatment programs, and documentation are all integrated to ensure a reliable irradiation service. The delivered and absorbed doses must be validated and documented to prove adequate processing and to comply with regulatory requirements. All of the plant safety systems must be closely monitored to ensure that the radiation source is in a safe position in the event of critical component failure during operation.

Figure 2 shows the setup of a gamma radiation facility with cobalt-60 as the radiation source at the Malaysian Nuclear Agency (NM) (Daud *et al.* 2005). The carrier is of hanging type. It is very important to segregate the processed product area from the unprocessed product area. A fence normally separates these areas.

Figure 3 shows the internal setup of an electron beam irradiator. The carrier is of conveyor type and can carry products on pellets, in totes, or in individual packages, depending upon the application and penetrating power. The photo shown is the scan horn of the electron beam machine available at NM.

Figure 4 shows a gamma cell used for the sterilization of tissue allografts as well as for the verification of radiation sterilization dose experiments of amnion and bone grafts (BATAN Research Tissue Bank, Jakarta).

Good Radiation Practice (GRP)

Good Radiation Practice (GRP) is an integral part of the overall manufacturing of any sterile medical product. GRP is in accordance with international standards (ISO 11137, 1995), and is as important as Good Manufacturing Practice (GMP) in the manufacturing line. It covers the following aspects:

- Irradiator
- Dosimeters

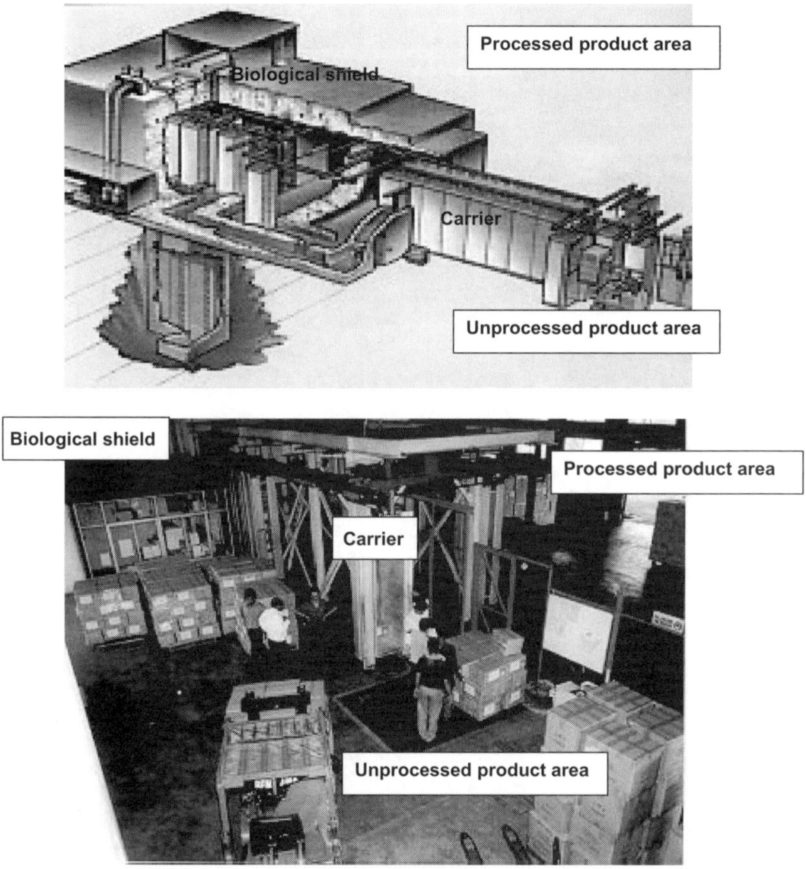

Fig. 2. Gamma irradiation facility (Mintec-Sinagama: diagram and photo).

- Dose mapping
- Material compatibility
- Product validation
- Routine process control

Irradiator

During plant commissioning, it is extremely important to characterize the magnitude, distribution, and reproducibility of the absorbed dose in products of a certain density as well as relate these parameters with operating

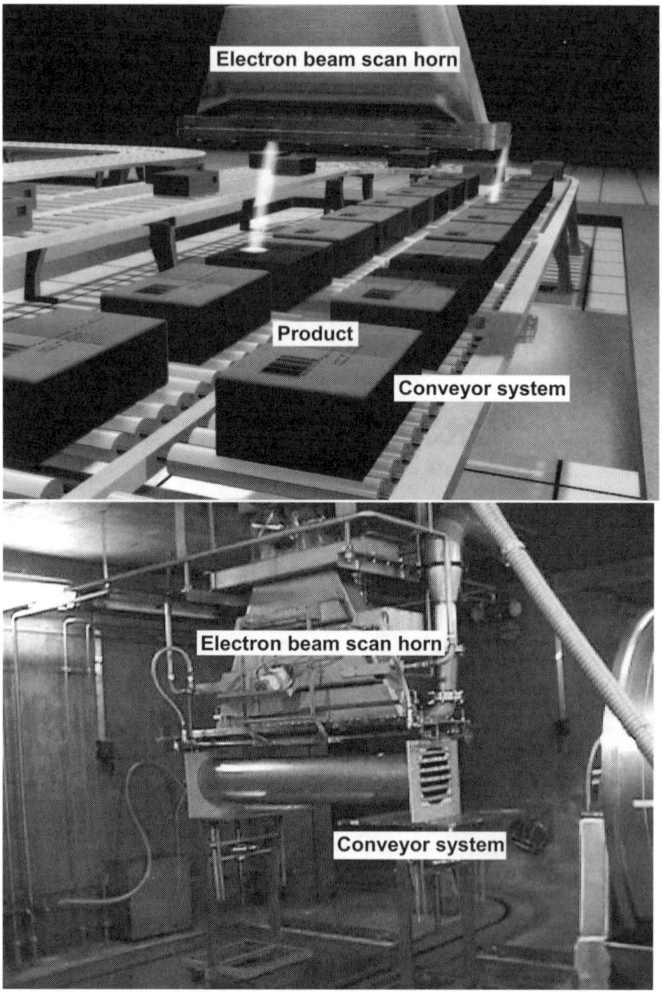

Fig. 3. Electron beam facilities (scan horn and conveyor system).

conditions. The plant operation must ensure that all systems are functioning correctly, calibrated, and reproducible.

Dosimeters

The primary (reference) dosimeter — e.g. Fricke (ferrous sulfate solution for gamma rays) or graphite calorimeter (for electron beams) — must be

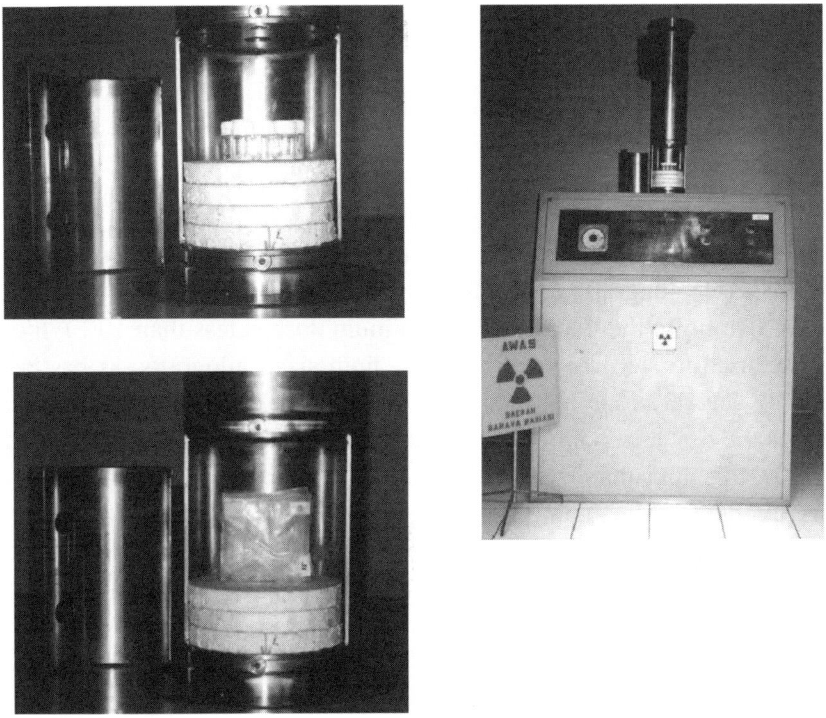

Fig. 4. Verification of radiation sterilization dose experiments of amnion and bone grafts. Ten uniform samples were irradiated at a dose rate of 2 kGy/h using a gamma cell (BATAN Research Tissue Bank, Jakarta.

used to compare the response of the routine dosimeter in the production environment. The routine dosimeter — e.g. ce/ce (ceric-cerous sulfate solution for gamma rays) or CTA (cellulose triacetate for electron beams) — is calibrated for use in the commissioning of irradiators and for routine operation. The dosimetry system must be tracable to an international comparison body, such as the International Dose Assurance Service (IDAS).

Dose mapping

Dose mapping is the placement of dosimeters throughout a representative product load during validation. The exercise identifies positions for placing routine dosimeters to trace the maximum and minimum doses. The ratio of the maximum to the minimum absorbed dose within an irradiation container can be determined as follows:

$$\text{Dose uniformity ratio (DUR)} = \frac{\text{Maximum dose}}{\text{Minimum dose}}$$

Gamma cell

A gamma cell of Co-60 can be used to validate the radiation sterilization dose of tissue allografts (ISO TIR 27), based on a dose uniformity ratio of nearly 1 (ratio of the maximum to minimum dose is less than 10%). It can also be used to sterilize small- and medium-sized allografts, as has been done by several tissue banks such as the Bangkok Biomaterial Center as well as the tissue banks in Padang and Jakarta, Indonesia (see chapters 16 and 17). It is not suitable to sterilize big and long bones because the size of the chamber is only about 2 L (see Fig. 4).

Routine process control

An irradiation plant must establish procedures to receive products for sterilization treatment, store the product, and return the irradiated products. Usually, the cartons are given a radiation batch number and routine dosimeters at selected locations. In addition, a radiation indicator is stuck to every carton. The indicator — commonly known as a go/no-go indicator — changes color after exposure to radiation, such as from yellow to red or from yellow to green, depending on the dye content. The indicator is not a dosimeter and will never record the absorbed dose. It is simply an indicator to guide the plant operator and later the users on whether the carton has been sent to the irradiation room.

After products have been irradiated, dosimeters are sent to the dosimetry quality control (QC) laboratory to measure the absorbed dose. All records of absorbed dose measurements are filed according to the international quality system for easy tracability. The plant then issues a certification for the minimum dose delivery (and also the maximum dose delivery, if required) for each radiation batch to the customer.

References

Daud M *et al.* (2005). *Nuclear Science and Technology*, NM, Bangi, Malaysia.

International Atomic Energy Agency (IAEA) (2004). Code of Practice for Radiation Sterilization of Tissue Allografts: Requirements for Validation and Routine Control, Project No. INT/6/052, IAEA, Vienna.
International Standards Organization (ISO) (1995). Requirements for Validation and Routine Control — Radiation Sterilization, ISO 11137, 1995(E), Switzerland.
Malaysian Nuclear Agency (NM) (2004). *Medical X-Ray*, NM, Bangi, Malaysia.

Chapter 9

Radiation Killing Effects on Bacteria and Fungi

Norimah Yusof

Malaysian Nuclear Agency (NM)
Bangi, 43000 Kajang, Selangor
Malaysia

Introduction

An important step in selecting radiation as the terminal sterilization of tissues is to understand the killing effect of radiation on microorganisms. Inactivation of bacteria and fungi are brought about partly by direct collision action in a sensitive part of the cell and partly by indirect action via highly reactive radicals produced in the cell liquid by the radiation (McLaughlin and Holm 1973). In the case of direct action, the incoming particles ionize a DNA molecule, an enzyme, or some other sensitive region, resulting in destruction of or significant changes to the cell. A sufficient amount of damage may result in complete changes or inactivation of a given viable organism. Radiation may damage the cell membrane; as a result, the cell life function may be profoundly changed or disturbed, the cell respiratory function may be affected, or cell division may be thwarted. In indirect action, the reactive radicals interact with cell constituents, leading to significant changes in the cell characteristics.

All microorganisms contain a certain amount of water. When radiation energy is deposited in an aqueous system, it leads to a chain of chemical reactions by which free radicals such as OH^* and H^* as well as molecules such as hydrogen peroxide (H_2O_2) are formed. These species are chemically highly reactive with vital constituents in the living organisms, thus indirectly causing lethal damage.

Microorganisms

Microorganisms are living organisms of primitive life forms. Most of them are unicellular, individually too small to be seen with the naked eye. The five major groups of microorganisms are bacteria, viruses, fungi (molds and yeasts), protozoa, and algae. Of these, bacteria and fungi are the most common microbes contaminating medical products.

Variations among the groups can be resolved into two principal types at the cellular level: eukaryotic and prokaryotic (Volk and Wheeler 1988). Eukaryotic microorganisms consist of the fungi (yeasts and molds) and the protozoa, while prokaryotic cell types consist of bacteria and cyanobacteria. Viruses are not cells, but consist primarily of nucleic acid surrounded by a protective coat. Viruses can replicate only when they are within a susceptible prokaryotic or eukaryotic cell.

As shown in Fig. 1, eukaryotic cells possess many intracellular membranes: endoplasmic reticula, Golgi apparatuses, ribosomes, mitochondria, microtubules, etc. In addition, eukaryotic cells possess a true nucleus composed of a number of DNA strands (chromosomes), all enclosed in a double-membrane structure (nuclear envelope) that separates the nucleus from the cytoplasm. Prokaryotic cells, on the other hand, have no separate membrane-bound organelles. Prokaryotic cells contain a single circular chromosome that is not enclosed within a membrane and does not break up into chromosomes during cell division.

In general, bacteria are most commonly found in and on medical products. Fundamental studies on the radiation effects on bacteria began immediately after the discovery of X-rays by Rontgens in 1895, and have become the basis for elucidating the mechanism of lethal action of radiation on cells.

Radiation Effects

Irradiation with gamma rays, X-rays, or accelerated electrons — all of which are ionizing radiations — has been recognized as a sterilization technique

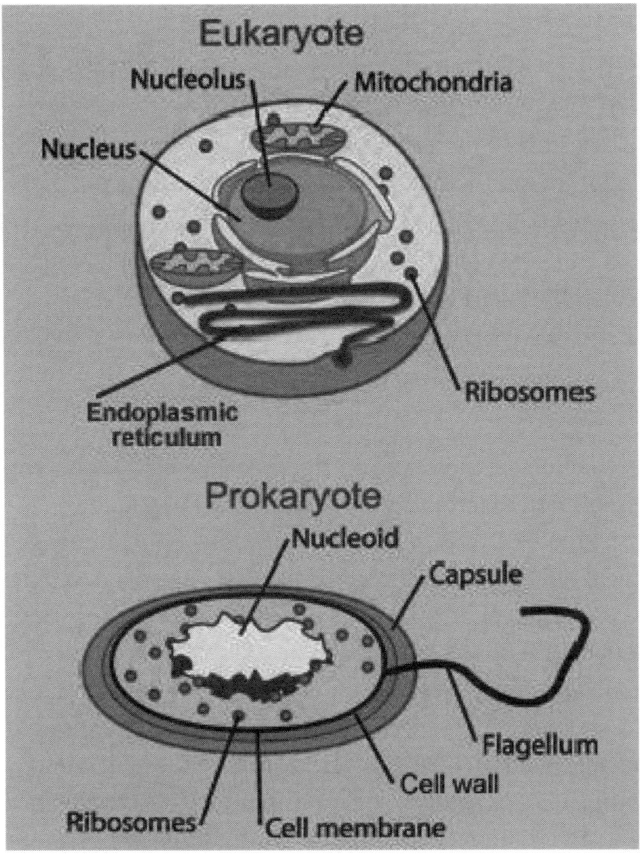

Fig. 1. Basic structure of eukaryotic and prokaryotic cells.

alongside heating, drying, and chemical usage. Ionizing radiations kill all types of microorganisms, and usually have enough energy for penetration into solids and liquids. Radiations do not significantly heat or wet materials, and are widely used for the industrial sterilization of heat-sensitive medical and laboratory equipment. Therefore, radiation can be considered for sterilizing tissues.

As mentioned earlier, the effects of radiation on cells can be divided into direct and indirect actions.

Direct action

The direct action of radiation involves the simple interaction between the ionizing radiation and critical biological molecules, resulting in excitation, lesion, and scission of the polymeric structure. High-energy photons pass through a cell, interact with atoms or molecules along the path, and break the DNA strands. Due to photon energy deposited on the DNA, a transient formation of ions occurs in the DNA molecules. The action damages the DNA structure, thus disrupting the normal cell functions (NM 2005). Direct action may involve the addition of hydrogen atoms to the opened bonds.

Indirect action

The indirect action of radiation on microorganisms can be considered in three stages, each of extremely short duration: ionization (10^{-16} to 10^{-17} s), radical formation (10^{-12} to 10^{-14} s), and biochemical changes (10^{-8} s). The biological effects of radiation are basically due to biochemical changes within the organism (Gardner and Peel 1986).

Due to the breakdown of water molecules, the interaction of radiation with the aqueous system results in excitation and ionization, as described in detail in chapter 7. The presence of substantial quantities of water in microorganisms leads to free radical formation when radiation photons interact with water molecules, ejecting many electrons at high velocities. Consequently, the indirect effect of radiation normally occurs as an important part of the total action of radiation, summarized as follows:

$$H_2O \rightarrow e^-_{aq} + OH^* + H^*$$

Aqueous electron (e^-_{aq}) and the free radicals (H^*, OH^*) are very reactive. They easily interact further among themselves, with water molecules, with their own reaction products, or with organic molecules within cell constituents (RH). The organic molecules RH also become directly ionized into the free radicals R^*, which react with biologically important cellular molecules (e.g. proteins, enzymes, amino acids, metabolites, nucleic material, etc.) and cause radiobiological damage. These chain reactions, which are called the indirect action of radiation, are generally held responsible for the radiation effects. Indirect action involves aqueous free radicals known as radiolytic products that act as intermediaries in the transfer of radiation energy to biological molecules.

Bacteria and fungi are affected by ionizing radiation in a similar manner, but very much related to the nature of the organism and especially to its complexity. Radiation damage is mainly associated with the impairment of metabolic reactions. Much evidence shows that the damage occurs more in DNA molecules compared to other critical sites including membranes and ribosomes of microorganisms. The main biological target, DNA, controls the genetic constitution and reproductive process of the cell. DNA is the most vital cell constituent, and it presents a relatively large volume in the microbial cell for absorption of radiation and a large surface for reaction with radiolytic products. Two types of DNA damage have been recognized: a break in one (single-strand break) or both (double-strand break) of the DNA strands, and a lesion in the nitrogenous bases.

Figure 2 shows some of the DNA damages. About 40% of the DNA damage is caused by direct action and 60% is caused by indirect ionization, which also causes injury to membranes (Hendry 2003). One active radical may cause a double-strand break if it is directly produced in the DNA molecule. Indirect action produces single-strand breaks; but if the damaged sections on the two strands overlap, then the effect would be the same as a double-strand break. Death of the cell may result from about 3 double-strand breaks in *Escherichia coli* to about 1400 in *Micrococcus radiodurans.* Following the DNA damages, the killing effect after irradiation is due to the loss of reproductive ability of bacteria and fungi.

Repair of Damaged DNA

Some microorganisms have a great capability to repair damaged DNA molecules. For instance, *Micrococcus radiodurans* and *Micrococcus radiophilus*, which are believed to be capable of repairing DNA damage, are more resistant than bacterial spores. Some strains of *Streptococcus faecium* are more resistant than any nonsporing bacteria. The efficiency of a repair system is often reflected by a large increase in the dose of radiation for inactivation. The ability of cells to recover and grow after irradiation reflects on their resistance. Bacteria and fungi are not killed immediately after a lethal dose has been absorbed. At the cellular level, death usually occurs during the first DNA replication.

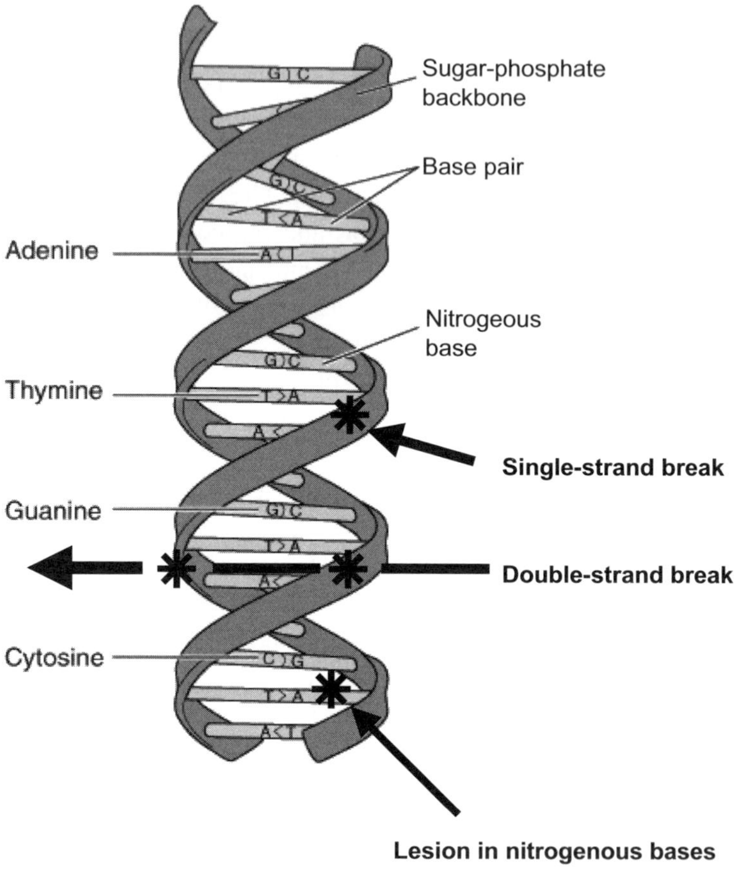

Fig. 2. DNA damages by radiation.

Radiation Response

The response of bacteria and fungi to radiation is conveniently expressed as D_{10} (kGy), the dose required to reduce one log cycle or kill 90% of the population. In practice, a number of equal-sized populations are exposed to different doses of radiation and different counts in the number of survivors. The counts, expressed as colony-forming units or cell survival fractions, are plotted on a log scale against the doses on a linear scale. The surviving cells' decreases against doses give rise to an inactivation or response curve.

In radiation sterilization, there are generally three types of radiation response curves or survival curves for any single-strain microbial

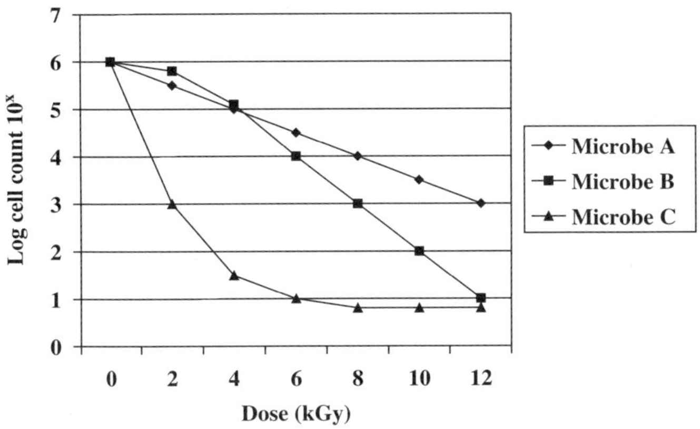

Fig. 3. Dose response curve for three microorganisms.

population. As shown in Fig. 3, the response curve can be linear, shouldered, or exponential. The response curve for microbe A is the most common, whereby the killing rate is directly proportional to the radiation dose given. The curve for microbe B — with a "shoulder" at lower doses — indicates that the microbe has the ability to repair some damage occurring at lower doses; but beyond a certain dose, the killing is again proportionate to the radiation doses. The gradient at the slope or straight line is determined as the D_{10} value. The curve for microbe C is very unlikely to be obtained for any pure culture. This type of survival curve can be from a mixed population made up of very sensitive and very resistant microbes.

The D_{10} value is calculated as the gradient of the linear part of the curve, or as follows:

$$D_{10} = \frac{D}{[\log N_0 - \log N]}$$

where

D is the radiation dose (kGy) required to reduce the population from N_0 to N
N_0 is the initial viable count
N is the viable count after dose D

As explained in chapter 2, the greater the D_{10} value, the more resistant the microbes are towards radiation.

Factors Influencing Response to Radiation

The D_{10} value or radiation sensitivity is influenced by many factors, including the type and species of microorganism, cell cycle stage, oxygen, water content, temperature during irradiation, chemicals and nutrients, and to a certain extent the dose rate. The D_{10} values of some common microorganisms are listed in Table 1.

Table 1. D_{10} values of some common microorganisms in various conditions.

Microorganism	D_{10} value (kGy)	Irradiated medium
Yeast		
Saccharomyces cerevisiae	0.5	Saline + 5% gelatin
Torulopsis candida	0.4	Saline + 5% gelatin
Molds		
Aspergillus niger	0.5	Saline + 5% gelatin
Penicillium notatum	0.2	Saline + 5% gelatin
Vegetative bacteria		
Salmonella typhimurium	0.2	Phosphate buffer
	1.3	Frozen in buffer
Escherichia coli	0.09	Phosphate buffer
Staphylococcus aureus	0.2	Phosphate buffer
	1.4	Ophthalmic ointment
Pseudomonas sp.	0.03–0.06	Phosphate buffer
Streptococcus faecium	2.6	Phosphate buffer
Micrococcus radiodurans	2.2	Phosphate buffer
Aerobic spore formers		
Bacillus subtilis	1.7–2.5	Paper disk
	0.6	Saline + 5% gelatin
Bacillus pumilus E601	1.7	Water
	2.0	Dried
	3.0	Dried (vacuum)
Bacillus sphaericus	10.0	Dried organic compound
Anaerobic spore formers		
Clostridium botulinum	0.8	Water buffer
	3.2	Frozen at −20°C
Clostridium welchii	1.2–2.0	Water
	2.7	Paper disk
Clostridium tetani	2.4	Water
Viruses		
Foot and mouth	13.0	Frozen at −60°C
Vaccinia	1.7	*In vacuo*

Types and species

In general, the radiation sensitivity of an organism is roughly inversely proportional to its size. Microorganisms are more resistant to radiation than other higher forms of life. Many bacteria are relatively more resistant compared to fungi. The viruses, the most minute living entities, are the most radiation-resistant, some surviving at as high as 100 kGy (10 Mrad); whilst man, approximately at the other end of the size range and complexity, suffers death with only 5 Gy (500 rad). Gram-negative vegetative bacteria are more sensitive compared to Gram-positive vegetative bacteria. The general order of increasing resistance is as follows:

Molds and yeasts $<$ Vegetative bacteria $<$ Bacterial spores $<$ Viruses

Bacterial spores are usually more resistant than vegetative bacteria. As in Table 1, *Bacillus subtilis* is resistant during spore forming (D_{10} = 1.7–2.5 kGy), but is almost similar to yeasts and molds when irradiated in saline + 5% gelatin with the D_{10} value reduced to 0.6 kGy. The protection mechanism may be related to the spore core and the nondividing stage.

The particular phase of growth at the time of irradiation might account for the observed differences, as high resistance is expected in the stationary phase and most sensitive in the dividing or vegetative stage. Radioresistancy may also be due to variation between genera, species, and strains. *Clostirium* sp., when irradiated in water, varies in resistance according to species. As in Table 1, *C. botulinum* (D_{10} = 0.8 kGy) is more sensitive than *C. welchii* (D_{10} = 1.2–2.0 kGy), which in turn is more sensitive than *C. tetani* (D_{10} = 2.4 kGy). The radioresistance of *Micrococcus radiodurans* (D_{10} = 2.2 kGy) and *Streptococcus faecium* (D_{10} = 2.6 kGy) is associated with their very efficient repair mechanisms. Fortunately, *M. radiodurans* is nonpathogenic and is unlikely to occur as a contaminant on tissue products. The radiation resistance of fungus spores is usually much less than the resistance of spore-forming bacteria. Therefore, a radiation dose sufficient to inactivate bacterial contamination on tissues will naturally eliminate fungal contamination (Hendry 2003).

Oxygen

Oxygen can enhance radiation damage. Oxygen may react either with e^-_{aq} and H^* to produce the perhydroxyl or superoxide radical or with organic radicals to give peroxy species. The resistance of microorganisms is usually increased two to five times if irradiated in nonaerated conditions. The spore of *Bacillus pumilus* has a D_{10} value of 2.0 kGy when dried in air and 3.0 kGy when dried in the absence of oxygen (Table 1).

Water

A high amount of water results in more radical formation due to radiolysis. The influence of water on microorganisms' susceptibility is interrelated with that of oxygen. The interaction of oxygen with free radicals in aqueous condition results in more radiation damage. As listed in Table 1, the D_{10} value of the *Bacillus pumilus* E601 spore decreases from 2.0 kGy when irradiated dried on paper disk to 1.7 kGy in water. The D_{10} value of *Clostridium welchii* decreases from 2.7 kGy on paper disk to 1.2–2.0 kGy in water.

Temperature

The radioresistance or D_{10} value reduces by as much as 50% when the temperature increases in the order of 10°C. A synergistic effect is observed when heat and irradiation are simultaneously applied; this effect is greater than the sum of the separate effects. An increase in the resistance of vegetative organisms is observed by freezing

When spores of *Clostridium botulinum* are irradiated in frozen phosphate buffer, there is a sharp increase in resistance from 0.8 to 3.2 kGy (Table 1). This is attributed to the reduction of indirect effect, as the active radicals produced in water are immobilized. The D_{10} value for *Salmonella typhimurium* in phosphate buffer increases from 0.2 to 1.3 kGy when irradiated in frozen buffer. The protective effect of low temperature is also observed in other vegetative organisms.

Nutrient or organic substrates

Protection against radiation damage is conferred when irradiated in an enriched environment such as dried serum broth, grease films, sucrose, and other complex substrates. As indicated in Table 1, the D_{10} value for *Staphylococcus aureus* increases from 0.2 kGy in phosphate buffer to 1.4 kGy in ophthalmic ointment. The D_{10} value for *Bacillus sphaericus* in dried organic compound is considered high, reaching 10 kGy.

Chemical agents

Some chemicals such as glycerol, thiourea, dimethyl sulphoxide, and cysteine tend to protect bacteria against radiation damage. They possibly scavenge free radicals, thus blocking radiolysis or using up oxygen and causing depletion during irradiation. On the other hand, other chemicals including iodoacetic acid and potassium iodide act as sensitizers, resulting in an increase in single-strand breaks through the reaction of iodine compound with radiolytic products of water or cell components. Some chemicals may influence the radiation effects after irradiation. The environment before, during, and immediately after irradiation influences the variation in radioresistance or D_{10} values for bacteria and fungi.

Dose rate

At very high dose rates, oxygen depletion occurs, resulting in greater resistance when a pure culture of bacteria is exposed to electron beams. The large dose rate difference between gamma and electron beams could be significant; however, the dose rate used in commercial plants has no significant effect on resistance. Dose-rate differences between gamma sources (acute and chronic) are too small to be of any significance with respect to bacterial inactivation.

Microbiological Quality Control

The number (bioburden) and type (resistancy) of microorganisms on the products are two important parameters to be considered in a microbiological quality control (QC) test of finished tissue products. This microbiological QC test must be designed to ensure that the procurement and processing conducted meet certain defined or stipulated standards, and that the radiation dose selected is able to achieve high-sterility assurance.

Bioburden

Bioburden refers to the total number or count of viable microorganisms on a packaged product prior to sterilization processing. The test also includes isolation and identification.

Sterility test

A sterility test is performed to determine if viable microorganisms are present on the sterilized product. The test is conducted for product release, and is applicable to sterilization methods other than radiation.

Conclusion

The damages by ionizing radiation that lead to killing effects in bacteria and fungi can occur via two main mechanisms, namely direct action and indirect action due to reactive products of water molecules. Microorganisms in principle are relatively resistant to radiation, simply due to their small size and target size of DNA compared to higher forms of life. The resistance is influenced by a number of factors, including the type, species, and cell cycle stage of the microbe; the presence of oxygen and water during irradiation; the temperature; the nutrient content; various radiation scavengers and radiation protectants; and the dose rate of radiation sources. By understanding the mode of action of the killing effects of radiation on bacteria and fungi as well as the factors influencing the effects, we can specify the best irradiation conditions in which radiation can effectively kill the microorganisms with little or no detrimental damage to the tissue products.

References

Gardner JF and Peel MM (1986). *Introduction to Sterilisation and Disinfection*, Churchill Livingstone, Edinburgh.

Hendry JE (2003). Protective effects on microorganisms in radiation sterilised tissues. In: Kennedy JF, Phillips GO, and Williams PA (eds.), *Sterilisation of Tissues Using Ionising Radiations*, CRC Woodhead Publishing, England, pp. 331–338.

Malaysian Nuclear Agency (NM) (2005). *Radiation Awareness*, NM, Bangi, Malaysia.

McLaughlin WL and Holm NW (1973). Physical characteristics of ionising radiation. In: *Manual on Radiation Sterilization of Medical and Biological Materials*, IAEA Technical Report Series No. 149, Vienna, pp. 5–12.

Volk WA and Wheeler MF (1988). *Basic Microbiology*, Harper & Row, New York.

Yusof N (1999). Quality system for the radiation sterilisation of tissue allografts. In: Phillips GO, Strong DM, von Versen R, and Nather A (eds.), *Advances in Tissue Banking*, Vol. 3, World Scientific, Singapore, pp. 257–281.

Chapter 10

New Emerging Infectious Diseases Caused by Viruses and Prions, and How Radiation Can Overcome Them

Nazly Hilmy and Paramita Pandansari

BATAN Research Tissue Bank (BRTB)
Center for Research and Development of Isotopes and Radiation Technology, BATAN
Jakarta 12070, Indonesia

Introduction

Despite remarkable advances in medical research and treatment during the 20th century, infectious diseases caused by viruses remain among the leading causes of death worldwide for three reasons: (1) the emergence of new infectious diseases, (2) the re-emergence of old infectious diseases, and (3) the persistence of intractable infectious diseases. Emerging infectious diseases caused by viruses, including human outbreaks of previously unknown or known disease, have significantly increased in the past two decades. Re-emerging diseases are known diseases that have reappeared after a significant decline in incidence. New emerging and re-emerging infectious diseases caused by viruses and prions are breaking and rebreaking out around the world.

Transmission of infectious diseases through contaminated blood, feces, and other body liquids from an unscreened donor onto an allograft, xenograft, or food product will increase the outbreak of infectious diseases. An allograft is a graft transplanted between two different individuals of the same species (e.g. from one human being to another human being), while a xenograft is a graft transplanted between two different species (e.g. from animals to human beings) (IAEA 2004).

Viruses are very small microbes that have DNA/RNA and are generally resistant to radiation, but they can be eliminated by radiation if the dosage is high enough. A prion is defined as a small proteinaceous infectious particle, which resists inactivation by procedures that modify nucleic acids (Prusiner 1996). Research on the elimination of their contamination on products by irradiation is limited. Prions and several viruses are responsible for human epidemics/pandemics: they have made the transition from animal host to human host, and now several of them are transmitted from human to human. The human immunodeficiency virus (HIV) is responsible for the AIDS epidemic, the severe acute respiratory syndrome (SARS) is suspected of being caused by the corona virus, and the bird flu or avian influenza is caused by the *Orthomyxoviridae* (H5N1) virus family. Other examples of emerging infectious diseases include mad cow disease and Creutzfeldt–Jakob disease, caused by prions (CDC 2003; WHO 2003; Pruss *et al.* 2005).

New infectious diseases continue to evolve and emerge. Changes in human demography by changing transmission dynamics to bring people into closer and more frequent contact with pathogens, human behavior, land use, etc. are contributing to new disease emergences. This may involve exposure to animal or arthropod carriers of these diseases. Zoonotic pathogens are more likely to be associated with emerging diseases than nonemerging ones (Murphy 1998).

The increasing trade in exotic animals as pets and food sources has contributed to a rise in opportunity for pathogens to jump from animal reservoirs to human beings. For example, close contact with exotic rodents imported to the United States as pets was found to be the origin of the recent US monkeypox outbreak, and the use of exotic civet cats for meat in China was found to be a route by which the SARS corona virus made the transition from animal to human hosts. In addition, the migration of birds was found to be a route for the outbreak of avian flu type H5N1 (CDC 2003; NIAID 2005; NCID 2005; WHO 2006).

Radiation technology has been used to sterilize medical devices as well as allografts, xenografts, and implanted devices used in surgeries without risk of infection. This chapter describes new emerging diseases, their possibility to contaminate allografts and xenografts, as well as the possibility to eliminate contaminated viruses and prions from tissue bank products either by irradiation or by combined treatment of irradiation and other methods for safe utilization.

Emerging Infectious Diseases and How Far They Can Affect the Allografts and Xenografts (Hilmy and Pandansari 2006)

Emerging infectious diseases caused by viruses and prions are defined as infections that have newly appeared in a population, or have existed but are rapidly increasing in incidence or geographic range. Within the past few years, many infectious disease outbreaks have been reported in some countries.

Viral diseases (Table 1)

The SARS corona virus (SARS Co-V) emerged in several Asian countries such as Hong Kong, China, Taiwan, and Singapore in 2003 (CDC 2003; Eastlund 2005).

The West Nile virus was first isolated in Uganda in 1937; today, it is most commonly found in Africa, West Asia, Europe, and the Middle East. In 1999, it was found in the western hemisphere for the first time in the New York City area; in the early spring of 2000, it appeared again in birds and mosquitoes and then spread to other parts of the eastern United States. By 2004, the virus had been found in birds and mosquitoes in every state except Alaska and Hawaii. Between January 1, 2004, and January 11, 2005, the West Nile virus was reported to have caused 2470 cases of disease, including 88 deaths (NCID 2005).

The Ebola virus (*Filoviridae* family) is an RNA virus that causes hemorrhagic fever. It has emerged in several countries in Africa, such as Zaire, Sudan, Gabon, and South Africa. The Marburg virus (*Filoviridae* family) is also an RNA virus that first emerged in Africa in 1967 and re-emerged in 2005 in Angola.

HIV, hepatitis B virus (HBV), and hepatitis C virus (HCV) are still emerging in Asia, Africa, and elsewhere. They can be transmitted through blood transfusions and organ or allograft transplantation (Conrad *et al.* 1995;

Table 1. Emerging and re-emerging diseases caused by viruses.

Virus	Diseases	Countries affected
West Nile virus (flavivirus)	Encephalitis, meningitis (neuroinvasive disease)	United States (1999–2005)
Corona virus	SARS	China, Hong Kong, Taiwan, Singapore, Canada, US (2003)
Bunyaviridae family	Rift Valley fever	Africa (1978, 1993), Madagascar (1991), Saudi Arabia (2000)
Monkeypox virus (orthopoxvirus group)	Monkeypox	Central & West Africa (1978), US (2003), Germany, Yugoslavia
Nipah virus	Encephalitis & respiratory illness	Malaysia, Singapore (1999)
HIV	AIDS	Worldwide
Hendra virus	Respiratory & neurological diseases	Australia (1994)
Hantaan virus	Hantavirus cardiopulmonary syndrome	Korea (1950), Finland (1980), New Mexico (1993)
Ebola virus (filovirus)	Ebola hemorrhagic fever	Zaire, Sudan, Uganda, Gabon (1976–2001)
Bird flu virus	Avian influenza (H5N1)	Hong Kong (1997), Vietnam, Indonesia (2004–2006)

O'Brien and Pomerantz 1996; Chisari and Ferrari 1997; Pruss *et al.* 2005; Eastlund 2005).

The Nipah virus (*Paramyxoviridae* family) has a single-stranded (ss) DNA, and emerged in Malaysia and Singapore in 1998–1999. The Hendra virus (*Paramyxoviridae* family) also has an ssDNA, and emerged in 1994 in Brisbane, Australia.

The Hantaan virus caused Korean hemorrhagic fever from 1950 to 1960. It re-emerged in Finland as the Puumala virus in 1980, and in New Mexico as the Sin Nombre virus in 1993.

Avian influenza or bird flu virus type H5N1 is caused by an RNA virus (*Orthomyxoviridae* family). It emerged in Hong Kong in 1997; Vietnam and

Indonesia in 2004–2006; Turkey in 2005; Macedonia and Romania in 2005; and most recently in Nigeria, Germany, and Austria in February 2006. This virus consists of two vital proteins: hemagglutinins, and neuraminidase. The virulent virus type H5N1, which jumps from birds/animals to humans, can cause a pandemic. As of February 2006, a total of 88 human deaths caused by avian influenza A (H5N1) have been reported, of which 18 were in Indonesia, 42 in Vietnam, 14 in Thailand, 4 in Turkey, and 4 in China. Millions of birds have been killed, and this practice is expected to continue year by year following their migration (WHO 2006).

If tissues obtained from screened donors are free of HIV and hepatitis B/C viruses (as stated in several tissue bank standards), but are infected by one of the new emerging infectious disease viruses without any process to eliminate them, then they might be transferred to the recipient through transplantation of the contaminated allografts or xenografts.

Prion diseases (Table 2)

Prion diseases are caused by infectious agents called prion proteins, which do not have a nucleic acid genome. A prion is a small proteinaceous infectious particle, which resists inactivation by procedures that modify nucleic acids (Prusiner 1996).

Prion diseases are often called spongiform encephalopathies because of the postmortem appearance of brains with large vacuoles in the cortex and cerebellum. Specific examples of prion diseases in animals include scrapie in sheep; transmissible mink encephalopathy in mink; chronic wasting

Table 2. Prion diseases in animals and humans.

	Diseases
Animals	Scrapie Transmissible mink encephalopathy Chronic wasting disease Bovine spongiform encephalopathy
Human beings	Creutzfeldt–Jakob disease (CJD), variant CJD Gerstmann–Straussler–Scheinker syndrome Fatal familial insomnia Bovine spongiform encephalopathy

disease in mule, deer, and elk; and bovine spongiform encephalopathy in cows. Humans are also susceptible to several prion diseases such as Creutzfeldt–Jakob disease, Gerstmann–Straussler–Scheinker syndrome, fatal familial insomnia, and bovine spongiform encephalopathy, which host-jumps from cows to humans (Prusiner 1995; Prusiner 1996; WHO 2003; Pattison 1998; Pruss *et al.* 2005).

Specific factors precipitating disease emergence can be identified in virtually all cases. These include ecological, environmental, and demographic factors that place people in increased contact with previously unfamiliar microbes or their natural host; human demography and behavior; international travel; technology and industry; microbial adaptation and change; and breakdown in public health measures (Murphy 1998; Woolhouse and Gowtage-Sequeria 2005).

Zoonotic Viruses

Many members of the *Flaviviridae* and *Bunyaviridae* families appear to be zoonotic viruses, which can be transmitted from animals to humans (HIV is a zoonotic virus that can also be transferred from human to human).

Zoonoses (i.e. diseases caused by zoonotic pathogens) can be broken down into two basic groups: those spread by direct contact with an infected animal, and those spread via an intermediate vector. Humans can be infected through many vectors; for example, members of the hantavirus genus are spread by rats, the West Nile virus by mosquitoes, and avian flu by pigs or direct contact with birds. All zoonotic members of the *Flaviviridae* and *Togaviridae* families are transmitted via an intermediate vector; while all zoonotic members of the *Arenaviridae, Paramyxoviridae*, and *Filoviridae* families are transmitted through direct contact.

Avian influenza A1 type H5N1 is a bird virus that jumps from birds to humans either via pigs or through direct contact with birds. The rapid migration of birds and movement of people around the globe today present such newly evolved emerging viruses with unparalleled opportunities to spread through the human species, perhaps with catastrophic consequences.

The Sin Nombre hantavirus, which caused an outbreak in New Mexico in 1993, is another example of a zoonotic virus. In this case, deer mice were thought to be the natural host and passed the virus through their urine and feces. The good growing conditions following an especially wet spring in 1993 allowed for an increase in the deer mouse population, which in turn resulted in more humans coming into contact with the infected material.

In 1999, the West Nile flavivirus (an African virus) emerged in the United States. The virus's normal host is birds, but humans may become infected when mosquitoes feed first on an infected bird and then on a person. The virus is rapidly spreading because it appears that numerous species of birds can serve as hosts and that the virus can be transmitted by a wide variety of different mosquitoes.

Some zoonotic viruses can be transmitted from human to human under special circumstances. The filoviruses that cause Ebola fever are zoonotic viruses, but their natural host and mode of transfer to humans have not yet been identified. Like other zoonotic viruses, the Ebola virus causes a severe disease with a very high mortality rate. Unlike most other zoonotic viruses, however, the Ebola virus can be transmitted via blood, tissues, or other body fluids from one person to another.

The Hendra virus is a member of the *Paramyxoviridae* family, and was first isolated in 1994 from specimens obtained during an outbreak of respiratory and neurological diseases in horses and humans in Hendra, a suburb of Brisbane, Australia. The human infections were due to direct exposure to tissues and secretions from infected horses. The Nipah virus, also a member of the *Paramyxoviridae* family, is related but not identical to the Hendra virus. The Nipah virus was initially isolated in 1999 upon examining samples from an outbreak of encephalitis and respiratory illness among adult men in Malaysia and Singapore. This virus was transmitted to humans, cats, and dogs through close contact with infected pigs.

The classification of viruses allows predictions about the details of replication, pathogenesis, and transmission to be made. This is particularly important when a new virus is identified. Without a classification scheme, each newly discovered virus would be like a black box. The current classification scheme allows most newly described viruses to be placed in a box with a label. In the best-case scenario, much can be assumed about the biology of the virus. Even in the worst-case scenario, a framework for investigation can be suggested because there are so few virus discoveries being made now that do not fit into the existing classification scheme. Indeed, most of the major groupings of viruses infecting humans and domesticated animals have been identified (Bruce 2002).

For a virus to multiply, it must obviously infect a cell. Viruses usually have a restricted host range (i.e. animal and cell type) in which this multiplication is possible. A comprehensive review by Murphy (1998) has identified zoonotic status as one of the strongest risk factors for a disease emergence. Roughly 75% of emerging pathogens are zoonotic, and zoonoses are twice as likely to be considered emerging than nonzoonoses.

The virus classification is shown in Fig. 1.

Viruses can be subdivided by genome type as follows:

- double-stranded (ds) DNA, e.g. *Herpesviridae* and *Picornaviridae*
- single-stranded (ss) DNA, e.g. *Parvoviridae*
- dsRNA, e.g. *Reoviridae*
- ssRNA, which can be divided into positive-sense RNA (e.g. *Picornaviridae*) and negative-sense RNA (e.g. *Paramyxoviridae*) (Bruce 2002)

Humans are infected by viruses and prions in two ways:

1. Animal to human
   Diseases can be transferred from animals to humans by direct contact with animal products as well as by close contact with animals and pets through feces, saliva, and the environment.
2. Human to human
   Diseases can be transmitted through the transplantation of human organs and tissues (e. g. kidney, liver, cornea, bone, soft tissue) as well as through blood transfusions, bone marrow transplants, and platelet transfusions.

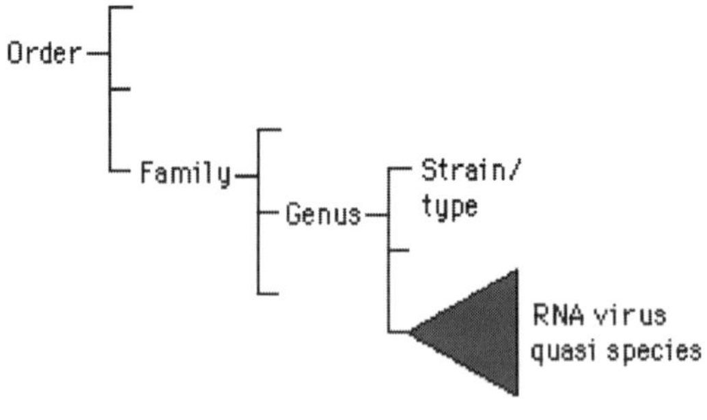

Fig. 1. Virus classification.

Diseases can also be transmitted through close contact with infected humans, e.g. in hospitals or at home.

The Possibility of Radiation to Reduce the Outbreak

Increasing international trade in animals and animal products has contributed to a rise in opportunity for pathogens to jump from animal reservoirs to humans and also from humans to humans. Products that can be contaminated by viruses or prions are meat and meat products, poultry products, dairy products, bone meal, eggs and egg powder, dried blood plasma and other blood products, xenografts, allografts, feathers (from birds), animal skin, etc.; they have a risk of spreading the disease to humans (Prusiner 1995; IAEA 2004; Eastlund 2005; WHO 2006).

To minimize and eliminate the risk of disease transmission from animal products to humans, proper processing of products should be done. This includes washing, drying, packaging, and then irradiation either at room temperature or at frozen state. In the case of allografts, strict donor screening combined with processing and irradiation are carried out at several tissue banks around the world (Pruss *et al.* 2005; Eastlund 2005; Hilmy and Lina 2001; Fideler *et al.* 1994). Allografts without terminal sterilization can be affected by viruses during the window period (Table 3). The window period is the period between the time of infection and the time the virus is detectable by screening tests.

Effects of Radiation on Viruses and Prions

It has been known that high-energy radiation of gamma rays and electron beams has the ability to generate reactive species during interaction with

Table 3. Window period (WP) of several viruses (Busch and Kleinman 2000).

Virus	HIV	HCV	HBV
WP (using FDA[a]-licensed test kit)	22 days (anti-HIV)	70 days (anti-HCV)	56 days (HBsAg)
WP (using nucleic acid test)	7–12 days	10–29 days	41–50 days

[a]Food and Drug Administration.

matter. This process involves ionization and excitation. Ionizing radiation can affect the materials in two ways, i.e. direct and indirect. Direct effects usually refer to the interaction of radiation with molecules, causing ionization or excitation and then followed by damage in the molecules. Indirect effects usually refer to the damage done to molecules by radiolytic products of irradiated water, oxygen, or other materials in the medium.

A virus is a subcellular organism with a parasitic intracellular life cycle and no metabolic activity outside the host cell. Therefore, it cannot actually stay alive outside the host cell. The antibiotics and chemotherapeutic agents that inactivate bacteria are generally ineffective against viruses. Viruses as a rule are considerably more resistant to radiation than either bacteria or bacterial spores.

The size of viruses ranges mostly from 20 nm to almost 14 000 nm. Genomes (DNA and RNA) are the major targets for the biological effects of ionizing radiation in killing the microbes. Depending on the size and type of genome, viruses can be very resistant or sensitive to irradiation. The main cause of virus inactivation is protein damage. The radiation dose required to inactivate an infectious virus or its nucleic acid is much greater under direct condition than under indirect condition. The damage of the viral nucleic acid appears to be almost solely responsible for the loss of infectivity. The sensitivity of the targets depends very much on their sizes. A large target is more sensitive to radiation compared to a smaller one. In general, a cell with a large nucleus and much DNA is more vulnerable than one with a small genome. Compared to genomes of bacteria, yeasts, and molds, viral genomes are very small, thus explaining their higher resistance to radiation.

The radiation resistance of different virus groups shows considerable differences. Viruses with single-stranded genomes are about 10 times more sensitive than viruses with double-stranded genomes, although the genomes are smaller. Viruses with large genomes may be five times more sensitive than viruses with small genomes. However, their resistance may vary as much as 10-fold depending on a number of factors, particularly the concentration of oxygen (O_2) and water, the organic materials in the suspending substrate, the temperature (frozen or room temperature), and the pH (which is unfavorable to microbes) during irradiation. Irradiation at the frozen state ($-70°C$ to $-80°C$) where water is immobilized, as well as in organic substrate (e.g. in a high concentration of protein and alcohol), will increase the radiation resistance of viruses. In contrast, radiation in wet condition at room temperature will increase the sensitivity of viruses compared to radiation in dry state. Although strand breakage has been reported as an important cause of radiation inactivation for single-stranded nucleic acid, the combination of base damage and intrastrand cross-link formation is also important. The alteration is lethal because the viruses cannot reproduce after damage to their nucleic acids.

Many D_{10} values of viruses exceed 5 kGy; in fact, some of them (e.g. foot and mouth disease virus) have D_{10} values of 13 kGy when irradiated at frozen state. The effects of radiation on microorganisms, including viruses, are exponential. The radiation sterilization dose used depends on the viral bioburden (Fideler *et al.* 1994; Hilmy and Lina 2001; Pruss *et al.* 2005). Table 4 shows several D_{10} values of viruses that can cause emerging diseases (Pruss *et al.* 2005). It can be seen that radiation does kill viruses. The amount of radiation dose required to accomplish a log reduction of viruses (i.e. D_{10} value) is higher than those of bacteria and mold/fungi, although some bacteria spores are very resistant to radiation (e.g. spores of anaerobic *Clostridium sordelli*) (Grieb *et al.* 2005).

Infectious risks of tissue and organ transplantation have often been identified after first being recognized as a blood transfusion–transmitted infection. Although the susceptibility of these viruses to gamma irradiation or other sterilants is unknown wholly, the routine use of sterilization may provide some protection from the transmission of diseases through tissue transplantation (Eastlund 2005).

Table 4. D_{10} value of envelope and nonenvelope viruses and bacteria (Hilmy and Lina 2001; Pruss *et al.* 2005).

Virus	D_{10} value (kGy)
HIV-1/2[a]	4–7.09
Bovine parvovirus[b]	7.27
Polio virus type 1[b]	7.13
Hepatitis A virus[b]	5.31
Pseudorabies virus[a]	5.29
Bovine viral diarrhoea virus[a]	<3.0
Bacteria, mold, yeast	<2.0

[a]Envelope virus.
[b]Nonenvelope virus.

Conrad *et al.* (1995) reported that the hepatitis C virus can be transmitted by processed unirradiated bone, ligament, and tendon, but no cases exist with irradiated bone of 17 kGy. In addition, studies on HIV transmission from window period donations were conducted in the USA from 1999 to 2003; the results stated that irradiation in sterilizing doses can significantly reduce the viral load and, in combination with appropriate donor screening and laboratory testing, will significantly enhance and improve the safety of tissues being used for transplantation (Strong 2005).

Unlike a virus, a prion is an infectious protein that is produced by modifying the structure of a specific prion protein (PrP) found on nerve cell membranes. The most common form of prion disease in humans is sporadic Creutzfeldt–Jakob disease (CJD) and variant CJD. Less than 1% of CJD cases are infectious, and most of them appear to be iatrogenic. Between 10% and 15% of prion disease cases are inherited, while the remaining ones are sporadic. PrP^{CJD} has been found in the brain of most patients who died of CJD. The term PrP^{CJD} is preferred by some investigators when referring to the abnormal isoform of human PrP in the human brain. PrP^{Sc} is always used after human CJD prions pass into an experimental animal.

At present, prions have gained wide recognition as extraordinary protein agents that cause a number of infectious, genetic, and spontaneous disorders (Prusiner 1995). Prions are very resistant to endogenous protease (which would normally destroy the protein), temperatures above 100°C, formalin, extremes of pH, nonpolar organic solvents, and years of burying. They are able to pass through 0.1-μm filters. The infectivity of prions can be destroyed by 0.1 N NaOH solution for 1 h at room temperature, or by 0.5% NaOCl solution for 1 h at 130° C. Since prion is a very small modified protein without any nucleic acid component that can be degraded by ionizing radiations, it is resistant to ultraviolet and gamma radiation, which break down nucleic acid. Up to now, no detailed findings have been reported on their D_{10} values. An irradiation dose of 25 kGy could not eliminate prions from lyophilized dura mater (CDC 1987; Hilmy and Lina 2001; Pruss *et al.* 2005).

Future Prospects of Using Irradiation to Eliminate Viruses and Prions

Since the new emerging infectious diseases caused by viruses and prions will always re-emerge year after year, along with the possibility of these diseases to jump from animals to humans, the risk of using products of animal and human origin (e.g. allografts and xenografts) will increase. If efforts to eliminate virues and prions from these products are not made, then we will face severe problems in health, global trade, and the economy. One solution to overcome these problems is by radiation. The application of radiation or a combined treatment of radiation and other technologies (e.g. washing process, lyophilization, freezing, pasteurization) will give the opportunity to eliminate such contaminations from allografts; however, the research in this field is currently limited. Research activities in this field should be increased and supported because the future prospect of using radiation to eliminate these contaminations is promising.

References

Bruce AV (2002). *The Biology of Viruses*, 2nd ed., McGraw Hill, Singapore, p. 341.

Busch MP and Kleinman SH (2000). *Transfusion* **40**:143–146.

Centers for Disease Control and Prevention (CDC) (1987). Update: Creutzfeldt–Jakob disease in a patient receiving a cadaveric dura mater graft. *JAMA* **258**:309–310.

Centers for Disease Control and Prevention (CDC) (2003). Update: outbreak of severe acute respiratory syndrome — worldwide, 2003. *MMWR* **52**:241–248.

Chisari FV and Ferrari C (1997). Viral hepatitis. In: Nathanson N, Ahmed R, Scarano FG, Griffin DE, Holmes KV, Murphy FA, and Robinson HL (eds.), *Viral Pathogenesis*, Lippincott-Raven, Philadelphia, PA, pp. 745–747.

Conrad EU, Gretch D, Obermeyer K, Moogk M, Sayers M, Wilson J, and Strong DM (1995). Transmission of the hepatitis-C virus by tissue transplantation. *J Bone Joint Surg* **77**:214–224.

Eastlund T (2005). *Sterilisation of Tissues Using Ionising Radiation*, Woodhead Publishing, Cambridge, p. 233.

Fideler BM, Vangsness CT, Moore T, Li Z, and Rasheed S (1994). Effects of gamma irradiation on the human immunodeficiency virus. *J Bone Joint Surg Am* **76**: 1032–1035.

Grieb TA, Forng RY, Lin J, Wolfinbarger L, Sosa Melgarejo J, Sharp C, Drohan WN, and Burgess WH (2005). In: Kennedy JF, Phillips GO, and Williams PA (eds.), *Sterilisation of Tissues Using Ionising Radiations*, CRC Woodhead Publishing, England, pp. 285–302.

Hilmy N and Lina M (2001). Effect of ionizing radiation on viruses, proteins and prions. In: *Advances in Tissue Banking*, World Scientific, Singapore, p. 358.

Hilmy N and Pandansari P (2006). New emerging diseases caused by viruses and prion. In: *14th International Meeting of Radiation Processing (IMRP) 2006*, Kuala Lumpur, Malaysia.

International Atomic Energy Agency (IAEA) (2004). Code of Practice for the Radiation Sterilization of Tissue Allografts — Requirements for Validation and Routine Control, IAEA, Vienna.

Murphy FA (1998). Emerging zoonoses. *Emerg Infect Dis* **4**(3):429–435.

National Center for Infectious Diseases (NCID), Centers for Disease Control and Prevention (CDC) (2005). Infectious Disease Information: Emerging Infectious Diseases, available at http://www.ncid.cdc.com

National Institute of Allergy and Infectious Diseases (NIAID) (2005). Emerging Infectious Diseases, available at http://www.niaid.nih.gov/dmid/eid/#top

O'Brien WA and Pomerantz RJ (1996). HIV infection and associated disease. In: Nathanson N, Ahmed R, Scarano FG, Griffin DE, Holmes KV, Murphy FA, and Robinson HL (eds.), *Viral Pathogenesis*, Lippincott-Raven, Philadelphia, PA, pp. 815–836.

Pattison J (1998). The emergence of bovine spongiform encephalopathy and related diseases. *Emerg Infect Dis* **4**:390–394.

Prusiner SB (1995). Prion disease. *Sci Am* **272**:48–57.

Prusiner SB (1996). Prion. In: Fields BN and Knipe DM (eds.), *Fields Virology*, Lippincott-Raven, Philadelphia, PA, pp. 2901–2949.

Pruss A, von Versen R, and Pauli G (2005). Viruses and their relevance for gamma irradiation sterilisation of allogeneic tissue transplants. In: Kennedy JF, Phillips GO, and Williams PA (eds.), *Sterilisation of Tissues Using Ionising Radiations*, Woodhead Publishing, England, pp. 235–254.

Strong DM (2005). Effects of radiation on the integrity and functionality of soft tissue. In: Kennedy JF, Phillips GO, and Williams PA (eds.), *Sterilisation of Tissues Using Ionising Radiations*, CRC Woodhead Publishing, England, pp. 163–172.

Woolhouse EJM and Gowtage-Sequeria S (2005). Host Range and Emerging and Reemerging Pathogens: Emerging Infectious Diseases, Centre for Infectious Diseases, University of Edinburg, UK, available at http://www.cdc.gov/eid

World Health Organization (WHO) (2003). Health Technology and Pharmaceutical Cluster: Guidelines on Transmissible Spongiform Encephalopathies in Relation to Biological and Pharmaceutical Products, WHO/BCT/QSD/13.01, Geneva.

World Health Organization (WHO) (2006). Epidemic and Pandemic Alert and Response (EPR): Disease Outbreak News, WHO, Geneva, available at http://www.who.int/

Chapter 11

Effects of Gamma Irradiation on the Biomechanics of Bone

Aziz Nather*, Ahmad Hafiz Zulkifly† and Shu-Hui Neo*

**NUH Tissue Bank*
Department of Orthopaedic Surgery
Yong Loo Lin School of Medicine
National University of Singapore
Singapore

†Department of Orthopaedics, Traumatology and Rehabilitation
Kulliyah of Medicine
International Islamic University Malaysia
Malaysia

Introduction

Lyophilized bone allografts are widely used nowadays for reconstructive surgery in various clinical disciplines. One major concern with such transplantations, however, is the risk of infectious disease transmission. To reduce the risk of transmission, a good method of terminal sterilization is needed. One currently employed method is to irradiate the graft with ionizing radiation (gamma irradiation), in which the dosage is dependent on the bioburden, the resistance of microorganisms to the sterilization procedure, and the sterility assurance level (SAL). Gamma irradiation is generally accepted as safe and effective.

While gamma irradiation may be effective in reducing the bioburden of microorganisms (especially that of viruses), many controversies have emerged regarding the effect of various dosages of gamma irradiation on the biomechanics of the bone allograft, especially at high doses where the ability of the bone allograft to play a structural role after transplantation is thought to be compromised. Currently, the recommended dosage for the sterilization of bone allografts is 25 kGy. This is practiced in tissue banks in the UK, the USA, and other countries around the world, with the exception of the Central Tissue Bank in Warsaw and other multitissue banks in Poland (where a dosage of 35 kGy is used). Another exception is in Australia, where 15 kGy has become the new gold standard.

Compressive Properties of Bone

Anderson *et al.* (1992) investigated the compressive mechanical properties of human cancellous bone after gamma irradiation at 10, 31, 51, and 60 kGy. Sections with a 2-cm thickness that were cut from the proximal tibiae of two male cadavers were irradiated at the abovementioned dosages of gamma irradiation. Sections that were not exposed to radiation served as controls. They found that there were no significant differences in compressive failure stress between the irradiated and control specimens, except for those irradiated at 60 kGy ($p = 0.03$). When the compressive strain, failure stress, and elastic modulus of sections were compared, there was no significant difference in compressive strain between all of the irradiated and control specimens. There was no evidence that gamma irradiation at 25 kGy affects the mechanical properties of proximal tibia allografts.

In a similar study conducted by Zhang *et al.* (1994) that investigated the force at failure, compressive strength, stiffness, Young's modulus, deformation, and strain of iliac crest wedges, there was no statistically significant difference between the irradiated (at 20–25 kGy) and nonirradiated deep-frozen and freeze-dried tricortical iliac crest allografts. The authors also recommended using 25 kGy for the secondary sterilization of human iliac crest wedges.

However, there has been contention over the results of Zhang *et al.* (1994) and Anderson *et al.* (1992). Cornu *et al.* (2000) investigated the biomechanical properties of bone after freeze-drying and gamma irradiation sterilization at 25 kGy. All of the treated specimens were rehydrated by immersion in saline solution and the frozen specimens thawed at room temperature prior to mechanical testing. Compression tests were then performed with a 100-kN screw-driven machine. The cancellous bone slices underwent *in situ* compression between two flat-nosed steel columns. Depending on the size of the bone, 8 to 12 compression tests were performed. The results of the study showed that after the freeze-dried bone was irradiated, ultimate stress declined sharply from −19% (without irradiation) to −43% (after irradiation). Irradiation was found to significantly weaken the bone.

Tensile Strength of Bone

In a study by Dziedzic-Goclawska (2000), whole femurs obtained from 20-week-old WAG male rats (lyophilized or fresh) were irradiated at doses of 25, 35, and 50 kGy. Nonirradiated femurs served as controls. Using an Instron Universal Testing Machine (Instron Corp., Canton, MA), the femurs were tested in three-point bending. The strength of the bone, or the maximum force needed to break the bone, was then calculated from the respective deflection curve. The study showed that in lyophilized femurs irradiated at 25, 35, and 50 kGy, the strength decreased by 43%, 57%, and 64%, respectively. In fresh femurs, the decrease was significantly lower, i.e. by 17%, 25%, and 34%, respectively. It seems that hydration can reduce undesirable, radiation-induced damage to the bone allograft.

Hamer *et al.* (1996) performed a similar study, showing that the bending strength of bone was reduced to 64% of control values after irradiation at 28 kGy and that the reduction in strength was dose-dependent. Femora were obtained from seven donors postmortem and were stripped of soft tissue. The femoral diaphyses were cut into 10–12 ring sections, approximately 1.6 mm thick, perpendicular to the long axis of the femur. Within each group from a particular donor femur, alternate rings were assigned to the treatment and control groups. Specimens were passed through a commercial plant twice to give a dose of 60 kGy, and once to give a dose of 28–30 kGy. A three-point bending jig was used to study the bending strength of the specimens. Each specimen was loaded and unloaded once within its linear elastic regions, and then loaded to failure. The bending strength was compromised at 28 kGy.

Another study by Triantafyllou *et al.* (1975) showed that the bending strength of bone was markedly reduced to 10%–30% of controls by a combination of lyophilization and radiation sterilization at a dose of 33 kGy. In a more recent study by Akkus and Belaney (2005), tensile monotonic tests were performed on bone tissue following gamma irradiation sterilization. The results are discussed in greater detail in the following section.

Fatigue Life of Bone

Akkus and Belaney (2005) studied the extent of degradation in the fatigue life of bone tissue following gamma radiation sterilization at a standard dose level of 36.4 kGy. High-cycle and low-cycle tests of control and irradiated human cortical bone tissue were performed. These simulate the dynamic nature of the physiological loading conditions experienced by allografts that cannot be found through monotonic loading. The authors showed that the elastic modulus and the yield stress were not affected by sterilization at 35 kGy. However, the energy to fracture, the postyield energy, and the fracture strain experienced significant reductions of 86.4%, 70.0%, and 60.5%, respectively.

In the low-cycle regime, the average fatigue life of control specimens was on the order of 10^5 cycles. The low-cycle fatigue life of irradiated specimens, on the other hand, was dramatically reduced by 99.5% to only on the order of 100 cycles to failure. In the high-cycle range, none of the control specimens failed within 300 000 cycles, while all of the irradiated specimens failed within 12 240–74 400 cycles. The mean fatigue life of high-cycle bone was reduced by 86.8% due to gamma radiation sterilization. Akkus and Belaney (2005) recommended that gamma radiation sterilization of the graft should be at the lower end of the standard dose range, i.e. 25 kGy, to minimize the impairment of mechanical and fatigue properties of the allograft.

Torsion of Bone

At a high irradiation dosage of 60 kGy, Bright and Burchardt (1983), Komender (1976), and Triantafyllou *et al.* (1975) all claimed that the specimens showed a reduction in bending, compression, and torsion strength. The torsion strength was decreased to 65% at a dose of 60 kGy, and to 70% by a combination of irradiation at 30 kGy and freeze-drying. Up to 30 kGy, though, 90% of torsion strength was maintained.

Nather *et al.* (2004) studied the biomechanical strength of freeze-dried, gamma-irradiated, cortical allografts using the tibial diaphysis of the adult cat. Large allografts (two thirds of the right tibial diaphysis) of 28 adult cats were procured, lyophilized to reduce the water content to 5%, and irradiated at a dose of 25 kGy. The allografts were transplanted back into the same 28 cats, four for each observation period of 4, 6, 8, 12, 16, 28, and 36 weeks. The corresponding segment of the unoperated left tibia served as the control for each cat. After the respective observation periods, the cats were sacrificed and the allografts were taken and embedded in rectangular jigs or molds of $3.2 \times 2.4 \times 3.2$ cm using quick-setting dental cement, leaving the central 2-cm portion free for torsion testing. The allografts were loaded to failure with an external rotation torsional force until an oblique fracture was produced.

The study showed that the maximum torque of freeze-dried, irradiated, cortical allografts was significantly weaker than that of deep-frozen, cortical allografts. At 24 weeks, the maximum torque was only about 12% of normal strength compared to 64% for deep-frozen allografts — one fifth of the strength of deep-frozen allografts. This difference was shown to be statistically significant in all of the observation periods (8, 12, 16, and 24 weeks), as shown in Fig. 1.

Nather *et al.* (2004) concluded that lyophilized, gamma-irradiated, cortical bone allografts — which only possess one fifth of the strength of large, deep-frozen, cortical bone allografts — are not suitable for use in massive reconstruction of the extremities, especially in the lower limbs where immediate weight-bearing is required. Instead, allografts that have been lyophilized and irradiated are useful as morselized bone grafts for packing cavities in bones such as simple bone cysts or in the maxillofacial region.

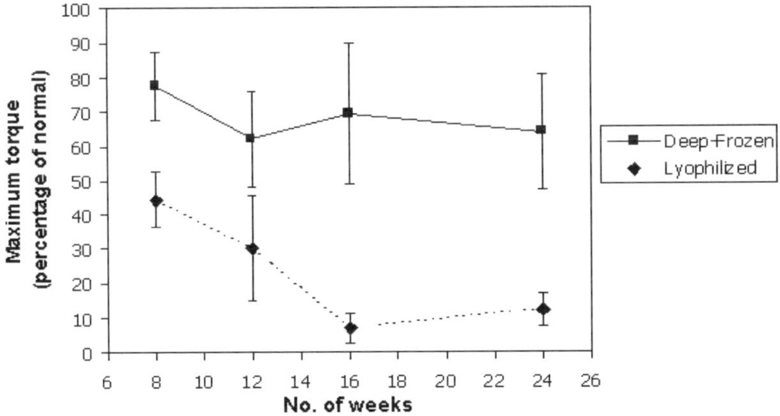

Fig. 1. Graph showing the maximum torque of deep-frozen and freeze-dried cortical allografts.

Fracture Toughness

In a study investigating the fracture resistance of gamma irradiated (27.5 kGy) cortical bone allografts by Akkus and Rimnac (2001), fracture toughness was found to be reduced, and the ability of bone tissue to undergo damage in the form of microcracks and to diffuse damage was significantly impaired. This might be because gamma irradiation induces immature intramolecular cross-links between collagen molecules and scission of tropocollagen α chains. Since allograft bone tissues are also used in various geometries like dowels, pins, and screws (which have stress concentrations present in the form of holes, ridges, and screw threads), the impaired fracture resistance of bone in the presence of stress concentration is a concern for radiation-sterilized allografts.

Summary

Table 1 summarizes the studies by various investigators on the effect of gamma radiation on the biomechanical strength of bone.

Table 1. Biomechanical studies of the effect of gamma radiation on bone.

Dosage of gamma irradiation	Author	Findings
25–30 kGy	Anderson *et al.* (1992), Zhang *et al.* (1994)	No effect on the biomechanics of bone at 20–25 kGy.
	Hamer *et al.* (1996)	The bending strength of bone was reduced to 64% of control values at 28 kGy. The reduction was dose-dependent.
	Nather *et al.* (2004)	At 25 kGy, the maximum torque of freeze-dried, irradiated, cortical allografts from cats was significantly weaker than that of deep-frozen, cortical allografts.
	Dziedzic-Goclawska (2000)	The bending strength was decreased by 43% at 25 kGy.

(*Continued*)

Table 1. (*Continued*)

Dosage of gamma irradiation	Author	Findings
	Akkus and Rimnac (2001)	The fracture toughness was reduced, and the ability of cortical bone to undergo damage in the form of microcracks and to diffuse damage was impaired, at 27.5 kGy.
	Triantafyllou *et al.* (1975), Komender (1976), Bright and Burchardt (1983)	Up to 30 kGy, 90% of torsion strength was maintained. The torsion strength was decreased to 70% by a combination of irradiation at 30 kGy and freeze-drying.
30–50 kGy	Triantafyllou *et al.* (1975)	The bending strength of bone was reduced to 10%–30% of controls by lyophilization and radiation sterilization at 33 kGy.
	Akkus and Belaney (2005)	At 36.4 kGy, the tensile fatigue life of cortical bone was reduced by two orders of magnitude. The fracture strain was reduced by 60.5%.
	Dziedzic-Goclawska (2000)	The bending strength was decreased by 57% and 64% at 35 and 50 kGy, respectively.
60 kGy	Triantafyllou *et al.* (1975), Komender (1976), Bright and Burchardt (1983)	At 60 kGy, the torsion strength was decreased to 65%.
	Anderson *et al.* (1992)	The compressive failure stress was significantly reduced at 60 kGy.
	Hamer *et al.* (1996)	The limit of proportionality was only compromised at 60-kGy irradiation.

Conclusion

The effect of gamma irradiation on the biomechanics of bone is very much dependent on the dosage employed. There has been much contention regarding the best dosage for bone irradiation in order to preserve the biomechanics and strength of bone (while also effectively reducing the bioburden and sterilizing the graft), so that it is safe for use.

References

Akkus O and Belaney RM (2005). Sterilization by gamma radiation impairs the tensile fatigue life of cortical bone by two orders of magnitude. *J Orthop Res* **23**:1054–1058.

Akkus O and Rimnac CM (2001). Fracture resistance of gamma radiation sterilized cortical bone allografts. *J Orthop Res* **19**:927–934.

Anderson MJ, Keyak JH, and Skinner HB (1992). Compressive mechanical properties of human cancellous bone after gamma irradiation. *J Bone Joint Surg Am* **74**(5):747–752.

Bright R and Burchardt H (1983). The biomechanical properties of preserved bone grafts. In: Friedlaender GE, Mankin HJ, and Sell KW (eds.), *Bone Allografts: Biology, Banking and Clinical Applications*, Little, Brown & Co., Boston, pp. 223–232.

Cornu O, Banse X, Docquier PL, Luyckx S, and Delloye C (2000). Effect of freeze-drying and gamma irradiation on the mechanical properties of human cancellous bone. *J Orthop Res* **18**:426–431.

Dziedzic-Goclawska A (2000). The application of ionizing radiation to sterilize connective tissue allografts. In: Phillips GO (ed.), *Radiation and Tissue Banking*, World Scientific, Singapore, pp. 57–99.

Hamer AJ, Strachan JR, Black MM, Ibbotson CJ, Stockley I, and Elson RA (1996). Biomechanical properties of cortical allograft bone using a new method of bone strength measurement: a comparison of fresh, fresh-frozen and irradiated bone. *J Bone Joint Surg Br* **78**(3):363–368.

Komender A (1976). Influence of preservation on some mechanical properties of human Haversian bone. *Mater Med Pol* **8**:13–17.

Nather A, Thambiah A, and Goh JCH (2004). Strength of deep-frozen versus lyophilized large biomechanical cortical allografts. *Clin Biomech* **19**:526–533.

Triantafyllou N, Sotiorpoulos E, and Triantafyllou J (1975). The mechanical properties of lyophilized and irradiated bone grafts. *Acta Orthop Belg* **41**:35–44.

Zhang Y, Homsi D, Gates K, Oakes K, Sutherland V, and Wolfinbarger L Jr (1994). A comprehensive study of physical parameters, biomechanical properties, and statistical correlations of iliac crest bone wedges used in spinal fusion surgery. IV. Effect of gamma irradiation on mechanical and material properties. *Spine* **19**(3):304–308.

Chapter 12

Physical and Mechanical Properties of Radiation-Sterilized Amnion

Norimah Yusof

Malaysian Nuclear Agency (NM)
Bangi, 43000 Kajang, Selangor
Malaysia

Nazly Hilmy

BATAN Research Tissue Bank (BRTB)
Center for Research and Development of Isotopes and
Radiation Technology, BATAN
Jakarta 12070, Indonesia

Introduction

Amniotic membrane has been used as an effective dressing for treating burns, superficial wounds, and soft tissue defects. One main advantage in using amnion is that no changing of dressing is necessary, thus requiring minimal nursing time (Hasim and Yusof 1991). Most importantly, the healing process is faster compared to conventional treatment and leaves no ugly scarring. Most of the tissue banks in the Asia-Pacific region have been routinely producing processed membranes since the early 1990s. During processing, amniotic membrane is washed and treated to inactivate any possible HIV contamination before drying. The purpose of the drying process is to reduce the moisture content to less than 10%, preferably 6%–7%. Amniotic membranes in final packaging are gamma sterilized at less than 25 kGy, depending on the microbiological quality (i.e. bioburden). Chapter 15 describes in detail the microbiological quality control of amnion products.

Radiation sterilization is recommended for increased safety of the final product. Therefore, further studies of efficacy pertaining to the change in mechanical properties, structural changes, changes in the content of active substances, and the beneficial effect of radioprotectants are needed. The application of higher doses of irradiation to soft tissues such as amniotic membrane can result in irreversible damage. Each tissue has different clinical applications that must be taken into account in order to assure effectiveness when high doses are applied.

Normally, an expiry date of 1 or 2 years is noted on the package; however, the membranes are mostly used up immediately after being supplied to hospitals. The shelf life of a product depends on product qualification tests demonstrating the functional stability after treatment and storage. There are two main physical properties that can be checked besides microbiological quality:

1. Test on physical properties, namely water content, water vapor transmission rate, and water absorption. Among these, the test on water content must be carried out as a routine product quality check on randomly picked samples to ensure that the samples are properly dried. Low moisture content is a prerequisite for two main purposes: to allow long-term preservation at ambient temperature, and to minimize the indirect effect of ionizing radiation during sterilization.
2. Test on mechanical properties, namely tensile strength and elongation of amnion after sterilization. This is not a routine quality control (QC) check, but it is useful to validate the processing procedure and to ensure that the radiation sterilization dose applied on the product has no major effect on tensile strength and elongation. Initial work can be carried out to determine the mechanical characteristics of the membrane after radiation sterilization and at various intervals throughout the storage period. The test assists tissue banks in setting the shelf life, and thus validates the expiry date of the amnion.

According to the European Association of Tissue Banks' (EATB) General Standards for Tissue Banking (1995), a maximum storage period with an expiration date should be assigned to each tissue product. The American Association of Tissue Banks' (AATB) Technical Manual (1992) recommends a 5-year shelf life for freeze-dried tissues packed in vacuum.

For those tissues not packed in vacuum packages, the shelf life must be determined by the maintenance of tissue sterility over the stated length of storage time, and they should be stored under appropriate conditions. Given that sterility is guaranteed as long as the integrity of the packaging is maintained, the shelf life very much depends on product qualification tests demonstrating functional stability after radiation doses (ISO 11137, 1995).

There have been very few publications describing the stability of amnions after irradiation and storage (Yusof 1997). Early work at the BATAN Tissue Bank, Indonesia, revealed that gamma irradiation up to 30 kGy did not have a significant effect on the biomechanical characteristics of freeze-dried amnions (Hilmy *et al.* 1987; Hilmy *et al.* 1992). A 50% reduction in the tensile strength and elongation of irradiated freeze-dried amnion was only observed after 1 year of storage. The radiation-stable packaging materials used, polyethylene and laminated aluminum foil, did not affect the biomechanical properties of amnions (Hilmy *et al.* 1988). Studies carried out at the Malaysian Nuclear Agency (NM) Tissue Bank indicated that air-dried amnions sterilized at 17 kGy maintained the mechanical properties up to 12 months of storage with no significant reduction in tensile strength and elongation (Yusof 1997). Products stored up to 20 months still had the properties similar to freshly processed amnions.

This chapter describes the procedures involved in testing the physical and mechanical properties of amnions, and how the expiry date or shelf life of air-dried amnions can be established based on the validation exercise.

Processing of Amniotic Membrane

Amniotic membrane procured from the placentae of healthy mothers must be individually washed and processed. Each tissue bank must develop and validate a specific processing procedure for amnion that conforms to any tissue banking standards to ensure that the processed amnions are appropriate for safe and efficient clinical use. Chapter 17 describes in detail how to conduct the validation exercise for amnion processing and radiation dose. Amniotic membranes can be dried either by freeze-drying using a lyophilizer (Hilmy *et al.* 1992), air-drying in laminar flow overnight (Yusof and Asnah 1995), or oven-drying at 40°C (Bari and Begum 1999). All of the steps involved must be validated to demonstrate the effectiveness of the drying procedures according to the International Atomic Energy Agency (IAEA) International Standards for Tissue Banks (2002) under item B3.1 10. Amnions are packed in triple packs.

Amnion samples are randomly picked for a water content test before sterilization. After sterilization, amnions are kept in a locked cabinet in a cool and dark place. According to the IAEA International Standards for Tissue Banks (2002) item B3.1 30, tests and procedures must be performed to measure, assay, or monitor the processing, preservation and storage methods, equipment, and reagents to ensure compliance with established tolerance limits. The results of such tests or procedures shall be recorded.

As mentioned in the IAEA International Standards for Tissue Banks (2002) item B3.9 00, expiry dates must be established for all tissues released from a tissue bank. Therefore, samples are taken for mechanical testing at time intervals during storage, provided there are enough samples to permit such a test, to eventually determine the expiry date. As required by the IAEA International Standards for Tissue Banks (2002) item B5.2 00, a label must be placed on each tissue container/package indicating the following: the nature of contents, product description, name and address of tissue bank, tissue identification number, and lastly expiration date.

Physical Properties

Moisture content

There are many ways to determine the water or moisture content. One of them is via the gravimetric method. In this method, the amnion sample is subjected to the following steps:

1. Dry a crucible in a 105°C oven, preferably overnight, until its weight is constant. Place it in a dessicator for about 20 min before weighing to stabilize the reading.
2. Place the amniotic sample (minimum weight, 0.1–0.2 g) in the crucible and weigh it.
3. Dry the crucible with the sample in an oven at 60°C for about 4 to 6 h (until the weight is constant), then transfer it to a dessicator and weigh.
4. Calculate the percentage of water content as follows:

$$\%\text{ water content} = \frac{W_\text{i} - W_t}{W_\text{i} - W_\text{c}} \times 100$$

where

W_i is the initial weight of crucible and sample
W_t is the weight of crucible and sample after drying for t h when the weight is constant
W_c is the weight of crucible

Water vapor transmission rate (WVTR)

In principle, the material to be tested is fastened over the mouth of a dish, which contains a desiccant. The assembly is placed in an atmosphere of constant temperature and humidity, and the weight gain or loss of the assembly is used to calculate the rate of water vapor movement through the sheet material under the selected conditions. The following procedure has been established according to the American Society for Testing and Materials (ASTM) E 96-66 (1972b):

1. Activate 30 g calcium chloride ($CaCl_2$) in a clean dish (e.g. pin bowl or crucible) at 200°C until the weight is constant.
2. Cover the dish as soon as possible with amniotic membrane; fasten with rubber band and use a sealant (e.g. plasticine or grease) to hold and avoid any leakage. Weigh the container with the sample and dry $CaCl_2$.
3. Place the dish in a humidity chamber or dessicator at 90%–95% humidity and 30°C temperature.
4. Measure the area of amnion ($22/7 \times r^2$, where r is the radius of amnion covering the dish).
5. Set up another assembly using cotton gauze instead of amnion as the control.
6. Calculate the WVTR (g/cm²/h) by calculating the increasing weight of $CaCl_2$, as follows:

$$\%\ \text{WVTR} = \frac{D_w}{W_c \times AH} \times 100$$

   where

   D_w is the increase in weight of $CaCl_2$
   W_c is the initial weight of $CaCl_2$
   A is the area of amnion covering the dish
   H is the exposure time (h) in humidity chamber

7. Plot a graph of WVTR against time (h).

Water absorption

Amnion as a wound dressing must have both absorption and water vapor transmission properties (Hilmy *et al.* 1987). To stimulate healing, amnion should also be permeable to gases, especially oxygen. The following procedure is established according to the ASTM E 96-66 (1972b):

1. Measure the initial weight of the amnion sample (minimum 5 cm $\times$ 5 cm).
2. Immerse or soak the sample in distilled water for 1, 2, 3, up to 24 h.
3. Remove the sample with forceps, and wrap it immediately with clean tissue paper to remove excess water.
4. Measure the final weight of the amnion sample.
5. Calculate the percentage of water absorption, as follows:

$$\% \text{ water absorption} = \frac{W_t - W_{\rm i}}{W_{\rm i}} \times 100$$

   where

   $W_{\rm i}$ is the initial weight of amnion sample
   W_t is the weight of amnion sample after soaked for t h

6. Plot the graph of water absorption against immersion hours. The actual water absorption is obtained when the curve is plateaued off.
7. Calculate the water absorption per h per 1 g or 1 cm of the amnion sample.

Results of physical properties

The water content was calculated after placing the amnion in an oven at 60°C for 4 h, as the weight of amnion reached the steady state after 3–4 h as shown in Fig. 1 (Yusof *et al.* 1994).

Table 1 presents the results of the physical property test conducted at the NM Tissue Bank, Malaysia, for amnion samples taken randomly from three processing batches with a minimum of three pieces from each batch (Hasim and Yusof 1994). The amnions were checked just before irradiation. The water content of freeze- and air-dried amnions was almost similar, i.e. around 6% either at 4 or 24 h — this is within the acceptable range of 4%–7%. The NM Tissue Bank used these findings to select the air-drying method as a routine process that allows the reduction of processing costs by 40% (Yusof and Asnah 1995).

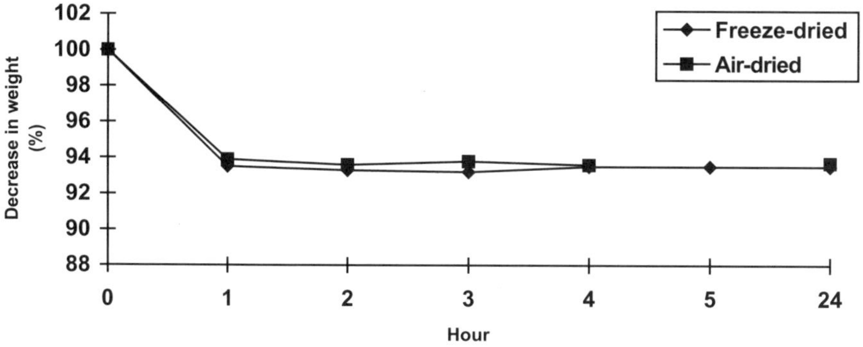

Fig. 1. Decrease in weight (%) of air- and freeze-dried amnions at 60°C over time.

Table 1. Physical properties of processed amnions prior to radiation sterilization.

	Air-drying	Freeze-drying
% water content		
(60°C, 4 h)	6.46 ± 0.83	6.41 ± 0.60
(60°C, 24 h)	6.34 ± 0.56	6.31 ± 0.55
Water vapor transmission rate (35°C)		
$g/m^2/h$	875.21	1286.02
$g/m^2/24\,h$	773.64	796.51
Water absorption (RT, 4 h)		
$\%/cm^2/h$	2.33 ± 0.43	2.72 ± 0.10

For the WVTR test, the weight of calcium chloride ($CaCl_2$) in a container covered with amnion increased proportionally with time, as shown in Fig. 2 (Yusof *et al.* 1994). According to Table 1, freeze-dried amnion had a higher WVTR compared to air-dried amnion, indicating that the well-preserved cell structure of amnion after freeze-drying would allow better water transmission through the membrane. However, the WVTR was not much different after 24 h. In clinical usage, both freeze- and air-dried amnions have comparable effectiveness as a wound dressing. The membranes are able to absorb and hold liquid, and are able to transfer the exudate of a wound away from the wound surface while keeping the wound bed

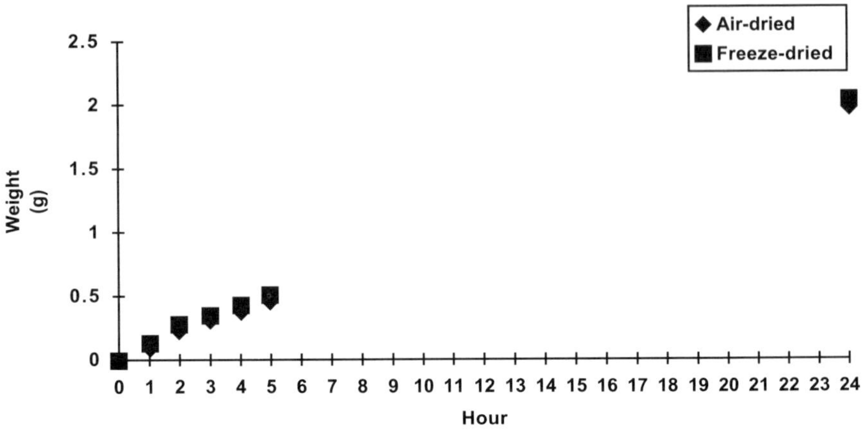

Fig. 2. Increase in weight due to water vapor transmission in irradiated amnion.

moist. In fact, with these properties, amnion (either freeze- or air-dried) can be an effective biological barrier to heat and protein loss.

For the water absorption test, the increase in weight tended to plateau off or decrease after 3–4 h, as shown in Fig. 3 (Yusof *et al.* 1994). As indicated in Table 1, after being soaked in water for 4 h, the freeze-dried amnion could absorb water ($2.72 \pm 0.10\%/cm^2/h$) slightly better than air-dried amnion ($2.33 \pm 0.43\%/cm^2/h$). This might be due to better-preserved cell structure by freeze-drying. Similarly, the total water absorbed per h ($g/cm^2/h$) or over 24 h ($g/m^2/24\,h$) was slightly higher in freeze-dried amnions.

Mechanical Properties

The determination of mechanical properties starts with a piece of amnion sample and includes, firstly, the preparation of the specimen in the shape of a dumbbell, ring, or straight piece of uniform cross-section; and secondly, the testing of the specimen. The following procedure is established according to the ASTM D 638-84 (1972a):

1. Take randomly irradiated amnion samples from the storage place.
2. Cut the amnion sample (without carrier) into a dumbbell shape with the size shown in Fig. 4. Obtain at least three pieces of dumbbell shapes from each processing batch.

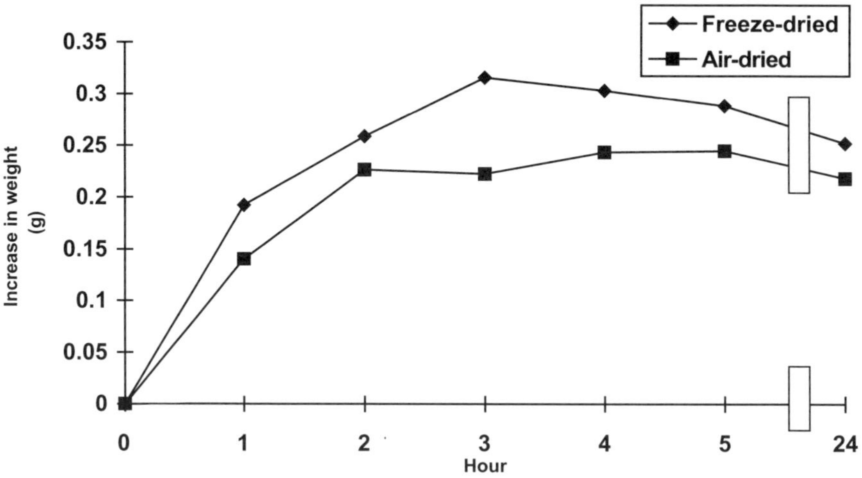

Fig. 3. Increase in weight (g) of irradiated freeze- and air-dried amnions due to water absorption over time.

3. Mark the narrow area and measure the width.
4. Measure the thickness at a minimum of five locations by using a thickness tester.
5. Place the sample in the holders of a universal testing machine.
6. Choose and set the speed and load of the test, and start the machine.
7. Record the load extension of the sample when the rupture has taken place.
8. Calculate the tensile strength (kg/cm^2) and elongation (%), as follows:

$$T_v = \frac{W}{A_o}$$

where

T_v is the tensile strength at break (kg/cm^2)
W is the load (kg)
A_o is the original cross-sectional area (cm)

$$\% \text{ EL} = \frac{L - L_o}{L_o} \times 100$$

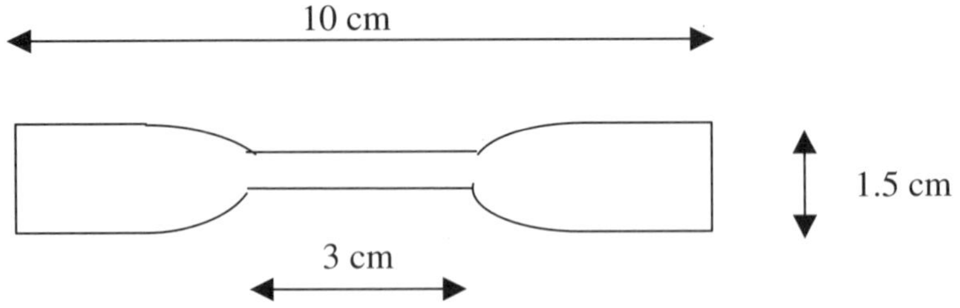

Fig. 4. Dumbbell specimen of amnion for tensile test.

where

% EL is the percentage of elongation
L is the distance between gauge marks at the moment of rupture
L_o is the original distance between gauge marks

At the NM Tissue Bank, amnion pieces were air-dried in laminar flow for 16 h before being packed into triple layers. The thickness of the amnion ranged from 0.0153 mm to 0.0209 mm. After radiation sterilization at the NM gamma irradiation plant (Type JS8900, IR-174), amnions — which were kept in a locked cabinet in the dark at room temperature (27°C ± 1°C) and a humidity of 69% ± 3% — were taken randomly for mechanical testing. The handling of amnion samples is quite difficult, as the amnion is very thin, fragile, and easily broken even at early stages of the test. The selection of sites for cutting and the number of pieces obtained from each piece were very much determined by the size and shape of the membrane. The orientation of the membrane to its original position was difficult to determine.

The tests were conducted using the Instron Universal Testing Instrument (Model 4301) with a load of 1 kN, crosshead speed of 20 mm/min, and grip distance of 50 mm. As shown in Table 2, there was no difference in the tensile strength and elongation of irradiated amnion when compared to the control after about 9 months of storage (Yusof 1997). Gamma irradiation at 17 kGy showed no significant effect on the tensile strength and elongation at $p < 0.05$.

In another study, monitoring was conducted immediately after irradiation even up to 20 months of storage, as presented in Table 3 (Yusof 1997). The tensile strength of irradiated amnion was not significantly different ($p < 0.05$) compared to that of the control except for 6 and 12 months, whereby the former was higher. The authors could not detect any reduction

Table 2. Effect of radiation (17 kGy) on mechanical properties of air-dried amnion.

Treatment (no. of donors)	No. of samples	Storage (month)	Tensile strength (kg/cm^2)	Elongation (%)
Nonirradiated (4)	25	9.0	329.71 ± 147.34	14.11 ± 4.70
Irradiated (3)	20	8.7	377.70 ± 127.10	11.67 ± 1.61

in both tensile strength and elongation, even though a 50% reduction in the properties of freeze-dried amnion after 12 months of storage was previously reported (Hilmy *et al.* 1992).

In determining the expiry date of air-dried amnions beyond 20 months, another study was conducted over more than 5 years on limited numbers of amnion available in storage (Yusof and Ozkara 2000). As shown in Table 4, the tensile strength of amnion stored from 2 years 10 months (34 months) to 6 years (72 months) varied from 64.39 to 205.43 kg/cm^2, while the elongation varied from 5.9% to 31.3%. The results were not statistically analyzed due to the limited number of specimens tested; however, all of the tensile strengths recorded were lower than those in Table 3. There was no relationship between the storage period and the mechanical properties of amnion; there was no reduction in mechanical properties with a prolonged storage period, even after 5 years. A large number of samples may be required to lessen the variation in measurements caused by considerable heterogeneity in thickness among the samples and within a single sample. No discoloration

Table 3. Effects of radiation (17 kGy) and storage at room temperature on air-dried amnions.

Storage (month)	No. of samples	Tensile strength (kg/cm^2)	Elongation (%)
0 (control)	31	209.00 ± 123.71	13.45 ± 4.13
4	7	304.97 ± 66.92	12.25 ± 4.10
6	8	405.51 ± 200.60	12.73 ± 3.96
8	5	239.00 ± 85.12	9.81 ± 3.91
12	7	488.60 ± 411.42	12.46 ± 5.26
16	3	279.89 ± 130.79	15.82 ± 4.76
18	5	327.27 ± 108.68	14.05 ± 4.71
20	14	267.50 ± 105.04	14.38 ± 3.89

Table 4. Mechanical properties of gamma-irradiated amnion after storage.

Storage (month)	No.of specimens	Thickness (mm)	Tensile strength (kg/cm^2)	Elongation (%)
34	1	0.0272	64.39	11.30
36	1	0.0438	78.90	31.30
49	3	0.0177	147.76	20.97
52	3	0.0210	158.78	20.07
54	3	0.0209	154.63	18.97
70	1	0.0224	102.87	5.90
72	9	0.0163	205.43	16.90
Control (0 month storage)	31		209.00	13.45

was visually observed among the stored samples when compared to freshly processed amnion.

When the results of tensile strength and elongation were plotted against the storage period (months) as in Figs. 5 and 6, no specific trend could be deduced. The mechanical characteristics of the samples were still comparable to those of the control, and the authors could not trace any detectable degradation in the physical appearance of the membrane. In clinical practice, amnion is usually removed directly from the package onto the wound after debridement without any prior rehydration in physiological solution.

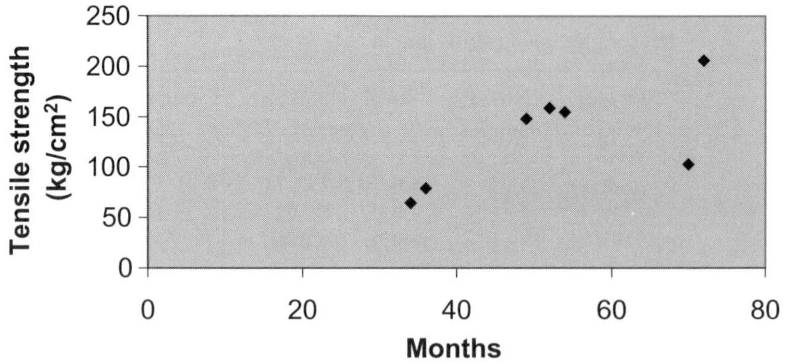

Fig. 5. Tensile strength of air-dried and gamma-sterilized amnion over storage.

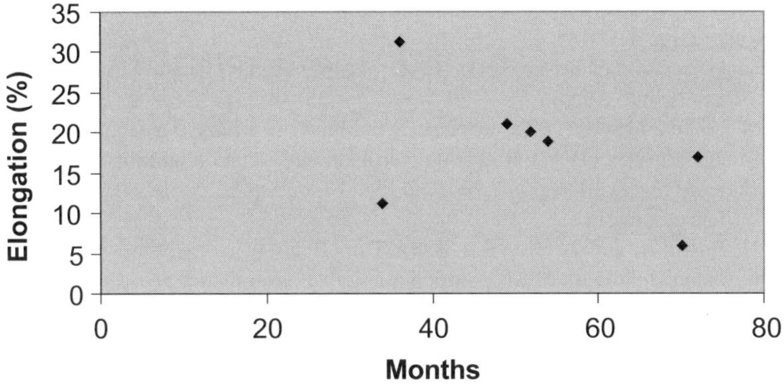

Fig. 6. Elongation of air-dried and gamma-sterilized amnion over storage.

Therefore, the mechanical properties need to be maintained for easy handling by nursing staff.

Conclusion

There was no relationship between the storage period and the biomechanical properties of amnion. We could not find any reduction in biomechanical properties with prolonged storage period, even up to 6 years. We could not observe any changes in the color and physical appearance of all the stored amnions when visually inspected and compared to freshly processed amnion. However, a large number of samples is required to lessen the variation in measurements caused by considerable heterogeneity in thickness among the samples and within a single sample. Based on the studies carried out, the expiry date of 2 years is reasonably acceptable and validated.

References

American Association of Tissue Banks (AATB) (1992). AATB Technical Manual, McLean, VA.

American Society for Testing and Materials (ASTM) (1972a). *Annual Book of ASTM Standards*, D 638-84, ASTM, Philadelphia.

American Society for Testing and Materials (ASTM) (1972b). *Annual Book of ASTM Standards*, E 96-66, ASTM, Philadelphia.

Bari MM and Begum R (1999). Use of radiation sterilised amniotic membrane grafts as temporary biological dressings for the treatment of leprotic ulcers. In: Phillips GO,

Kearney JN, and Strong DM (eds.), *Advances in Tissue Banking*, Vol. 3, World Scientific, Singapore, pp. 477–483.

European Association of Tissue Banks (EATB) (1995). EATB General Standards for Tissue Banking, Vienna, Austria.

Hasim M and Yusof N (1991). Tissue banking in Malaysia. *Malays J Nucl Sci* **9**(2):127–131.

Hasim M and Yusof N (1994). Radiation sterilization of amnion and its clinical use. *Proceedings of the IAEA Meeting on Radiation Sterilization of Human Tissues*, October 4–7, Vienna, Austria.

Hilmy N, Basril A, and Febrida A (1988). The effects of storage and irradiation doses on mechanical strength of freeze-dried amnion chorion membrane. *Proceedings of the IAEA/RCM on Radiation Sterilization of Human Tissues*, November 7–11, Taiyuan, China.

Hilmy N, Basril A, and Febrida A (1992). Effects of procurement, packaging, storage time and irradiation dose on physical properties of amnion membranes. *Proceedings of the IAEA/PFM on Radiation Sterilization of Tissue Grafts*, April 1–3, Manila, Philippines.

Hilmy N, Siddik S, Gentur S, and Gulardi W (1987). Physical and chemical properties of freeze-dried amniochorion membranes sterilized by gamma irradiation. *Atom Indones* **13**(2):1–14.

International Atomic Energy Agency (IAEA) (2002). International Standards for Tissue Banks, IAEA, Vienna.

International Standards Organization (ISO) (1995). Validation and Routine Control — Radiation Sterilization, ISO 11137, 1995(E), Switzerland.

Yusof N (1997). Effect of gamma irradiation and storage on biomechanical properties of human amniotic membrane. *Proceedings of the 9th International Conference on Biomedical Engineering*, December 3–6, Singapore.

Yusof N and Asnah H (1995). Processing cost for routine production of radiation sterilised amnions. *Proceedings of the Malaysian Science and Technology Congress*, Vol. 3, Kuala Lumpur, pp. 76–83.

Yusof N, Hasim M, Asnah H, Norshamsuria O, and Salahbiah AM (1994). Microbiological aspect of radiation sterilisation of amnion graft. *Proceedings of the 5th Meeting of the Asia-Pacific Association of Surgical Tissue Banking*, June 1994, Suzhou, China.

Yusof N and Ozkara T (2000). Biomechanical properties of gamma irradiated amnion after storage. *Proceedings of the 8th International Conference on Tissue Banking*, Bali, Indonesia.

PART IV.

PROCESSING AND QUALITY CONTROL

Chapter 13

Dosimetry and Requirements for Process Qualification

Noriah Mod Ali

Secondary Standard Dosimetry Laboratory (SSDL)
Malaysian Nuclear Agency (NM)
Bangi, 43000 Kajang, Selangor
Malaysia

Introduction

One of the principal advantages of ionizing radiation as an industrial tool is the ability to achieve precise chemical and biological effects through the delivery of known doses of radiation. Since the absorbed dose is the quantity, which is directly related to the desired effect in radiation application, the need for suitable and accurate dose measurement techniques must not be underestimated. This is best appreciated by realizing the consequences of using inadequate techniques: underexposure or overexposure of the product, and loss of confidence in the irradiation process.

For any given irradiation condition, it is necessary to specify the absorbed dose in the particular material of interest because different materials have different radiation absorption properties. The regulatory body or any group responsible for the acceptance of products requires information demonstrating that every part of the process load under consideration has been subjected to dose limits within the acceptable range. The objective of such formalized procedures is to establish documentary evidence that the irradiation process has achieved the desired results.

The key element of such activities is inevitably a well-characterized, reliable dosimetry system that is traceable to national and international dosimetry standards. Only such dosimetry systems can help establish the required documentary evidence. In addition, industrial radiation processing such as the sterilization of healthcare products and the irradiation of foodstuffs are both highly regulated, in particular with regard to dosage. Some of these technologies do not need exact doses, but in most cases knowledge of the dose applied to achieve the necessary effect is needed. This information is also required to avoid damage to the product. For example, processing of healthcare products such as tissue allografts requires a radiation dose corresponding to very precise specifications. The minimum doses required for the sterilization of tissue allografts are in the order of 10–30 kGy, but the actual dose depends on the regulatory requirement and on the level of initial microbiological contamination. Once the sterilization dose for a specific product has been determined, it must be accurately delivered.

All products must receive at least the sterilization dose, but there is also a requirement to limit the maximum dose to the product in order to avoid deleterious effects on the materials, as the economics of the process will also be affected by an unnecessarily high dose. Taken together, these considerations lead to the need for tight dosimetric control of the process. Because of the implications for human health, the radiation sterilization process is under strict regulatory control. A number of international and national standards govern the practices and the required level of documentation (e.g. EN 1994, ISO 1995). The approval for the sale of radiation sterilization healthcare products depends on several factors, such as the official registration of the radiation facility, the use of good manufacturing practice and proper inventory control, and above all the accurate measurement of the radiation dose in the product.

Radiation dosimetry thus provides ultimate, independent control of the radiation process. It is a common requirement that dosimetry is traceable to national standards, and that the measurement uncertainty is known and documented. A well-characterized, reliable dosimetry system that is traceable to the international measurement system is the key element to provide proof that the radiation processing is done according to the required specifications.

Dosimetry System

Dosimeters are devices that are capable of providing a quantitative and reproducible measurement of dose through a change in one or more of the physical properties of the dosimeters in response to the exposure to ionizing radiation energy. A dosimetry system consists of dosimeters, measurement instruments and their associated reference standards, and procedures for the system's use. The measuring instrument must be well characterized, so that it gives reproducible and accurate results. Any radiation-induced effect (also called the dosimeter response), which is reproducible and quantifiable, can in principle be used for dosimetry.

The selection of an appropriate dosimetry system depends on a variety of factors, including the dose range needed to achieve a particular technological objective, cost, availability, and ease of use. A variety of dosimetry systems are available.

Classes of dosimeters

Dosimetry systems can be classified on the basis of their intrinsic accuracy and applications. Such a classification and the traceability chains are shown in Fig. 1. The figure also represents a traceability chain in that it outlines how primary standard dosimeters are used to calibrate reference standard dosimeters, which in turn are used to calibrate the routine dosimeters used for day-to-day measurements.

Primary standard dosimeters enable an absolute measurement of the absorbed dose to be made with reference only to the SI base units and fundamental physical constants. They do not need to be calibrated. This type of dosimetry system is generally maintained and operated by national standards laboratories, and is used to provide the basic standard for use in the country. There are two types of primary standard dosimeters: calorimeters and ionization chambers.

Reference standard dosimeters are dosimeters of high metrological quality that can be used as reference standards to calibrate other dosimeters. In turn, they need to be calibrated against a primary standard, generally through the use of a transfer standard dosimeter. They must have a radiation response that is accurately measurable, and this response must have a well-defined functional relationship with the absorbed dose. The effect of various parameters, such as irradiation temperature and postirradiation stability, on the dosimeter response must be well characterized and capable of expression in terms of simple correction factors. Commonly used reference dosimeters include Fricke, ceric-cerous, dichromate, ethanol-chlorobenzene (ECB), and alanine dosimeters.

Standards laboratory—national standards

Calorimeters, ionization chambers

|

(D_{carbon})

|

D_{water}

|

Reference class dosimeters

Fricke, ceric-cerous,
dichromate, ECB, alanine

|

Routine dosimeters

PMMA, radiochromic films, cellulose triacetate,
dyed plastics

Fig. 1. Typical traceability chain for high-dose dosimetry.

Routine (or working) dosimeters are used in radiation processing facilities for dose mapping and for process monitoring for quality control. They must be frequently calibrated against reference or transfer dosimeters, as they may not be sufficiently stable and independent from environmental or radiation field conditions. In addition, they may show significant variation from batch to batch. Commonly used routine dosimeters include polymethylmethacrylate (PMMA), radiochromic, cellulose triacetate (CTA), dyed plastics, ceric-cerous, ECB, and alanine dosimeters. A dosimetric accuracy of the order of 5%–10% is generally considered to be necessary for effective control of the sterilization process. Table 1 lists these three classes of dosimeters.

Calibration of routine dosimeters

Reliable dosimetry requires knowledge of the level of accuracy and precision of the dosimetry system used. This can be achieved by carrying out suitable calibration procedures for both the dosimeter system and the instrumentation used to evaluate the irradiated dosimeter, thereby assuring

Table 1. Useful dose ranges for various routine, reference standard, and primary standard dosimeters (classes: R, routine; S, reference standard; P, primary standard).

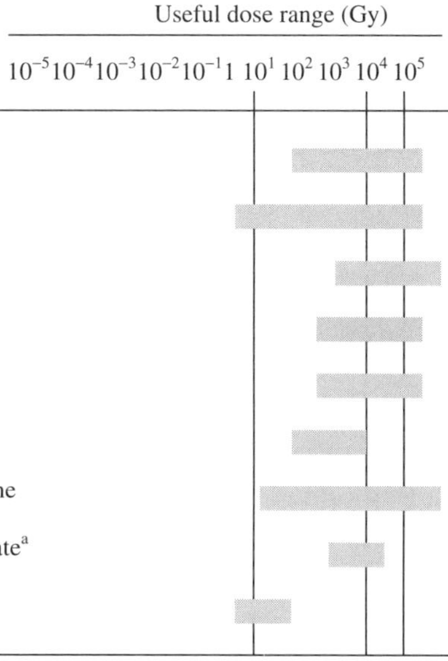

Dosimeter	Class
Calorimeter	P
Alanine	SR
Cellulose triacetate	R
Ceric-cerous	SR
Clear PMMA[b]	R
Dyed PMMA[b]	R
Ethanol-chlorobenzene	SR
Ferrous-cupric sulphate[a]	R
Ferrous sulphate[a]	S

[a]Aqueous solution.
[b]PMMA stands for polymethylmethacrylate.

measurement traceability to appropriate national standards. The main aim of the calibration is to establish a relationship between the absorbed dose and the dosimeter response. Calibration can be carried out in (1) a calibration laboratory, (2) an in-house calibration facility, or (3) a processing facility (in plant calibration).

The accuracy of a dosimeter can be significantly affected if the routine irradiation conditions of the dosimeter are different from the calibration conditions. Therefore, the present trend is to calibrate dosimeters under conditions that are as close as possible to those of regular application (processing condition) by applying in-plant calibration whenever possible. In principle, the dosimeters used for electron irradiation should be calibrated in an electron beam. However, the response for a large majority of dosimeters is similar for the two radiation types (i.e. electron and gamma), at least over a limited dose range. Nevertheless, before using dosimeters that are calibrated in a gamma field for electron dose measurements, it is necessary to confirm that its behavior is similar in the dose range of interest.

Since dose gradients are much steeper for electron beams than for gamma fields, the dosimeters should be thin for precise measurements. A somewhat thicker dosimeter may be used at the position of the peak of depth–dose distribution, since the dose here changes only slightly with depth in the product. The response of the dosimeter must be relatively independent of the spectral energy because the energy spectrum also changes with depth in the material.

Elements of Process Qualification

The design and construction of irradiation facilities are linked to the physical nature of the radiation emission (Fig. 2) (IAEA Technical Reports Series 409, 2002). Radionuclide sources emit radiation equally in all directions. Hence, to absorb the emitted radiation energy most effectively, the process loads must be distributed around the source leaving as small a

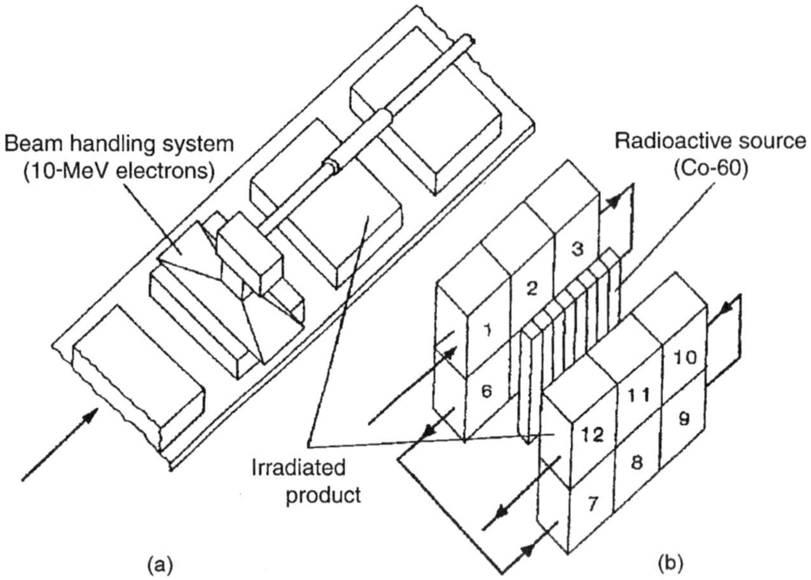

Fig. 2. Schematic diagram of (a) an electron facility, in which process loads are brought into the radiation field one at a time; and (b) a radionuclide facility, in which several process loads surround the radiation source and are thus irradiated together.

gap as possible. Machine sources, on the contrary, emit a unidirectional beam; even when converted into *bremsstrahlung*, the forward direction is predominant. Consequently, the process loads to be irradiated have to be brought before the beam exit window of the accelerator. Besides, an electron beam must be widened by technical means (scanning or scattering) for a homogeneous dose distribution over process loads of extended size. However, both types of irradiation facilities have in common the need for movement of the process load in process to compensate for differences in locations, thus making the resulting dose distribution more homogeneous.

The major considerations in the design of an irradiator are the uniformity of the absorbed dose in the irradiated product, efficient utilization of the radiation energy, and cost-effectiveness based on minimizing the combined capital and operating costs. The physical nature and quantity of the product to be treated determine the general design principles, and the desired effect determines the magnitudes of the minimum and maximum doses to the product. The margins of free choice of dose distribution are rather narrow, especially at radiation sterilization. The minimum dose delivered in a particular place in a box of healthcare products must be higher than the sterilization dose, determined by the required level of inactivation of microorganisms. The maximum dose in the site receiving the highest dose must be higher than the sterilization dose, allowed by the resistance of a material of the device towards radiation. The limits are set in accordance with the process specifications and governmental regulatory requirements.

The actual minimum dose D_{min} and maximum dose D_{max} as measured in the product must be within these limits. The dose uniformity ratio U, which is defined as the ratio of D_{max} to D_{min}, is a useful concept to verify that the doses are uniform in the irradiated products. The case of gamma irradiation is comparatively simple, as it deals with a relatively high homogeneity of dose distribution. This is the case when the unit operation of irradiation is done in large installations, where the objects of irradiation move around the sources, collecting and averaging the absorbed dose. The situation is more complicated in the case of electron beam irradiations, where practically only a one-step irradiation is made. Split-dose or double-sided irradiations are possible only in exceptional cases.

Dosimetry for Process Control

Radiation treatment of the product must be performed in well-characterized irradiation plants. This means that the plants are able to deliver a certain dose of radiation to a product, and that the key parameters for controlling and maintaining the dose are well known and can be reported within the specified limits. The measurement of the relationship between the absorbed dose and the plant's key parameter, as well as the measurement of the dose distribution in reference homogeneous products, enables global characterization of the radiation plant to be attained. From a dosimetric point of view, the relationship between maximum and minimum doses and the dose at an easily accessible position are also determined in order to facilitate subsequent monitoring of the process.

These can be determined through a product facility qualification exercise, which includes dose mapping of a new irradiation facility, validation of the new product in an established facility, and use of dosimetry for quality control in the routine operation of the process. The techniques used are generally the same for gamma facilities and electron accelerators, but differences exist due to the different nature and technical details of the plant as discussed above. Properly applied dosimetry in these three phases provides assurance that the process is carried out properly, economically, and within prescribed dose limits. It is a form of a quality control procedure to guarantee the safety or reliability of the irradiated product.

Dose mapping

Dose mapping is the measurement of dose distributions throughout a reference product package in its complete passage. It is also known as plant commissioning, and is carried out at a new facility to demonstrate that it is delivered and installed in accordance with specifications. It is carried out at regular intervals or after changes that can influence the dose or dose distributions to demonstrate that the facility can consistently deliver the radiation process. One of the aims of this procedure is to characterize the irradiation facility in terms of relating plant parameters to the absorbed dose. For gamma radiation, it is normally performed by distributing dosimeters throughout a simulated product that has a density near to the highest density normally accommodated during the actual process.

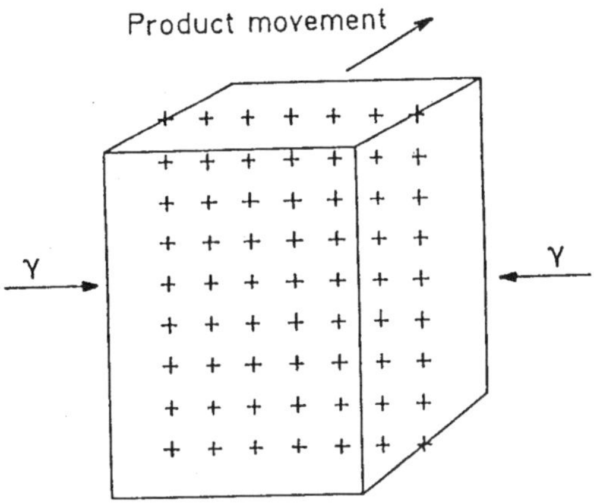

Fig. 3. Grid pattern for placing dosimeters in the dose mapping exercise in gamma facilities.

The positioning of dosimeters for process qualification dose maps is generally not in a regular grid layout. It is not possible to place dosimeters everywhere in the device box; instead, the dosimeters are concentrated in locations most likely to receive extremes of dosage, based on knowledge of the irradiator and previous dose maps of a similar product. Figure 3 shows an example of a grid pattern for the placement of dosimeters for dose distribution measurements in one plane against gamma radiation. More planes may be used and more dosimeters may be placed where gradients are anticipated. The initial measurements enable the determination of the dose distribution and the location of minimum and maximum doses (Fig. 4). They also determine the timer setting required to achieve the desired minimum dose for the actual product.

For electron beams, the characterization of a radiation field is done along the *x*-, *y*-, and *z*-axes of the beam (Fig. 5). It includes measuring the mass energy of the electron beam, the beam profile, and the scan width. A typical dose distribution along the scan width measured with strips of film dosimeters is shown in Fig. 6. Instead of measuring the surface dose along the *x*- and *y*-axes, depth–dose distribution along the *z*-axis is needed to plan for an effective irradiation process. The depth–dose distribution of electrons may be checked using a stack of CTA film dosimeters that cover the whole range of depth material; alternatively, an aluminium step wedge may be used (Fig. 7). Figure 8 shows a typical depth–dose distribution in

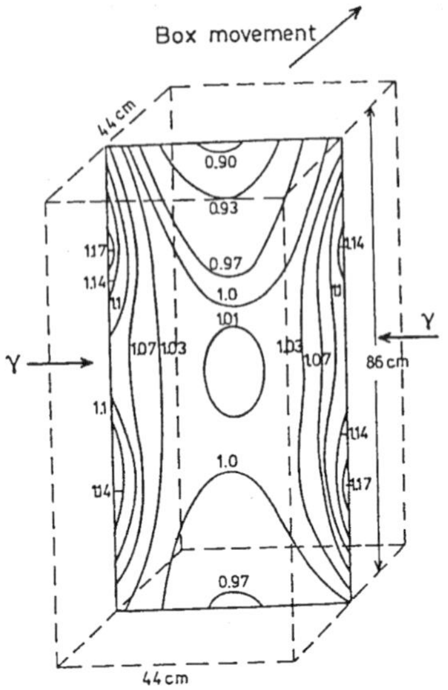

Fig. 4. Isodose curves on a horizontal plane with the dosimeter placed perpendicular to the source plaque.

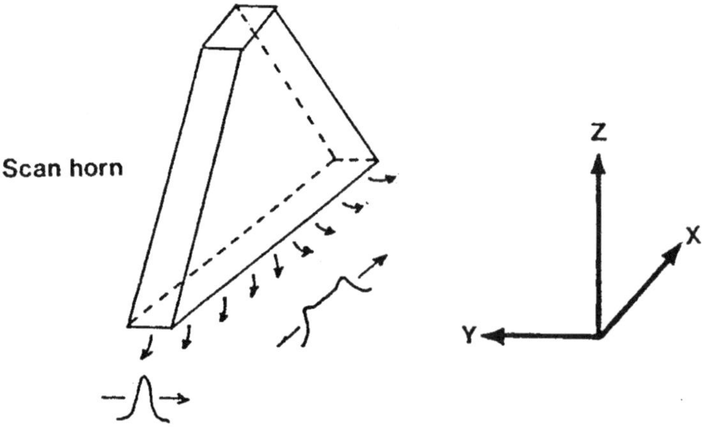

Fig. 5. Three-dimensional coordinate system for characterizing the radiation field of an electron accelerator.

matter. A useful range parameter is determined from these distributions, and is used to minimize the possibility of any overdose and to maximize the beam penetration. The relationship between the nominal dose and the conveyor speed is then determined.

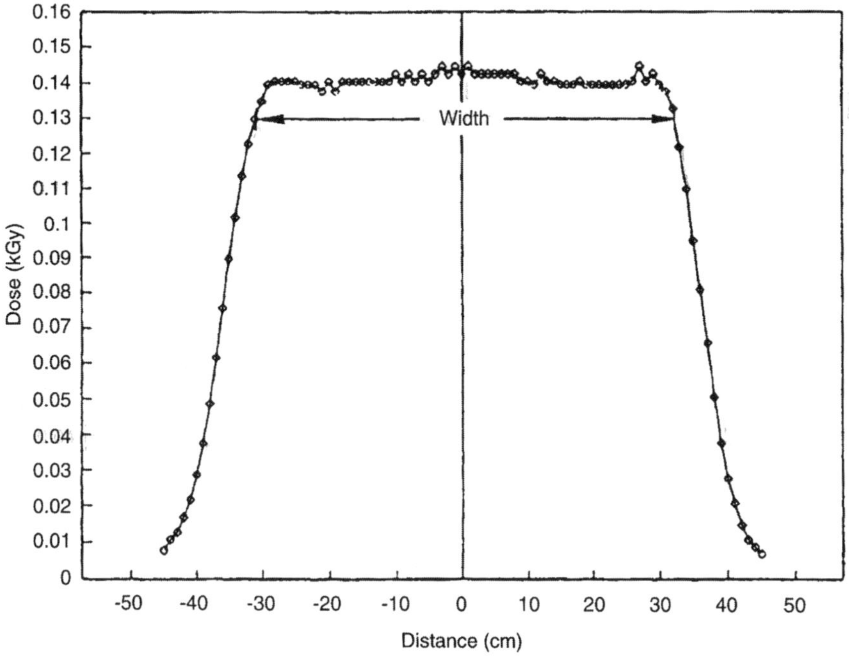

Fig. 6. A typical dose distribution along the scan direction for an electron irradiator (x-axis).

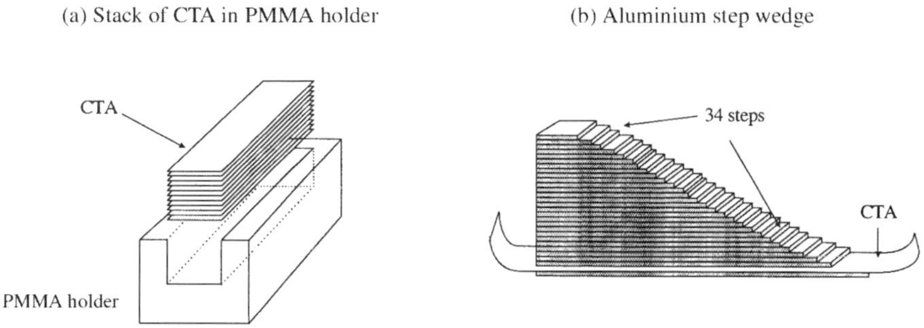

Fig. 7. Measurement of distribution along the z-axis.

The information obtained during dose mapping in facility qualification regarding the maximum and minimum dose zones can be useful, and can provide guidance as to where to place the dosimeters for this exercise (Figs. 9 and 10). Significant dose variation can occur over short distances, especially in electron beam irradiators, and so considerable skill is required to locate

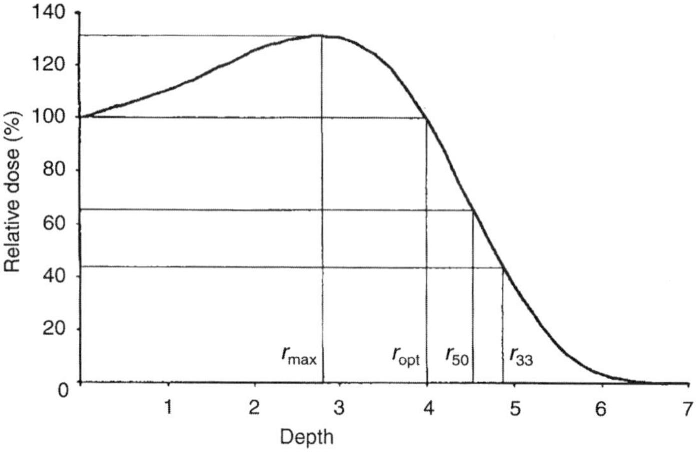

Fig. 8. Typical depth–dose curve for electrons, where the entrance (surface) dose is 100%. The various ranges are identified as follows: r_{max} is the depth at which the maximum dose occurs, r_{opt} is the depth at which the dose equals the entrance dose, r_{50} is the depth at which the dose equals half of the maximum dose, and r_{33} is the depth at which the dose equals one third of the maximum dose.

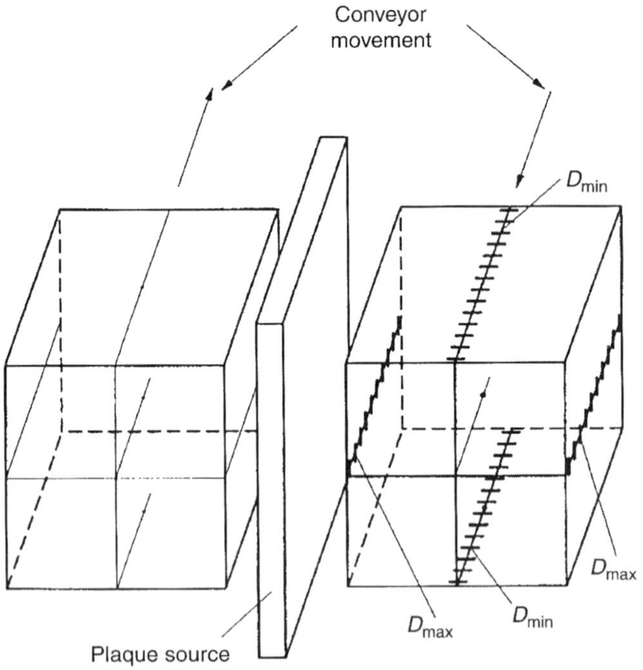

Fig. 9. Typical regions of the minimum and maximum doses of two single-direction passes of a rectangular package, with one on each side of a stationary gamma ray plaque source.

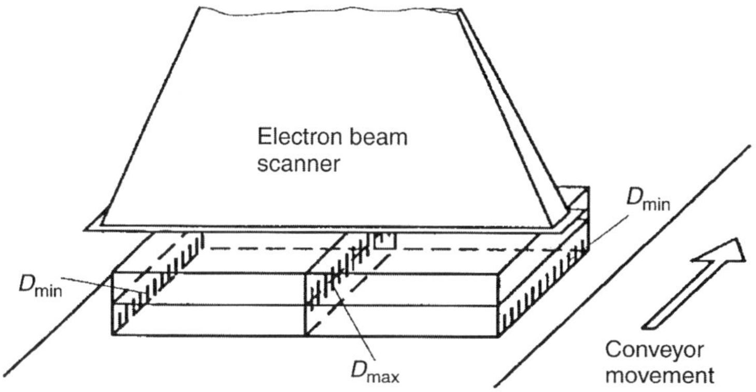

Fig. 10. Typical regions of the minimum and maximum doses for a single-pass, single-direction electron beam irradiation.

the true maximum and minimum positions. Particular attention should be given to inhomogeneous product distribution, orientation of the product relative to the direction of the radiation, voids, local differences in specific density, and interfaces. Previous experience may also prove indispensable. The problem of defining the proper placement of dosimeters is most pronounced for electron irradiation, which because of a monoenergetic energy distribution and a well-defined direction of the electron beam is known to produce large dose gradients.

The maximum and minimum doses and their locations are determined in this exercise, but the dose map should be carried out in more than one product box in order to determine the measurement uncertainty. Simultaneous with the measurements of the maximum and minimum doses, the parameters of the irradiation facility must be recorded and a reference dose must be measured. The reference dose is the parameter that is used to monitor the output of the irradiation facility, and it is used for routine process control.

Product validation

When a plant is fully characterized, the next step is to analyze more specifically the product to be routinely processed. To this end, dosimetry must give evidence that the minimum dose required has actually been exceeded and that the maximum dose deposited causes no degradation of the products. For this purpose, the product to be processed is submitted to a validation exercise that makes it possible to pinpoint the areas with maximum and minimum doses as well as variations of the absorbed dose in the same area. From this data, a nominal dose value and a set of control parameters of the radiation plant can be determined so as to guarantee routine radiation processing within the specified dose limits.

The product validation of healthcare products is more straightforward than the product validation of tissue allografts, which by their nature are more variable in their physical characteristics. In particular, the density of tissue allografts may vary depending on their water content. In addition, some tissue allografts may be heterogeneous in their distribution of density within the product, requiring an appropriate number of dosimeters for the product validation exercise. A consideration of these factors affecting the actual absorbed dose in tissue allografts must be undertaken so that the level of accuracy in delivering a dose can be determined.

Product validation is an exercise that is aimed at obtaining documented evidence that each product irradiated under a given set of conditions receives an absorbed dose within specified limits.

Routine dose control

This involves monitoring of the dose received by the product during processing. The important parameters are the minimum and maximum doses received, but these very often occur at inaccessible locations within product boxes. Therefore, the dose at a convenient monitoring location is measured, and is related to the minimum and maximum doses by the ratios obtained during process qualification dose mapping. Routine dose control provides final confirmation of all the processing parameters. Therefore, routine dosimeters are fixed to or placed inside the product boxes during normal processing. The dose which is read will be used as a guideline for the release of the irradiated product for public use.

The frequency of routine dosimetric measurements depends on a number of factors that are specific to the particular irradiator and product, but it is always a balance between the cost and effort involved and the consequence of finding a reading outside specifications. Evidence for correct processing, including the adherence to any legal or technological dose limits, depends on the maintenance of full and accurate records by the irradiation facility.

Prior to the release of a product, the dosimetry records and recorded values of process parameters should be examined to verify the compliance with specifications. For each production run, the dose delivered to the product should be certified.

Conclusion

Radiation processing should be carried out within documented dose limits to ensure that the products are produced with parameters that are in accordance with specifications. The procedures for providing the documentation are specified in some cases; and in others, not. For example, the procedures for documenting the required minimum dose for the sterilization of tissue allografts are specific; but for measuring the minimum dose in a dose mapping exercise, the procedures are not specific and choices have to be made. The basis for these choices must always be that no product may be irradiated outside specifications.

The main components of a quality assurance plan in an industrial irradiation unit have been detailed above. Characterization of the radiation field of the facility, validation of the product, and routine process control by means of traceable dosimeters to national or international standards are the three most important contributions of dosimetry to the quality control of irradiation processes. The training of laboratory staff and the compilation of a dosimetry laboratory operations guide also enable the operator of an irradiation facility to guarantee the quality of its dosimeter measurements and, consequently, of the performed radiation treatments.

Taking into account the present situation in radiation processing dosimetry, it can be concluded that standardized and well-characterized dosimeter systems and procedures are available for process control. However, due to stricter requirements to improve quality assurance and the introduction of new technologies, both improved and new dosimetry systems, procedures, and methods are needed for process control under standardized conditions.

References

International Atomic Energy Agency (IAEA) (2002). Dosimetry for Food Irradiation, IAEA Technical Reports Series 409.

Kovacs A and Miller A (2004). Present status and expected progress in radiation processing dosimetry. Emerging Applications of Radiation Processing, IAEA-TECDOC-1386.

McLaughlin WL, Boyd AW, Chadwock KH, McDonald JC, and Miller A (1989). *Dosimetry for Radiation Processing*, Taylor & Francis, London.

Miller A, Sharpe P, and Chu R (2000). Dosimetry of industrial radiation processing. International Commission on Radiation Units and Measurements (ICRU) News, June 2000.

Mod Ali N (1993). Dosimetry for radiation processing in Malaysia. *Radiat Phys Chem* **42**:4–6.

Chapter 14

Validation of Radiation Dose Distribution in Boxes for Frozen and Nonfrozen Tissue Grafts

Norimah Yusof

Malaysian Nuclear Agency (NM)
Bangi, 43000 Kajang, Selangor
Malaysia

Introduction

The use of ionizing radiation for the sterilization of tissue grafts — a practice that began in the early 1950s — is becoming increasingly popular among many tissue bankers. In fact, the development of radiation as a sterilizing technique for bone allografts has paralleled the popularity of bone transplantation (Tomford 2005). Radiation sterilization does not substitute, but rather complements the strict donor screening, good processing practices, appropriate packaging, and proper storage of tissue products. Sterilization is required to provide an additional safety measure against infection. Radiation has been reported to inactivate the human immunodeficiency virus (HIV), which is related to the acquired immunodeficiency syndrome (AIDS) and the hepatitis C virus (HCV) (Czitrom 1993; Tomford 2005). Some have postulated that the HIV virus could be noninfectious at as low as 2.5 kGy (Spire *et al.* 1985), but others have claimed that it requires as high as 36–50 kGy (Conway *et al.* 1990). The current practice is to use radiation with pretreatment of grafts in dealing with viruses and resistant bacteria.

Ionizing radiation is an effective sterilizing method, yet many who currently use this technique know little about its advantages over other sterilization methods. These include the following:

- No significant increase in temperature to cause any physical or chemical changes, thus allowing tissues to retain their clinical properties
- High penetration of gamma rays, thus enabling hard and soft tissues to be sterilized in their final packaging in containers/boxes
- No toxic residues, thus requiring no quarantine period and allowing the tissues to be used immediately after sterilization
- Exposure time to radiation as the only variable, thus enabling precise and simple process control

Further comparison among the three most commonly used sterilization techniques is summarized in Table 1.

Radiation seems to be a safe and effective method to sterilize tissues. Tissues in final packages can be sent to any irradiator for sterilization. Most commercial irradiators use gamma rays emitted from a radioactive source, cobalt-60, in providing contract sterilization. Chapter 8 discusses the different types of irradiation and radiation facilities that are available for routine sterilization.

Table 1. Comparison of sterilization methods of tissue grafts.

Considerations	Autoclave	Ethyleneoxide (EtO)	Radiation
Tissue materials	Mainly damaged	NA	Only at high doses
Packaging	Special	Special	NA
Parameters to control	Vacuum Pressure Temperature Humidity Time	EtO concentration Vacuum Pressure Temperature Humidity Time	Time
Residues	NA	Yes	NA
Quarantine	NA	7–14 days	NA
Poststerilization test	Desirable	Required	Not necessary
Reliability	Good	Good	Excellent
Continuous operation	No	No	Yes
Environmentally friendly	Good	Poor	Good
Occupational safety	Good	Poor	Good

NA: not applicable.

Radiation sterilization is an integral part of the overall processing of tissue products. Therefore, Good Radiation Practice (GRP) in accordance with international standards is as important as Good Manufacturing Practice (GMP) in processing of tissues. As mentioned in chapter 8, Good Radiation Practice (GRP) comprises the following parameters (IAEA 1990):

- Irradiator
- Dosimeters
- Dose mapping
- Material compatibility
- Product validation
- Routine process control

Chapter 8 describes the irradiator and its components for the sterilization process, while chapter 13 describes the rest of the parameters towards establishing process control. Requirements for the validation and routine control of the sterilization process for medical devices are described in the international standard ISO 11137-1 (2006). The use of biological indicators for validation and process monitoring is not recommended for radiation sterilization because the relationship between microbiocidal action and radiation dose is well established.

This chapter describes the practical experience of the Malaysian Nuclear Agency (NM) in conducting dose mapping of tissue products and validation of product loading for gamma sterilization in order to develop a standard procedure for routine process control. Radiation dose distribution in a box must be established to ensure that all grafts in the box receive the required sterilization dose.

Dose Mapping and Validation

Tissue products are generally produced in either a dried (air- or freeze-dried) or frozen state. They are of different shapes, sizes, and densities. Therefore, it is of utmost importance to establish the radiation dose distribution in a box packed with packages of tissue products for a particular irradiation facility (batch type or continuous type) prior to routine sterilization service. The dose distribution is very much influenced by the type of tissue product (material, density, size) and the product configuration (homogeneity) in a box.

In a dose mapping exercise, the dose distribution throughout a box or container is characterized using either the actual product or a simulated tissue-equivalent material called a "dummy". For instance, a wooden stick can be used to replace a long bone because of their almost similar densities, and a piece of paper to replace amniotic membrane. Garcia *et al.* (2005) used dog food as surrogate material to simulate dry ice for dose mapping in the validation of irradiated frozen bone allografts.

Dosimeters

Dosimeters to measure the absorbed dose can be classified into two groups:

- Primary (reference) dosimeter — e.g. Fricke (ferrous sulfate solution for gamma) or graphite calorimeter (for electron beam) must be used to compare the response of the routine dosimeter in the production environment.
- Routine dosimeter — e.g. ce/ce (ceric-cerous sulfate solution for gamma) or CTA (cellulose triacetate for electron beam) is calibrated for use in the commissioning of the irradiator and routine exposure.
- The dosimetric findings must be tracable to international standards, such as the International Dose Assurance Service (IDAS). As shown in Table 2, there are several dosimeters that are commonly used in gamma irradiation facilities.

Ce/ce and Red Perspex dosimeters are commonly used in the validation work of sterilization because they can measure doses in the range of 10–50 kGy and 5–50 kGy, respectively. Even though a dose of 25 kGy is generally used by many tissue banks, there is a tendency now to use lower doses (especially for soft tissues) while some banks prefer to use higher

Table 2. Dosimeters for high-dose measurement at the NM gamma irradiator.

Dosimeter	Range of doses (kGy)
Ferrous sulphate (Fricke)	0.04–0.4
Ceric/cerous (ce/ce)	10–50
Ethanol-chlorobenzene	0.01–100
Red Perspex	5–50
Amber Perspex	1–30
Clear Perspex	3–20

doses of 30–36 kGy for irradiating frozen bones. In our validation work, we use the ce/ce dosimeter for two reasons: it is less sensitive to high humidity in tropical climates; and it can be continuously supplied by our Secondary Standard Dosimetry Laboratory, NM. The same dosimeter is also used in routine process control for tissue sterilization.

In conducting the validation work, many dosimeters are required for placement in between the products as well as inside and outside the box. However, the placement of dosimeters for a container of frozen bones packed in dry ice at −80°C is not possible because the ce/ce dosimeter will freeze and lead to erroneous readings; instead, the validation work is conducted at room temperature with the product configuration and density similar to the container with the actual frozen bones. One has to remember that for routine process control of frozen bones, dosimeters are placed at limited points, i.e. confined to the outside of the container. It is not advisable to open the container full of frozen bones just to place the dosimeters; in fact, such a container must not be opened at all prior to irradiation so as to avoid any increase in temperature. The container, preferably of insulated type, must be able to maintain the frozen temperature of the tissues throughout the irradiation period until they are despatched back to the tissue bank. For an ordinary box containing dried tissue products, a few dosimeters are normally placed inside the box prior to irradiation in order to measure the absorbed dose under routine process control.

The absorbed doses obtained from the dosimetric readings identify the zones of minimum and maximum doses. The dose uniformity ratio (DUR) is calculated as follows:

$$\text{Dose uniformity ratio (DUR)} = \frac{\text{Maximum dose } (D_{\text{max}})}{\text{Minimum dose } (D_{\text{min}})}$$

The locations of D_{max} and D_{min} are identified as the dose monitoring locations for routine process control. Dosimeters must be placed at these two locations during routine irradiation.

Irradiation personnel should be able to assist in characterizing the magnitude, distribution, and reproducibility of the absorbed dose in products of a certain density, and relate these parameters with the cycle time and operating conditions. The cycle time — the length of time that a product spends in an irradiation room to receive the minimum required sterilization dose — is set depending on the overall product bulk density, load (product) configuration of the box, and conveyor path of the irradiation facility. Irradiation personnel must also ensure that all of the systems in the radiation facility are functioning correctly, calibrated, and reproducible.

Material Compatibility

As part of product validation, tissue bankers must conduct material compatibility tests after irradiation, particularly for the following:

- To evaluate the tissue stability by conducting physical and chemical analyses
- To evaluate its packaging materials and the sealing condition, as sterility can only be guaranteed when the packaging is intact or not damaged

Packaging materials that are radiation-compatible must be selected for packing tissue grafts. A general guide on packaging material is given in ISO 11137 (1995), of which several radiation-stable thermoplastic materials are listed in Table 3. However, due to rapid developments in polymer science, it is recommended that tissue bankers refer to plastic manufacturers for new radiation-stable packaging materials.

Table 3. Radiation stability of thermoplastics (ISO 11137, 1995).

Thermoplastics	Radiation stability
Polystyrene	Excellent
Polyethylene	Excellent
Polyamides	Excellent
Polyimides	Excellent
Polysulfone	Excellent (natural material is yellow)
Polyphenylene sulfide	Excellent
Polyvinylchloride (PVC)	Good (antioxidants and stabilizers prevent yellowing)
Polyvinylchloride–polyvinylacetate	Less resistant than PVC
Polyvinylidene chloride	Less resistant than PVC
Polyvinyl formal	Less resistant than PVC
Polyvinylbutyral	Less resistant than PVC
Styrene acrylonitrile (SAN)	Good
Polycarbonate	Yellow (mechanical properties not greatly affected)

Dose Mapping

The following methodology, based on the procedure set up by the NM Tissue Bank, describes how to validate the dose distribution of frozen and nonfrozen tissue grafts. An ordinary paper carton/box is used to pack air-dried amnion and freeze-dried bone grafts, while an ice container (Coleman PolyLite 54) measuring 59 cm (L) × 33 cm (W) × 41 cm (H) is used to pack about 10–15 pieces of frozen long bones. Validation work is carried out at room temperature, as the ce/ce dosimeter (glass ampoule containing 5 mL of cerous sulfate solution) cannot be used in frozen state.

1. Place ce/ce dosimeters inside the box/container (i.e. inner walls of the box/container) at five positions on each wall, as shown in Fig. 1(a). Place preferably three ampoules at each position.
2. Pack the box/container with the tissue or tissue-equivalent material in their final packs. For long bones, use wooden sticks 13–18 inches in length and individually wrapped in three layers — plastic, linen, and finally packed in a plastic bag — to simulate packed frozen bones. Small bones are replaced with wooden blocks, while empty three-layered plastic bags are adequate for simulating amnions. The box/container is then packed with used newspaper to attain the same density of the box/container packed with the actual tissue products. To simulate an ice container packed with dry ice, more wood pieces may be required as dummies. Finally, check the density of the box.
3. Place ce/ce dosimeters at three points at each of the three levels — i.e. upper, middle, and lower layers — in between the dummies inside the box/container, as shown in Fig. 1(b).
4. Place ce/ce dosimeters on the outside of the box/container, i.e. the center point on each wall (front, back, left side, right side, and top), as shown in Fig. 1(c).
5. Send the box/container to the gamma irradiator and irradiate at 25 kGy.
6. After irradiation, release all of the dosimeters from the box/container and send for absorbed dose measurement.
7. Identify the locations of maximum dose (D_{max}) and minimum dose (D_{min}). They are usually among those positions inside the box.
8. Calculate the dose uniformity ratio (DUR). It is important to know the D_{max} that will be delivered by the irradiator after the D_{min} required to

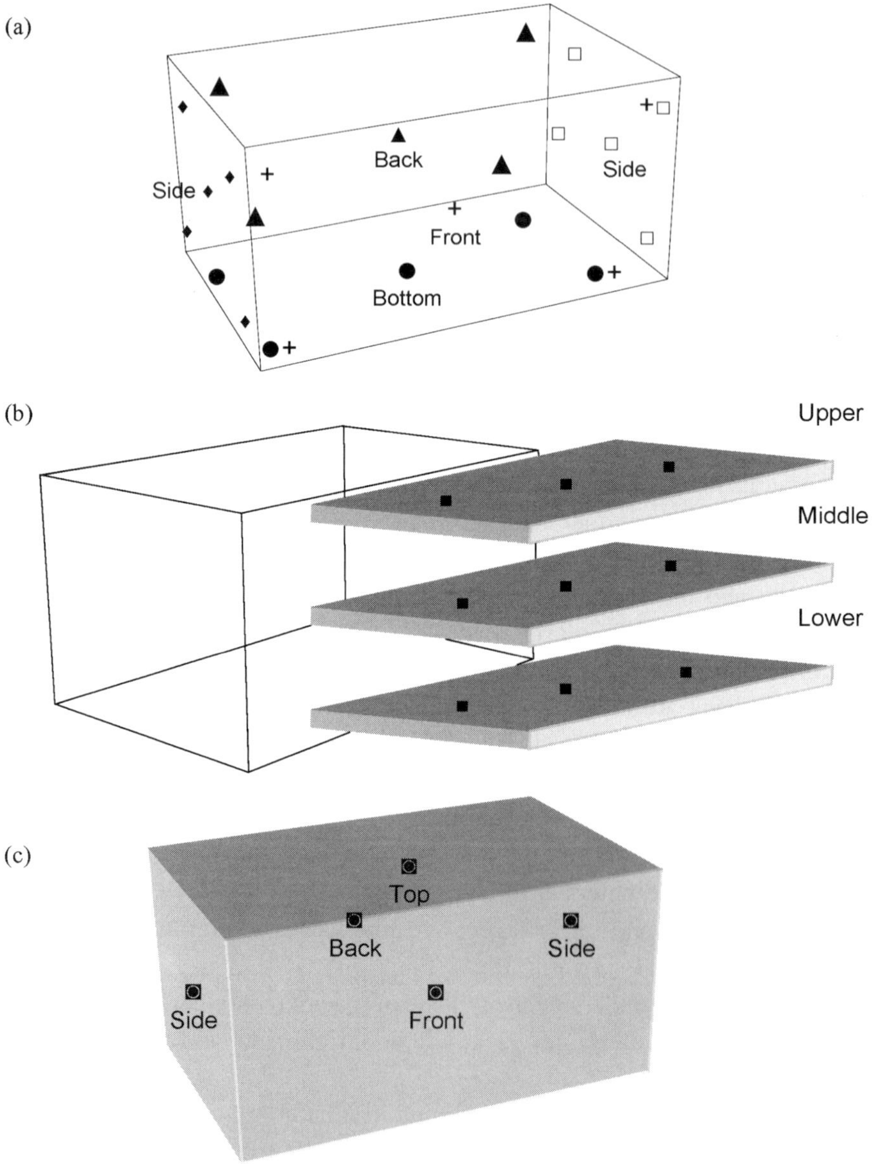

Fig. 1. Placement of dosimeters for dose mapping experiment. Dosimeters are attached (a) to the inner wall of the box/container, (b) to three layers inside the box/container, and (c) to the outer wall of the box/container.

sterilize the tissue products is achieved. The DUR recommended by the AAMI Guidelines (1992) is in the range of 1.0 to 1.05. Such a low DUR can be achieved by reducing the container size and/or rotating the container during irradiation or by doing more passes in the irradiation room (Yusof 1994).

9. For a container with frozen bones, the correction factor must be identified by comparing the D_{min} outside the container with the D_{min} inside the container.

In a previous study by the author (Yusof 1994), the DUR for a container with a density of 0.18 g/cm^3 was in the range of 1.13 to 1.15 when irradiated simultaneously with commercial medical products in the carrier. However, a better DUR of 1.06 to 1.07 was obtained when irradiated without any commercial routine medical products in the carrier. From three validation exercises, the positions of D_{max} and D_{min} were not consistent, and so not a single position was selected. In isodose studies conducted by the irradiator on boxes of medical items, most results indicated that the minimum dose was absorbed right in the center of the box. Therefore, it is recommended that for routine irradiation, dosimeters should be placed at several locations outside the box and one dosimeter right in the middle of the box. However, for frozen bones, given that dosimeters are not placed inside the container, the correction factor to the D_{min} (obtained from among the dosimeters placed outside of the box) needs to be applied. From the validation work, it was found that the D_{min} outside the container was 1.03 higher than the D_{min} absorbed by the bones inside the container. For example, to ensure that the D_{min} inside the container is 25 kGy, the D_{min} outside the container must be around 26 kGy.

Some tissue banks have or can get access only to a self-shielded gamma cell, which has a cylindrical irradiation chamber of limited size (normally 15 cm in diameter and 20 cm in height). In this case, dosimeters can only be placed at a few locations and smaller-sized dosimeters such as Red Perspex should be considered.

Routine Process Control

Having conducted the validation work, a standard procedure in handling a box/container of tissue grafts before irradiation is then established. The NM

Tissue Bank has identified positions to place dosimeters for routine absorbed dose measurement. Staff of the NM Tissue Bank place ce/ce dosimeters at these identified positions.

Nonfrozen (air- or freeze-dried) tissue products

As illustrated in Fig. 2(a), dosimeters are placed at five positions inside the cylindrical container when tissues are irradiated in a self-shielded gamma cell:

1. Top — at center point on top of the tissue packages
2. Center (at middle level) — in between the tissue packages
3. Front (at middle level) — on the container wall
4. Back (at middle level) — on the container wall
5. Bottom — at center point before filling up the container with the tissue packages

As illustrated in Fig. 2(b), dosimeters are placed at seven positions inside a paper carton/box containing packages of dried tissue products before being sent to the NM gamma irradiation facility:

1. Top — at center point on top of the tissue packages
2. Center (at middle level) — in between the tissue packages
3. Bottom — at center point before filling up the container with the tissue packages
4. Front (center of middle level) — on the wall
5. Back (center of middle level) — on the wall
6. Right side (center of middle level) — on the wall
7. Left side (center of middle level) — on the wall

Frozen tissue products

As illustrated in Fig. 2(c), before being sent to the NM gamma irradiation facility, dosimeters are placed at five positions outside of an insulated container containing packages of frozen bones:

1. Top — at center point on top of the container
2. Front (center of middle level) — on the wall

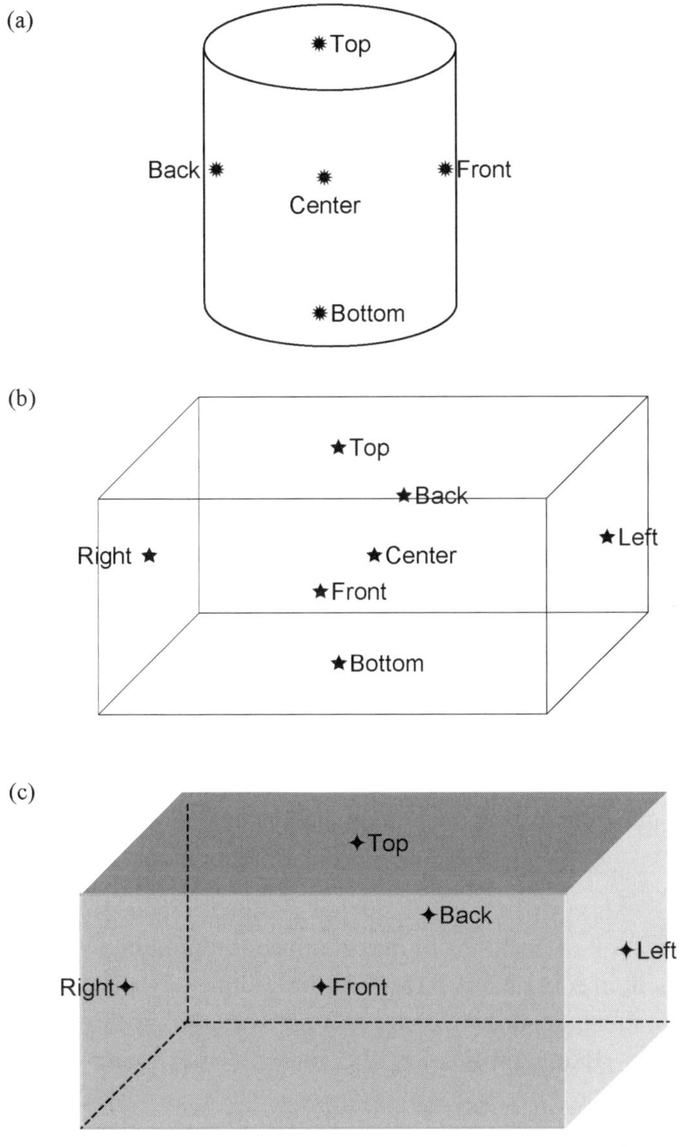

Fig. 2. Placement of dosimeters for routine process control. (a) Cylindrical container of self-shielded gamma cell; (b) paper carton/box; and (c) insulated container of frozen bones.

3. Back (center of middle level) — on the wall
4. Right side (center of middle level) — on the wall
5. Left side (center of middle level) — on the wall

The personnel at the irradiation facility, upon receiving the box/container, implement four main steps under routine process control:

1. Record the receiving, storing, and returning of products.
2. Paste a color change (go/no-go) indicator and an irradiation batch number on every box/carton.
3. Record the absorbed dose measurements.
4. Release the certification for the minimum dose delivery.

During routine irradiation, besides dosimeters, the go/no-go indicator is pasted on each tissue package. Unlike dosimeters, this irradiation indicator cannot measure the absorbed dose. It is just an indicator to differentiate the products after sterilization process through color changes, for instance from yellow before irradiation to red after irradiation.

In addition to the minimum dose, the NM Tissue Bank also requests for reports on the maximum dose and DUR for record keeping.

Conclusion

The dose mapping exercise involving the placement of dosimeters throughout a representative product load during validation is crucial, and leads to the following:

- Identification of positions of maximum and minimum doses through the placement of routine dosimeters during routine process control
- Identification of dose distribution or variability through the dose uniformity ratio (DUR), i.e. the ratio of maximum dose/minimum dose

Validation for the product loading pattern should be established for each type of tissue product within the container/box to achieve the best DUR. The minimum dose will ensure that each tissue receives the required absorbed dose to sterilize it; while the maximum dose will assist us to avoid overdosing, which is detrimental to tissue properties.

References

Association for the Advancement of Medical Instrumentation (1992). AAMI Guidelines for Radiation Sterilization, Arlington, VA.

Conway B, Tomford WW, Hirsch MS, Schooley RT, and Mankin HJ (1990). Effects of gamma irradiation on HIV-1 in a bone allograft model. *Trans Orthop Res Soc* **15**: 225–230.

Czitrom AA (1993). Principles and techniques of tissue banking. In: Heckman J (ed.), *American Academy of Orthopaedic Surgeons — Instructional Course Lectures*, Vol. 42, American Academy of Orthopaedic Surgeons, USA, pp. 359–362.

Garcia R, Harris A, Winters M, Howard B, Mellor P, Patil D, and Meiner J (2005). Improved method for gamma irradiation of donor tissue. In: Kennedy JF, Phillips GO, and Williams PA (eds.), *Sterilisation of Tissues Using Ionising Radiations*, CRC Woodhead Publishing, England, pp. 331–338.

International Atomic Energy Agency (IAEA) (1990). Guidelines for Industrial Radiation Sterilization of Disposable Medical Products, IAEA-TECDOC-539, Vienna.

International Standards Organization (ISO) (1995). Sterilization of Health Care Products — Requirements for Validation and Routine Control, ISO 11137, 1995(E), Switzerland.

International Standards Organization (ISO) (2006). Sterilization of Health Care Products — Radiation, ISO 11137-1 Part 1, Switzerland.

Spire B, Dormont D, Barre-Sinoussi F, Montagnier L, and Chermann J (1985). Inactivation of lymphadenopathy-associated virus by heat, gamma rays, and ultraviolet light. *Lancet* **1**:188–189.

Tomford WW (2005). Effects of gamma irradiation on bone — clinical experience. In: Kennedy JF, Phillips GO, and Williams PA (eds.), *Sterilisation of Tissues Using Ionising Radiations*, CRC Woodhead Publishing, England, pp. 133–140.

Yusof N (1994). The use of gamma irradiation for sterilisation of bones and amnions. *Malays J Nucl Sci* **12**(1):243–251.

Chapter 15

Importance of Microbiological Analysis in Tissue Banking

Norimah Yusof and Asnah Hassan

Malaysian Nuclear Agency (NM)
Bangi, 43000 Kajang, Selangor
Malaysia

Introduction

Microbiological quality control is the application of microbiological tests designed to ensure that the process meets certain defined microbiological quality standards. Microbiological analysis, as discussed in other chapters, is a useful tool for the quality control of processed tissues, in addition to physical tests such as the one for water content. Under the microbiological quality control (QC), microbiological analysis on the microbial count of each batch of tissue production indicates whether the tissue has been properly processed. The microbial count of a product before it undergoes sterilization is known as the bioburden. Bioburden estimation is an important tool not only to determine the hygienic level of tissue products, but also to determine the effectiveness of radiation doses for sterilization. The bioburden must be kept low, preferably less than 10 counts per graft, before the product is accepted for sterilization in order to achieve a high sterility assurance level (SAL).

In line with the quality system of tissue banking, each tissue bank should make an effort to establish and validate standard operating procedures (SOPs) or work instructions (WIs). This is because only grafts produced according to the established procedures will meet the required quality. Microbiological analysis can be used in the validation work to verify each step of tissue processing by taking random samples of tissues and washing solutions. Proper processing, together with Good Manufacturing Practice (GMP), is necessary to ensure that the quality of processed tissue will be consistently high. Through continuous microbiological analysis on processed tissue, tissue bankers can keep on improving the processing and handling procedures. Tissues with a low bioburden will ultimately be sterilized at doses lower than 25 kGy to attain the required high sterility assurance level (SAL) of 10^{-6}. Lowering the radiation dose may help to minimize the detrimental effects of radiation on the physical and biological properties of tissues (Yusof 1994).

The many uses of microbiological analysis include the following:

- Validation of processing procedures
- Routine monitoring of tissue products (product QC)
- Monitoring of incoming materials (tissues, packaging materials, etc.)
- Monitoring of environment where the processing takes place
- Validation and routine control of sterilization

This chapter will address the first two aspects of microbiological analysis, with case studies on amnion and bone for the following:

1. Validation of processing procedures (process validation)
2. Product QC (bioburden)

Methods of Estimating Microbiological Colonies

The international standard ISO 11737-1 (1995) describes in detail the methodologies, recommended diluents, and media used to conduct validation, as well as how a laboratory can establish its own working procedures. Three methods commonly used to estimate the microbiological colonies of any sample are as follows:

1. Pour plate method — the sample is mixed with melted, cooled agar so that microbial colonies will grow within and on the surface of the agar medium.
2. Spread plate method — the sample is spread over the surface with a sterile spreader so that colonies will grow on the surface of the agar medium.

3. Filtration method — the sample is filtered through a membrane and then the membrane is transferred onto the agar medium. This method is more sensitive and is particularly useful for products of low bioburden.

Only a microbial count between 30 and 300 colonies per plate is acceptable for the pour plate and spread plate methods. Therefore, for samples with very low bioburden (i.e. less than 30 counts), the filtration method is most suitable. Figure 1 describes the steps involved in conducting a microbiological test using the filtration method. The colony-forming unit (CFU) per sample product can be estimated.

The sample can be of raw material (after procurement), taken from any of the processing steps, or processed (finished tissue products). Samples taken

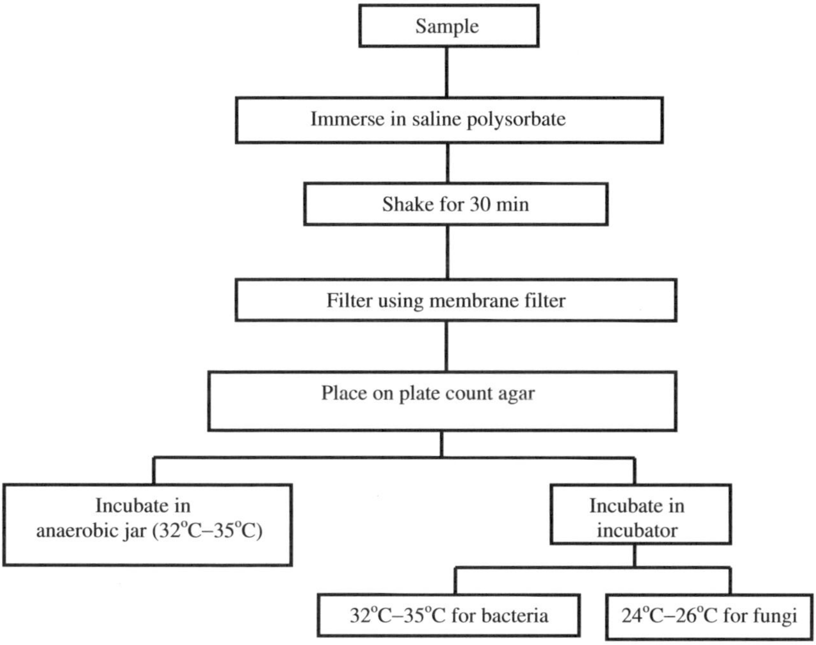

Fig. 1. Steps involved in conducting a microbiological test. Microbial colonies on plates are counted within 5–7 days after incubation, and the result is expressed as the colony-forming unit (CFU) per unit product.

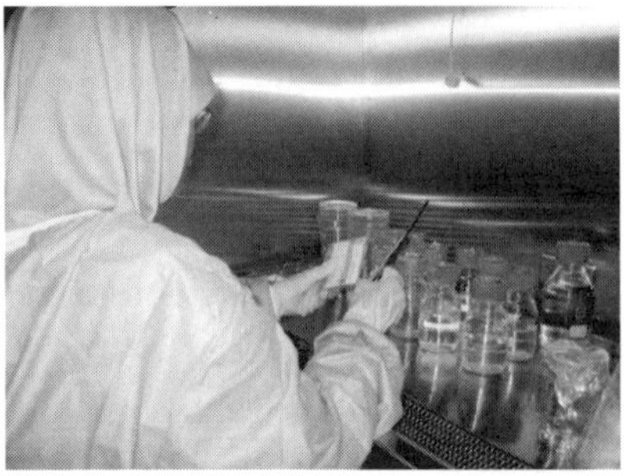

1. Disinfect package with 70% alcohol.

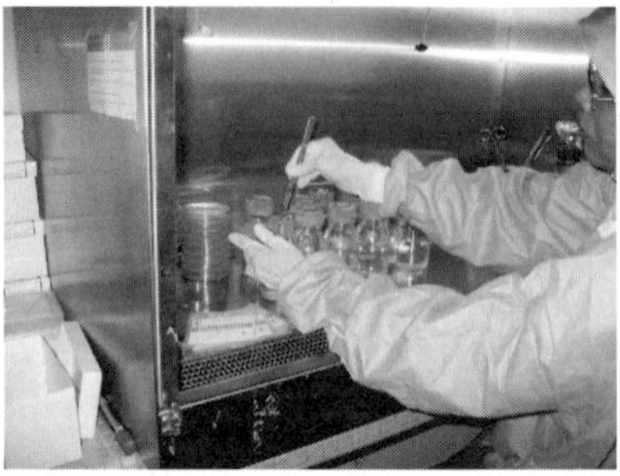

2. Immerse amnion into 0.01% sterile saline polysorbate.

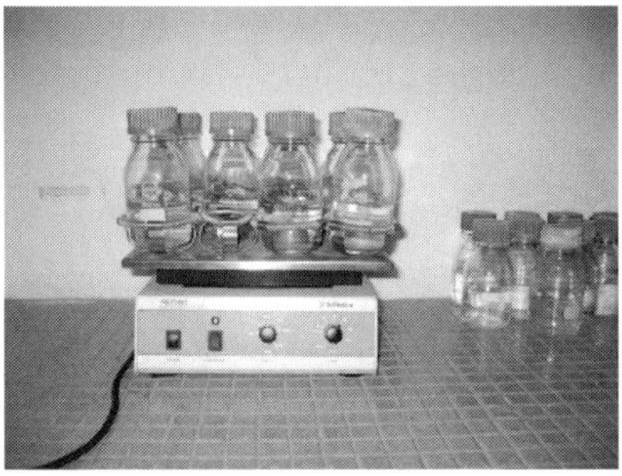

3. Mix for 15–20 min.

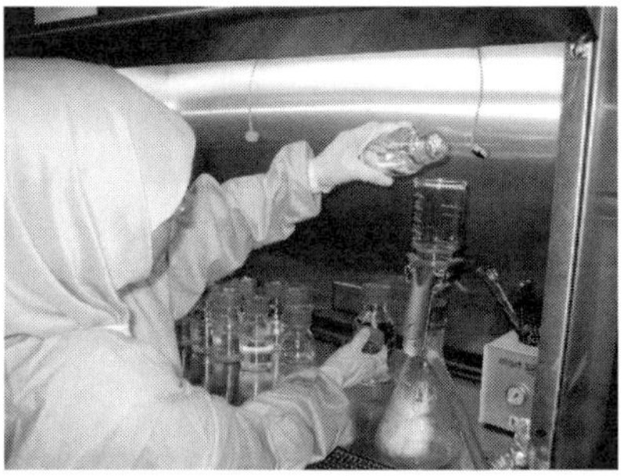

4. Filter aliquot through a 0.2–μm membrane filter.

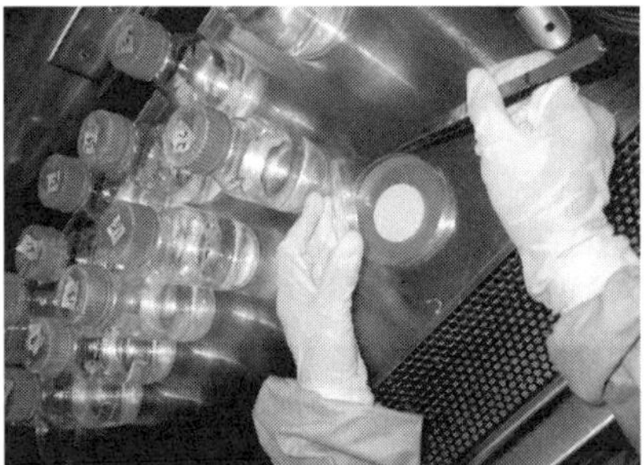

5. Place filter on agar plate.

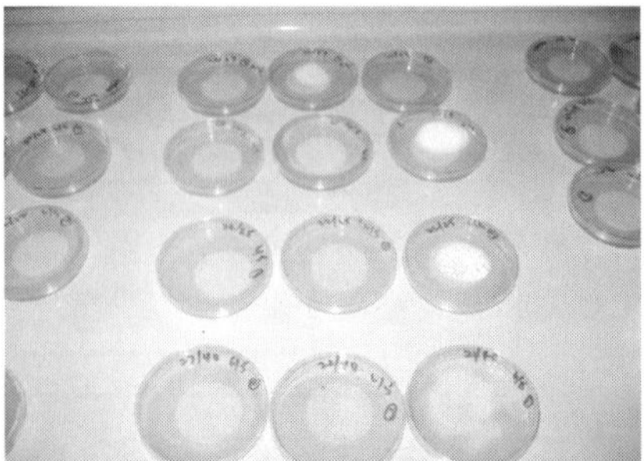

6. Incubate plates at 32°C–35°C for 5–7 days.

Fig. 2. Bioburden analysis on amnion using the filtration method.

from any of the processing steps can either be tissue or washing solutions. For those samples suspected of containing a high microbiological count, serial dilution is required and the first two methods (i.e. pour plate and spread plate) can be considered.

It should be stressed here that microbiological tests on tissues that are normally conducted by hospitals immediately upon procurement are merely for the screening of any positive growth, especially pathogenic microbes. The tests do not provide results on colony count.

Bioburden

Bioburden is the total number or count of viable microorganisms (bacteria, yeast, mold) on a packaged product prior to the sterilization process. Properly processed tissues usually have low bioburden. Therefore, the bioburden is determined using the filtration method. The work instruction (WI) established by the NM Tissue Bank, Malaysia, for conducting the bioburden test is simplified below, and can be used as a guide for other tissue banks to establish their own WI. Figure 2 shows pictures during the analysis.

NM Tissue Bank work instruction: bioburden analysis of tissue products

Instruments and tools

Table 1. Instruments and tools.

Laminar flow cabinet	Filtration unit (sterile)	Media bottles
Water distiller	Vacuum pump	Beakers
Incubator	Forceps and scissors (sterile)	Cotton gauze
Autoclave	Vortex mixture/Orbital shaker	Petri dishes (sterile)
Hot plate and stirrer	Gloves and lab gown	Anaerobic jar
	Membrane filters (sterile)	
	Pore size: 0.2 μm or 0.4 μm	
	Diameter: 4.7 mm	

Solutions

Table 2. Solutions.

Disinfectant	Alcohol 70%	
Diluent	Saline polysorbate solution (0.01%):	
	Sodium chloride	9.0 g
	Polysorbate solution (Tween 80)	0.1 mL
	Distilled water	1000 mL
Preparation	Mix the ingredients well by stirring on hot plate. Dispense 150 mL into 200-mL bottle (for amnion) and 100-mL bottle (for bone). Autoclave at 121°C for 15 min.	

Media

Table 3. Media.

Agar plate	Ready-mixed tryptone soya agar powder	40 g
	Distilled water	1000 mL
Preparation	Place the ingredients into beaker. Heat the mixture on hot plate and stir. Boil until the agar dissolves completely. Dispense into 1-L bottle or conical flask. Cap the bottle or plug the conical flask, and autoclave for 15 min at 121°C. Pour ~15–20 mL of media into sterile petri dishes aseptically (carried out in laminar flow cabinet). Allow to solidify. Incubate the plates upside down in incubator at 32°C–35°C for 24 h. Discard plates with growth.	

Sampling procedure

1. Pick random samples of amnion/bone for testing from each processing batch.
2. Weigh the bone and measure the size of the amnion.

Method

1. Switch on laminar flow cabinet at least 20 min before working. Disinfect the cabinet with 70% alcohol.
2. Assemble all of the instruments needed in the laminar flow cabinet.
3. Disinfect the outside of the packaging with 70% alcohol.

4. Cut the packaging, and transfer the sample into saline polysorbate solution using sterile forceps.
5. Mix for 5 min on vortex mixture/orbital shaker. Repeat if necessary. Leave to stand for a short while (5–15 min).
6. Place the sterile filter on the filtration unit with sterile forceps. Filter a certain volume of aliquot, depending on the preset results (conduct bioburden test on new samples by filtering aliquot at various volumes — 5, 10, 15, 20, 30, 40, 50 mL — and choose the volume that can give less than 100 CFU per filter). Pour sterile water to wash down the aliquot.
7. Remove the filter with sterile forceps. Roll the filter slowly onto surface of agar plate from the edge to eliminate air bubbles. Label the plates.
8. Rinse the filtration unit with sterile water after each filtration and before filtering the next sample.
9. Incubate the plates inverted for 5–7 days at 32°C–35°C for total aerobic bacteria (TB) and at 22°C–24°C for total fungus, yeast, and mold (TFYM). Place in anaerobic jar and incubate at 32°C–35°C for 5–7 days for total anaerobic bacteria (TAB). Count the colonies that appear on the filter. Calculate total count per sample according to the volume of the aliquot filtered, and/or apply dilution factor when applicable. In cases when TFYM and TAB are very small, incubate the plates for TB only.
10. Isolate the most commonly found microorganisms. For pathogenic bacteria such as *Streptococcus* sp., *Pseudomonas* sp., *Staphylococcus* sp., *Coliform* sp., and *Escherichia coli*, isolate them using selective media. If coliform bacteria and *E. coli* are found in the sample, then all of the grafts from that particular donor should be discarded.

Calculations

Calculate the total microbial count (TMC) as follows:

$$\text{TMC} = \text{TB} + \text{TFYM} + \text{TAB}$$

For example, when a tissue sample is immersed in 100 mL of diluent, the microbial number per tissue is calculated as follows:

$$\text{CFU per tissue product} = \frac{\text{TMC}}{\text{mL of diluent filtered}} \times 100\,\text{mL}$$

Microbiological Analysis of Amnion

Case 1: Process validation

Amnion procured from a maternity hospital was processed as illustrated in Fig. 3 (Hasim and Yusof 1991; Yusof *et al.* 1994a). Washing solution from each step (about 150 mL) was collected and analyzed for microbiological count. The experiment was repeated for processing with a 10-min (instead of 20-min) shaking time for salines I, II, and III in order to reduce the processing time. The processed amnions (surface area ranging from 120 cm^2 to 180 cm^2), freeze- or air-dried, were taken from each processing batch and subjected to microbiological analysis. Some common natural contaminants were identified.

The results presented in Table 4 show that the microbial count during the initial washing was high in all cases, and gradually reduced in the subsequent processing steps (Yusof *et al.* 1994a). When the shaking time for salines I, II, and III was shortened by 10 min, the number of microbes removed from the amnion into the washing solution for each step was less than that for 20 min of shaking; thus, a high number of microbes were still attached to the amnion, resulting in high bioburden. The results indicated that the shaking time of 20 min for salines I, II, and III should be maintained. Irrespective of the count in each washing solution, the microbial count or bioburden on amnion after drying was acceptably low (approximately 5 CFU/piece) after 20 min of shaking. Based on the microbiological analysis, the processed amnion in Fig. 3 was validated with the option for drying either by freeze-drying (lyophilization) or air-drying in laminar flow. A minimum of three washings in sterile saline is a prerequisite to remove any sodium hypochlorite residue.

Case 2: Bioburden

Amnions processed for routine production by the National Tissue Bank at the University of Science, Malaysia, were monitored over the first 4 years of its operation (Yusof *et al.* 1994a). Samples were randomly taken from several processing batches sent for sterilization. As shown in Table 5, the overall average bioburden for the first 3 years was high, around 100 colony counts per piece. In the fourth year, the bioburden was lowered to less than 10 after the bank improved its processing procedures and the operator was well trained.

Procure amnion from placenta of screened mother

↓

Wash with filtered water

↓

Rinse and keep in sterile normal saline

↓

Transfer to Tissue Bank in ice container at –4°C

↓

Shake in sterile water for 10 min

↓

Shake gently in 0.05% sodium hypochlorite for 10 min

↓

Shake in sterile saline (I) for 10 or 20 min

↓

Shake in sterile saline (II) for 10 or 20 min

↓

Shake in sterile saline (III) for 10 or 20 min

↓

Clean further with sterile gauze in laminar flow

↓

Stretch across over sterile cotton gauze

↓

Cut into pieces (~120–180 cm^2)

↓

Deep-freeze and freeze-dry (–40°C for 24 h)

or

Air-dry in laminar flow (room temp. for 16 h)

↓

Triple-pack in PE pouches and heat seal

↓

Label

↓

Radiation sterilize at 25 kGy

↓

Store in dark and cool place or despatch to hospitals

Fig. 3. Processing of amnions at the NM Tissue Bank.

From this case study, it is suggested that through microbiological analysis, a bank will be able to know if tissues have been properly processed; in addition, the bank must improve its processing-related activities/procedures. Improvements can be in the form of trained manpower, a clean environment, and hygienic practices such as proper handling and packaging. Amnion with gauze was also found to give a high count, as gauze (like any other biological material) provides a favorable environment for microbes to grow.

Table 4. Microbiological analysis of washing solutions from the processing steps of amnions (CFU/mL), and bioburden of the processed amnion (CFU/piece).

	Colony-forming unit (CFU)/mL					
Sample	A5	A6	A9	A23	A24	A25
Saline	TNTC	TNTC	TNTC	1336	413	695
Distilled water	TNTC	670	TNTC	112	469	184
Sodium hypochlorite	530	430	3335	14.5	43.5	102
Saline I	130	360	2975	4.8	19.4	34
Saline II	110	80	2620	14.5	4.3	29
Saline III	80	60	1795	0	0	4.8
Bioburden for processed amnion (CFU/piece)	5.3	5.3	5.9	112	530	NA

Samples were named by donor identification number.
Samples A5, A6, and A9: salines I, II, and III were shaken for 20 min.
Samples A23, A24, and A25: salines I, II, and III were shaken for 10 min.
TNTC: too numerous to count.
NA: not available.
All amnions were air-dried, except A5 (freeze-dried).

Table 5. Overall average bioburden of amnion grafts prior to irradiation (colony counts/graft) processed by the National Tissue Bank, Malaysia (Yusof *et al.* 1994a).

	Overall average bioburden (CFU/piece)
1990	85.2 (8)
1991	133.0 (8)
1992	84.5 (17)
1993	9.3 (28)

Numbers in brackets indicate the number of batches tested for that year.

Therefore, it is recommended that gauze must be radiation sterilized or autoclaved before use.

In another study, the bioburden of amnions from routine production by the NM Tissue Bank and the National Tissue Bank, Malaysia, was monitored from 1994 to 2003. The results are shown in Table 6 (Yusof *et al.* 2005). The findings suggested that bioburden as microbiological QC is a useful

Table 6. Average bioburden of amnions randomly taken from at least three processing batches per year.

Year	Bioburden (CFU/product unit)	
	NM Tissue Bank	National Tissue Bank
1994	21.7 ± 34.7	6.5 ± 7.1
1995	2.9 ± 3.8	7.7 ± 1.2
1996	2.7 ± 1.6	6.9 ± 4.2
1997	11.6 ± 18.6	NA
1998	NP	NA
1999	NP	NA
2002	NP	14.5 ± 12.7
2003	NP	15.6 ± 7.5

NP: amnion was no longer processed for routine production, only for R&D.
NA: not available.

tool to ensure that tissues produced by the banks are consistent in quality. The amnion processing procedure established by the NM Tissue Bank (and adopted by the National Tissue Bank) was further improved for routine production. In fact, the product quality was consistent over the years due to several factors: the skills acquired by the tissue bank operators, well-maintained equipment, a cleaner environment, and more efficient processing procedures. The variation in bioburden through the years may have also been due to variation in product sizes (ranging from 80 to 200 cm^2). The most commonly found contaminants on the amnions isolated over the years were identified as *Bacillus* sp., *Micrococcus* sp., *Corynebacterium* sp., and *Rhodotorula* sp. Bioburden monitoring can therefore be used as an audit on routine processing in tissue banks.

Microbiological Analysis of Bones

Case 1: Process validation

Femoral heads were procured during hip replacement surgery (Yusof *et al.* 1994b). The donors were screened according to the living donor exclusion criteria. Those with potentially serious transmissible diseases, such as hepatitis, malignancy, human immunodeficiency virus (HIV), osteoporosis, and rheumatoid arthritis, were excluded. The bones were quarantined at −30°C by the hospital while waiting for the results from serological and microbiological tests. Only the bones with negative results were released and either kept as deep-frozen at −80°C or released to the NM Tissue Bank for processing as freeze-dried bones.

At the tissue bank, the bones were processed according to Fig. 4. Washing was carried out until the bones looked clean and the washing solution was clear. Washing solution (100 mL) was randomly collected from any of the

Procure bone from screened healthy donor
↓
Deep-freeze at –30°C for at least 1 week (quarantine)
↓
Send to NM Tissue Bank
↓
Deep-freeze at –80°C for 1 week
↓
Cut and trim
↓
Wash,
shake for 30 min*
&
repeat until water is clear
↓
Pasteurize at 57°C for 3 h
↓
Wash,
shake for 30 min*
↓
Wash,
shake for 30 min*
↓
Deep-freeze at −80°C for 18–20 h**
↓
Freeze-dry for 18–20 h***
↓
Package
↓
Label
↓
Sterilize at 25 kGy
↓
Store in dark and cool place
or
Despatch

* Washing solutions are taken for microbiological analysis.
** Bone samples are taken for microbiological analysis both before and after deep-freezing.
*** Bone samples are taken after freeze-drying for microbiological analysis.

Fig. 4. Processing of bones at the NM Tissue Bank.

processing steps. Bone samples were collected at three steps — i.e. before deep-freeze, after deep-freeze, and after freeze-dry — for microbiological count using the filtration method.

Results of the monitoring of six processing batches are presented in Table 7. The microbiological count of the first washing solution was high in all of the samples tested. A total of 25 and 20 washings were done for LD9 and LD10, respectively, until the solution was clear before the bones were pasteurized; while for the rest, only up to 5 washings were done. In LD9 and LD10, the microbial count initially reduced with the washing steps, but went back up after the 9th and 13th washings, respectively. Surprisingly, no colony growth was observed in all of the washing solutions immediately

Table 7. Microbiological analysis of washing solutions from the processing stages of femoral heads (Yusof *et al.* 1994b).

	Microbiological count (CFU/100 mL) on sample					
Washing sequence	LD9	LD10	LD11	LD12	LD13	LD14
1st	TNTC	TNTC	2730	520 (pasteurized at 5th)	TNTC	1060 (pasteurized at 4th)
5th	TNTC	TNTC	40 (pasteurized at 9th)	0	20 (pasteurized at 8th)	0
10th	68	500	0	0	0	0
15th	184	10700	0	—	0	—
20th	39200	TNTC (pasteurized at 25th)	0	—	—	—
25th	2141 (pasteurized at 26th)	0	0	—	—	—
30th	0	0	0	—	—	—
35th	0	0	0	—	—	—
40th	0	0	0	—	—	—
Total no. of washings	41	40	33	13	17	10

Samples were named by donor identification number.
TNTC: too numerous to count.

after the bone was pasteurized at 56°C–58°C. Therefore, in the subsequent batches, the pasteurization was conducted much earlier, i.e. after the fourth to nineth washing whenever the washing solution was almost clear.

The findings showed that the pasteurization treatment of 56°C for 30 min, which is meant for inactivating HIV, could inactivate microorganisms as well. Table 7 shows a clear reduction of microbes in all of the samples immediately after pasteurization, regardless of how many washing steps were carried out earlier. It was obvious that the washing steps after pasteurization could be minimized as pasteurized bones seemed to require less washing, thus reducing processing time and cost. Based on the analysis, it is recommended that pasteurization is carried out after the fifth washing, followed by another three to five washings. According to Spire *et al.* (1985), a 100% inactivation of the lymphadenopathy-associated virus, which is possible of causing AIDS, could be achieved when the virus was heated at 56°C for 30 min. Therefore, as a safety precaution for tissue bank operators, it is advisable that the pasteurization of bones be carried out as early as possible. Make sure to remove bloodstains, as they may become darker due to pasteurization. From our observations, pasteurization can also remove some amount of fat from the bones.

Case 2: Bioburden

The bone weight was recorded before the microbiological analysis/bioburden test was conducted. The results of samples LD10, LD12, and LD14 at three different stages are shown in Table 8. No growth of microbes was detected in all of the stages. This clearly indicated that strictly adhering to the processing procedure results in high-quality bones with low bioburden.

The bioburden of freeze-dried bones processed by the NM Tissue Bank and National Tissue Bank over several years was compiled as in Table 9 (Yusof *et al.* 2005). Unlike amnion production, only a small number of bones were processed per year; therefore, only a few samples could be taken for bioburden estimation. Although no growth was observed on bones after pasteurization as in Table 8 for validation work, microbial count was obtained on processed bones from routine production. The contaminants may have come from the environment or during handling.

Table 8. Microbiological analysis of bones at different stages of processing.

	Microbiological count (CFU/g)* on sample		
	LD10	LD12	LD14
Before deep-freeze	NA	0	0
After deep-freeze	NA	0	0
After freeze-dry	0	0	0

*3 replicates per bone sample.
Samples were named by donor identification number.
NA: not available.

Table 9. Bioburden estimation of bones using the filtration method (average bioburden of samples randomly taken from processing batches per year).

Year	Bioburden (CFU/product unit or item)	
	NM Tissue Bank	National Tissue Bank
1993	88.4 ± 110	NA
1994	13.6 ± 26.6	7.0 ± 5.0 (human)
		9.8 ± 9.1 (bovine)
1995	21.4 ± 22.0	1.5 ± 1.5 (human)
		6.7 ± 8.9 (bovine)
1996	11.5 ± 11.6	10.8 ± 4.0 (human)
1997	4.0 ± 1.9	NA
1998	NP	NA
1999	NP	16.0 ± 10.0 (bovine)

NP: bone was not processed for routine production, only for R&D.
NA: not available.

The high count in 1993 suggested that the procedure was not yet in place and that the operators were being trained (Yusof *et al.* 2005). After several years in operation, the bioburden could be maintained at a low level, mainly around 10 CFU/item.

To show whether different types of processing — namely deep-freezing, freeze-drying, and demineralization — have any effect on bioburden, another test using rabbit bones without pasteurization was conducted. The results as shown in Table 10 indicated that freeze-drying significantly

Table 10. Bioburden of bone samples after different types of processing.

	Deep-freezing	Freeze-drying	Demineralization and freeze-drying
No. of samples	10	10	5
Bioburden	148.2	10.9	10.2

reduces the bioburden compared to deep-freezing. Demineralization might not further reduce the microbes.

Conclusion

Under the tissue banking quality system, all of the procedures in a tissue bank should be verified and validated. Microbiological analysis is a very useful tool in validating new procedures, besides being used as the quality control of the processed tissue grafts. The analysis is also used to monitor routine processing, from the starting material (i.e. the quality of the procured tissues) to the final tissue product. Other than microbial count, microbiological techniques such as the open plate method are used as monitoring tools to check the cleanliness of the processing area and its environment, while the sterility test is used to confirm the sterility of a product. Recently, microbiological analysis is being used in dose-setting experiments to verify the radiation sterilization process. It is therefore advisable for any tissue bank to have an in-house microbiology laboratory with competent personnel in order to conduct the various methods of microbiological analysis.

References

Hasim M and Yusof N (1991). Tissue banking in Malaysia — amniotic membrane. *Malays J Nucl Sci* **9**(2):127–131.

International Standards Organization (ISO) (1995). Sterilization of Medical Devices — Microbiological Methods — Part 1: Estimation of Population of Microorganisms on Products, ISO 11737-1, 1995, Geneva.

Spire B, Dormont B, Barre-Sinoussi F, Montagnier L, and Chermann JC (1985). Inactivation of lymphadenopathy-associated virus by heat, gamma rays, and ultraviolet light. *Lancet* **1**:188–189.

Yusof N (1994). The use of gamma irradiation for sterilization of bones and amnions. *Malays J Nucl Sci* **12**:243–251.

Yusof N, Abdul Rani S, Hasim M, Asnah H, Ang CY, and Muhamad Firdaus AR (2005). Bioburden estimation in relation to tissue product quality and radiation dose validation.

In: Kennedy JF, Phillips GO, and Williams PA (eds.), *Sterilisation of Tissues Using Ionising Radiations*, CRC Woodhead Publishing, England, pp. 319–329.

Yusof N, Hasim M, Asnah H, Norshamsuria O, and Salahbiah AM (1994a). Microbiological aspect of radiation sterilisation of amnion graft. In: *Proc 5th APASTB International Conference*, Suzhou, China.

Yusof N, Nor Azlan MA, Selamat SN, and Lee CM (1994b). Radiation sterilised freeze dried bone allograft — process validation. In: *Proc 8th International Conference on Biomedical Engineering*, National University Singapore, Singapore, pp. 303–305.

Chapter 16

Validation for Processing and Irradiation of Freeze-Dried Bone Grafts

Nazly Hilmy, Basril Abbas and Febrida Anas

BATAN Research Tissue Bank (BRTB)
Center for Research and Development of Isotopes and Radiation Technology, BATAN
Jakarta 12070, Indonesia

Introduction

The most common allogeneic freeze-dried bone grafts currently prepared at the BATAN Research Tissue Bank (BRTB) are freeze-dried bone allografts, demineralized and freeze-dried bone allografts, and frozen bone allografts. The processing and safety aspects of bone allografts have many similarities with the preparation of pharmaceuticals and medical devices by the manufacturing industry, in particular the safety aspects. Tissues from which virulent microorganisms have been isolated are not acceptable for transplantation, unless the procedure has been validated to effectively inactivate the microorganisms without causing potentially harmful effects (AATB 2002; EATB 1997; IAEA 2002).

According to the American Association of Tissue Banks (AATB), validation is the process of establishing documented evidence which provides a high degree of assurance that a specific process will consistently produce the predetermined outcome. The aim of this chapter is to describe the process validation of processing, pasteurizing, washing, demineralizing, lyophilizing, and packaging bone allografts (i.e. part of the validation of the presterilization process), as well as the process validation of the amount of the radiation sterilization dose (RSD) used to sterilize bone allografts for safe clinical use at the BRTB.

Preparation of Bone for the Validation Process

Tissues are retrieved, processed, and distributed according to the International Atomic Energy Agency's (IAEA) International Standards for Tissue Banks (IAEA 2002), the IAEA/National University of Singapore (NUS) learning module (1997), and the BRTB's procedural manual (Hilmy *et al.* 2003). Harvesting of bones should be done with a surgical kit in aseptic condition. All tissues are procured aseptically at the hospital from both live and cadaver donors, according to donor selection criteria designed to eliminate the risk of transfer of transmissible diseases, malignancy, etc. The processing procedures are designed to follow the Guide to Good Manufacturing Practice for Medicinal Products (PIC/S 2000).

Screened donor

Blood donors are screened according to the minimum blood test criteria of the IAEA International Standards for Tissue Banks (2002). These include screening for HIV-1/2 antibody (HIV-1/2 Ab), hepatitis B virus surface antigen (HBs Ag), hepatitis C virus antibody (HCV Ab), and syphilis. All test results should be negative.

Retrieval/Procurement

The retrieval of bone tissues is done at hospitals based on a memorandum of understanding (MoU) between the BRTB and the hospital. When all of the required bones have been procured, they are transferred into a container (Fig. 1). This container is constructed of metal or plastic, and is identical to the containers used for transporting tissue products. The transportation container is chilled using prefrozen slabs and is then transferred to the BRTB. Documentation relating to the donor's past medical records and serology testing are usually sent to the tissue bank separately (but should ideally be sent at the same time).

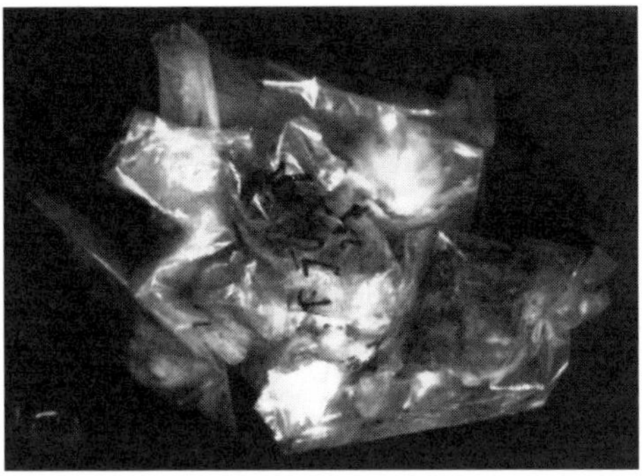

Fig. 1. Femoral heads procured from a live donor. Tissues from different donors should be packed and treated separately.

All bone tissues that arrive at the BRTB are documented. The documentation, storage, and processing of tissues from different donors should be separated (IAEA 2002). Donor details are recorded in the Donor Record Form. At this stage, the bones are individually identified by a tissue bank reference number. These files will be kept for 10 years or so, depending on the BRTB's policy. After documentation, tissues are stored at the quarantine stage and marked with a yellow color at −40°C until the results of the donor screening and swab test arrive. If the results are favorable, then the tissues are removed from the quarantine stage, marked with a green color, and processed.

The preparation steps of bones for the validation process are shown in Fig. 2.

Processing of Bone for the Validation Process

The processing steps of bone allografts consist of swab test, pasteurization, elimination of soft tissues, cutting, washing, lyophilization, demineralization (if needed), packaging and labeling, radiation sterilization, storage, and lastly distribution. Before distribution to hospitals or potential users, the quality of allografts should be evaluated by the quality control (QC) department (see chapter 20). Each processing step should be validated, documented, and conducted according to written standard operating procedures (SOPs). The degree of consistency of the validation results is used

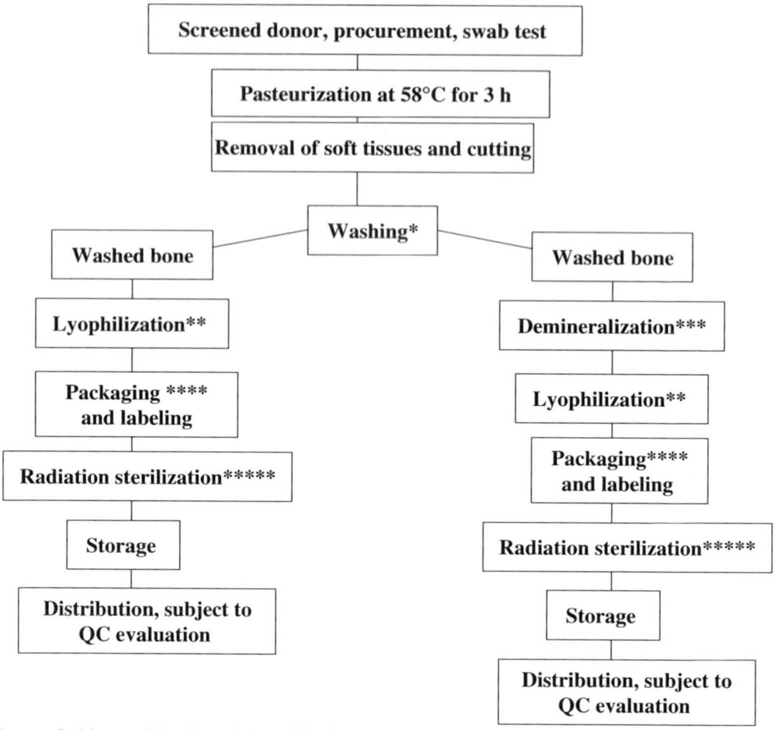

* Subject to blood particle validation.
** Subject to moisture content validation.
*** Subject to calcium content validation.
**** Subject to validation of packaging.
***** Subject to validation of radiation sterilization dose of 25 kGy or lower according to the IAEA Code of Practice (2004).

Fig. 2. Flow chart of bone processing and radiation sterilization.

to set up the SOPs. Screening of donors and retrieval of bone tissues are carried out at the hospital, based on the MoU between the hospital and the BRTB.

Microbiology swab test

Swab tests are done according to ISO 11737-1 (1995b). Pathogenic bacteria such as *Streptococcus* sp., *Pseudomonas* sp., *Staphylococcus* sp., coliform bacteria, and *Escherichia coli* are isolated by using selective media. If these pathogenic bacteria are found in the sample, then the sample should be discarded.

Pasteurization

The bone is removed from the deep freezer and is placed in an appropriate-sized glass beaker. The beaker is filled with sterile distilled water until the entire bone is submerged. The beaker is covered with clean aluminum foil, and then placed in an oven preheated to 58°C. The preheat time (i.e. the time taken for the temperature inside the bone to reach 58°C) should be validated, usually less than half an hour depending on the size of the bone. The pasteurization cycle is deemed to have been completed after 3 h. The temperature is monitored throughout the process. At the end of the cycle, the beakers are removed from the oven and the water is decanted. The soft tissues and cartilage are removed from the bone. These soft tissues are disposed in a special plastic bag and then buried. The bone is placed into a sterile plastic bag, sealed, and labeled using a permanent marker. The packed bone is then placed in a freezer at a temperature of −40°C overnight.

Cutting

Only authorized personnel are permitted to use a band saw (Fig. 3). The operator must wear a disposable gown, mask, cap, glasses, and sandals when operating the band saw. The exhaust fan is switched on during the processing. The band saw is disinfected using 70% ethanol prior to use.

The pasteurized bone is removed from the deep freezer and thawed under a laminar airflow cabinet (LAFC) for about 30 min. This bone is cut into appropriate sizes and shapes, and placed in a sterile screwed bottle. Waste tissues generated during the phase are collected and placed in a plastic bag, sealed, and taken to be buried. Immediately after the cutting procedure has been completed, the band saw is thoroughly cleaned and disinfected with an appropriate disinfectant solution. The band saw is subject to an evaluation of microbe contamination.

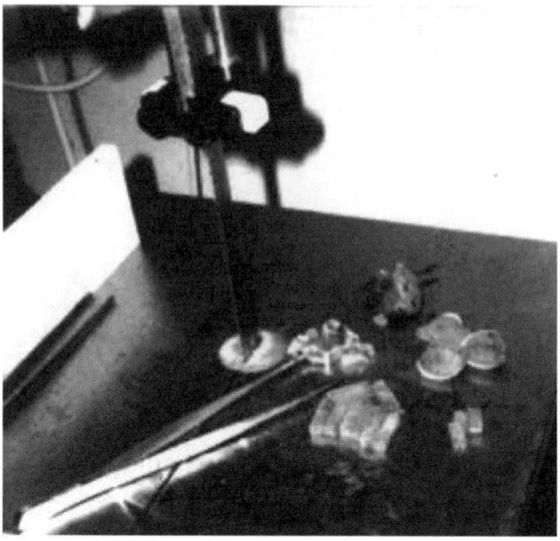

Fig. 3. Band saw for bone cutting.

Washing

The cut bones are transferred from the bottle into a metal wire basket. Warm water from a water heater is squirted with pressure to the bone for 10 min or more to remove the bone marrow. The bones are then transferred back into the bottle and filled with approximately 3 mL of 3% H_2O_2 solution until the bones are submerged. The bottle is covered and placed under an LAFC clean bench for 1 h. After 1 h, the solution is changed with sterile distilled water. The bones are washed three times with 300 mL of sterile distilled water, and are shaken well each time with gentle agitation on a shaking machine for 15 min. The distilled water is then changed with 300 mL of 70% propanol-2 solution before being placed under the LAFC overnight.

The next day, the 70% propanol-2 solution is changed again with sterile distilled water. The bone is washed three times with 300 mL of sterile distilled water, and is also shaken each time with gentle agitation on a shaking machine for 15 min. The last water solution is subject to validation: it should be free of blood particles, microbe contamination, and residue of chemicals used, and should have a pH of around 7 (IAEA/NUS 1997; Hilmy *et al.* 2000; Hilmy *et al.* 2003; Hilmy *et al.* 2006). After washing, the bone should be clean and free of blood particles (Fig. 4).

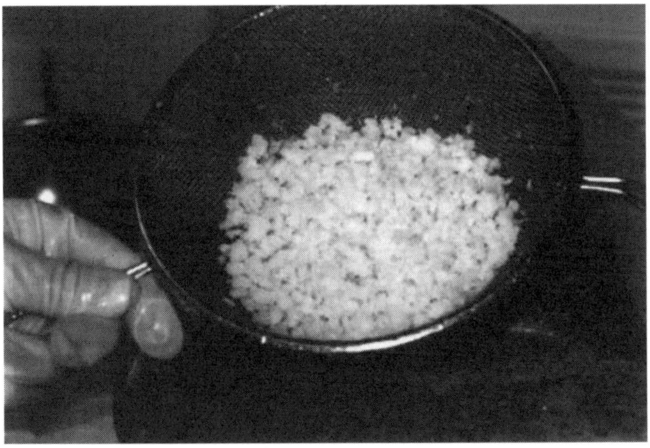

Fig. 4. Cancellous bones after the washing process.

Process validation: validation of blood particles, microbe contamination, and residue of chemicals used

The 300 mL of the last water solution is separated into 200 mL for the microbiology examination and 100 mL for the blood particle examination (microscopy examination).

1. Microbiology examination
   The technique for removing microbes from bone grafts is done according to ISO 11737-1 (1995b), i.e. by using the membrane filtration method. In this method, 200 mL of washed water is filtered and then the filtered paper is incubated at 30°C on trypticase soy agar (Difco) for 2 weeks. The results should be free of contaminating microbes. If microbes do exist, then they should be evaluated.
2. Blood particle/Red blood cell examination
   About 60 mL of the washed water is centrifuged by a Fisher Scientific centrifuge at a speed of 3000 rpm for 15 min. The sediments are observed for red cell/blood particle residues via a microscopic examination.

Results of validation experiments

The validation results of 10 washing process samples are shown in Table 1.

Table 1. Results of contaminating microbes after washing of bone.

Parameters	No. of sample									
	1	2	3	4	5	6	7	8	9	10
Total no. of microbes	0	0	0	0	0	0	0	0	0	0
Residue of blood particle	0	0	0	0	0	0	0	0	0	0

Freezing

The cleaned bone is placed on a sterile gauze in a sterile dish. The dish is then placed on a metal plate and left overnight in a deep freezer at −40°C to −80°C.

Lyophilization (freeze-drying)

Freeze-drying has emerged as one of the most satisfactory methods of preserving and storing human bone allografts for subsequent transplantation. The process consists of removing water from the frozen bone by sublimating it in a vacuum condition. The bone is lyophilized for 60 h (subject to validation). The routine procedure for operating the freeze-drying apparatus is followed. The bone is taken from the deep freezer and placed in a freeze-drying chamber, which has been precooled to −40°C (samples from different donors should be placed on separate racks). The duration of the freeze-drying cycle varies according to the amount, type, and size of the bone to be processed; typically, the process takes 1–3 days. A separate log book for the freeze-drying apparatus is maintained, and the chamber is disinfected at each freeze-drying cycle.

The water content of finished products should be less than 7% or less than 5%, depending on the BRTB's policy. After the freeze-drying cycle has been completed, the freeze-dried bones are selected to be used as allografts; only good-quality bones can be used.

Validation of moisture content of bone chips/blocks

During the freeze-drying process, the residual moisture content of the freeze-dried bones is measured by the gravimetric method in order to determine the efficiency of the lyophilization process and set up the SOP.

The gravimetric method for determining the residual moisture in freeze-dried products is specified by the regulations pertaining to biological products intended for use in humans. This method involves measuring the maximum weight loss of the weighed sample or until its weight is constant. First, a crucible is dried in an oven at 60°C, preferably overnight, until its weight is constant. Next, one or two bone graft sample pieces are placed in the crucible and weighed. The crucible with the sample is then placed in a 60°C oven overnight. After that, the crucible and sample are transferred from the oven to a weighing room, placed in a desiccator, and weighed. Further heating at 60°C is required until the sample weight is constant. The percentage of residual water is calculated as follows:

$$\frac{W_{\mathrm{i}} - W_t}{W_{\mathrm{i}}} \times 100$$

where

W_{i} = initial weight of sample
W_t = sample weight after heating for t hours

The validation results of residual moisture content are shown in Fig. 5. It can be seen from the figure that it takes about 50–60 h of lyophilization to reach a moisture content of 5% (Basril *et al.* 2006).

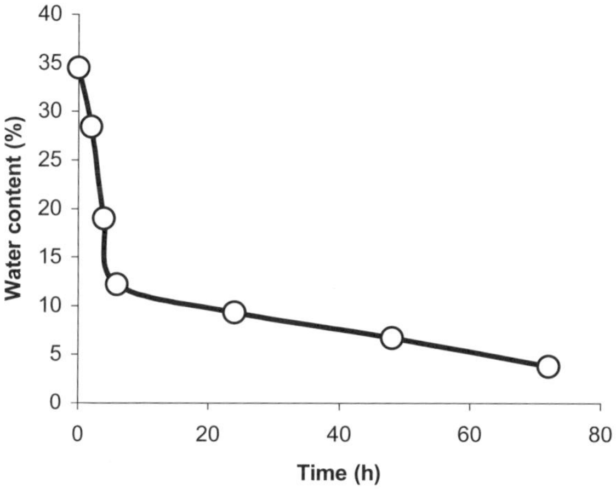

Fig. 5. Lyophilization time vs. residual moisture content of processed bone chips.

Demineralization

The bones are demineralized in an acid solution of 0.6 N HCl, and shaken with gentle agitation on a shaking machine for 1 to 6 h (depending on the size and type of bone) at a pH less than 2. Next, the bones are shaken three times with sterile distilled water on a shaking machine for 15 min. The solution is then changed with sterile phosphate buffer, and the bones are kept in a 37°C oven for 72 h. After that, the bones are shaken three more times with sterile distilled water on a shaking machine for 15 min. During the demineralization process, the pH of the acid solution has to be controlled because the mineral component of bone (primarily hydroxyapatite) is soluble only at a pH value below 4. At the end of the process, some bones are taken for validation. The demineralization process is stopped if the calcium (Ca) content is 8% or less (AATB 2002; Basril *et al.* 2006).

Validation process of demineralized bone by calculating the Ca content

The Ca content is determined via the titrimetric assay method as follows:

1. Weigh a bone sample of approximately 150 mg and transfer it into a glass beaker, and then add 5 mL of 4 N HCl into the beaker.
2. Heat the beaker until the sample is dissolved, and boil for 2 min to remove CO_2. Dilute the sample solution with 200 mL of distilled water, add two drops of methyl red indicator, and leave it in a water bath for 1 h at 90°C.
3. Add 20 mL of ammonium oxalate solution drop by drop into the beaker while shaking it. Add the ammonia solution until the color changes.
4. Heat the precipitate in water bath for 1 h.
5. Filter the precipitate, and wash it with water containing some drops of acetic acid solution with a pH of up to 7.
6. Place the filter paper with precipitate in a flask. Dilute the precipitate with 4 N H_2SO_4 solution and heat it in a water bath at 70°C.
7. Titrate with 0.1 N $KMnO_4$ solution.
8. Calculate the calcium content (%) as follows:

$$\%\,\mathrm{Ca} = \frac{V \times N \times 20}{W} \times 100$$

where

V = volume of $KMnO_4$ (mL)
N = concentration of $KMnO_4$
20 = equivalent weight of Ca
W = weight of sample

Measurement of the Ca content of the bone can also be done using other methods such as X-ray diffraction method (Basril *et al.* 2000).

Packaging

Packaging materials should be validated for their resistance to radiation. After freeze-drying, the bones are packed into polyethylene pouches with a thickness of 0.1 mm or into other materials as stated in ISO 11137 (1995a) and sealed with a heat sealer under a laminar airflow cabinet. The graft is triple-packed in sleeves from polyethylene pouches. Each layer is heat-sealed. A label is placed on the second-layer surface.

The validation results of the quality of packaging materials are presented in Table 2, which shows the water content of bone allografts up to a storage time of 12 months at room temperature. The table indicates that a storage time up to 12 months does not have a significant effect on the moisture content of the allografts.

Labeling

The label of the products should at least display the following:

- Date, name, and address of the tissue bank
- Graft name and code number (including frozen, freeze-dried)
- Size/volume of product
- Irradiation indicator (go/no-go)
- Expiration date
- Accompanying note that states "do not use if package is damaged"

Validation of radiation sterilization dose (RSD) (chapter 19; Hilmy et al. 2006)

The three methods used here are the three methods stated in the IAEA Code of Practice (2004). These include method A1, which is a modification

Table 2. The water content of bone allografts — cancellous (can) and cortex (cort) chips — in triple-layer polyethylene pouches up to 12 months of storage time (Basril *et al.* 2006).

Dose (kGy)	Month									
	0		3		6		9		12	
	Can	Cort	Can	Cort	Can	Cort	Can	Cort	Can	Cort
0	3.47 ± 0.48	3.32 ± 0.13	3.48 ± 0.19	3.22 ± 0.03	3.43 ± 0.08	3.46 ± 0.08	3.48 ± 0.08	3.22 ± 0.28	3.40 ± 0.06	3.40 ± 0.02
10	3.71 ± 0.13	3.83 ± 0.12	3.61 ± 0.26	3.86 ± 0.26	3.81 ± 0.06	3.85 ± 0.07	3.82 ± 0.26	3.84 ± 0.13	3.17 ± 0.25	3.82 ± 0.23
20	3.71 ± 0.14	3.77 ± 0.11	3.38 ± 0.25	3.84 ± 0.15	3.66 ± 0.88	3.61 ± 0.07	3.48 ± 0.35	3.88 ± 0.11	3.49 ± 0.47	3.75 ± 0.11
30	3.69 ± 0.03	3.65 ± 0.24	3.68 ± 0.16	3.56 ± 0.06	3.84 ± 0.70	3.55 ± 0.02	3.69 ± 0.08	3.54 ± 0.01	3.68 ± 0.14	3.62 ± 0.02

of method 1 of ISO 11137 (1995a); method B, which is related to ISO 13409 (1996); and method C, which is related to AAMI TIR 27 (2001). Twenty samples with a sample item portion (SIP) of one are needed for each experiment, i.e. 10 samples for bioburden determination and 10 samples for the verification dose (VD) experiment at a sterility assurance level (SAL) of 10^{-1}. Bioburden determination is done by shaking and then filtration, according to ISO 11737-1 (1995b); while the sterility test at the verification dose is conducted according to ISO 11737-2 (1998). If the VD experiment is successful, then the radiation sterilization dose to achieve an SAL of 10^{-6} can be either 25 kGy (methods B and C) or lower than 25 kGy (method A1; see Table 2b of the Code).

Bioburden determination

The bioburden load and bioburden estimate are determined according to ISO 11737-1 (1995b), using 10 samples with SIP = 1 and bacterial media of trypticase soy agar. The incubation temperature and time are 30°C and 14 days, respectively. Treatment to remove microbes from tissues is done by shaking the samples without glass beads in a 40-mL sterile saline solution for 10 min. Transfer of the tissue samples to a culture medium is done by using the membrane filtration method for lyophilized and demineralized samples, and the swabbing method for frozen bones (e.g. femoral heads, rings, struts). Gram staining and D_{10} value determination are done for all of the contaminated microbe colonies obtained.

1. Bioburden estimate
   The bioburden estimate establishes the number of microorganisms comprising the bioburden by applying a correction factor compensating for the recovery efficiency to a viable count. The correction factor technique for removing microbes from products is done by using inoculated methods with spores of *Bacillus pumilus* E 601, according to ISO 11737-1 (1995b). Spore suspension in water, which consists of about 100 spores per 0.1 mL, is prepared 1 day before usage, and then 0.1 mL of the suspension is dropped on the bone chip (SIP = 1) and dried for 12 h under a laminar flow bench. After that, the bone chip is shaken in 40 mL of sterile saline solution for 10 min to determine the bioburden (wash 1). Trypticase soy agar is used as bacterial media.

The correction factor and bioburden estimate are calculated as follows:

$$\text{Correction factor} = \frac{\text{Number of inoculated spores}}{\text{Wash 1}}$$

$$\text{Bioburden estimate} = \text{bioburden} \times \text{correction factor}$$

Any treatment used during the bioburden estimation should be reproducible and should avoid conditions that affect the viability of contaminating microbes.

2. Correction factor determination for irradiated tissue
The average number of five replicates of inoculated *Bacillus pumilus* E 601 spores on cancellous bone is 98 (minimum 90 and maximum 112 spores), and the average number of cells/*Bacillus pumilus* E 601 obtained from wash 1 is 40. Therefore, the correction factor of recovery is $98/40 = 2.5$; this number is used to calculate the bioburden estimate for all of the samples observed.
3. Calculation of bioburden estimate
The average bioburden of 10 cancellous bone chip samples with SIP = 1 is 0.77 ± 1.12 CFU/packet, with a minimum of 0 and a maximum of 2 CFU/packet. The bioburden estimate is $0.77 \times 2.5 = 1.95$ CFU or 2 CFU/packet. For demineralized bone powder grafts, the average bioburden with SIP = 1 is 0.76 ± 1.06 CFU/packet with a minimum of 0 and a maximum of 1 CFU/packet. The bioburden estimate is $0.76 \times 2.5 = 1.90$ CFU or 2 CFU/packet.

Verification dose (VD) experiment

All of the tissue samples are irradiated at room temperature in a gamma cell of Co-60 irradiator with a dose rate of about 2 kGy/h for freeze-dried cancellous/bone allografts as well as for freeze-dried and demineralized bone allografts, and at frozen state in dry ice (around −40°C) for frozen samples. The absorbed dose variation between the samples should be less than 10%. Clear Perspex dosimeters are used to measure the absorbed dose (IAEA 2004).

The results of the VD experiment are shown in Table 3. It can be seen in the table that at the same number of bioburden, the VD of method C is higher than those of methods A1 and B; thus, the possibility of success of the VD experiment will be higher for method C too. The calculation of the

Table 3. Results of verification dose (VD) experiment and radiation sterilization dose (RSD): cancellous chips and demineralized bone powders.

Method	Bioburden/ packets at SIP = 1	VD exp. (SAL 10^{-1})	Results	Table 2b*	Accepted RSD (kGy)
A1: ISO 11137 (1995a)	2 CFU	Table 2a*: 1.7 kGy	Success	15.2 kGy	15.2
B: ISO 13409 (1996)	2 CFU	Table 3*: 1.65 kGy	Success	—	25
C: AAMI TIR 27 (2001)	2 CFU	Table 4*: 5.2 kGy	Success	—	25

*These Tables are stated in the IAEA Code of Practice (2004).

VD in AAMI TIR 27 (2001) follows the method VD_{max} by Kowalski and Tallentire (1999).

In this experiment, most of the contaminating microbes were Gram-positive aerobic bacteria. No Gram-positive or Gram-negative spore-forming bacteria, mold, or yeast were found in all of the samples observed from January 2004 to August 2005. The D_{10} value of the contamination in dry state was less than 0.5 kGy.

Extrapolation of the reference microbial resistance distribution to produce an SAL of 10^{-6} at 25 kGy for bioburden levels less than 1000 CFU allows the use of a higher VD than would be predicted by method A1 and method B — hence, a greater probability of a successful VD experiment (VD_{max}). This AAMI method takes into account how the VD for a standard distribution of resistance (SDR) varies with the bioburden level for a given SAL, assuming that an SAL of 10^{-6} is achieved at 25 kGy. Depending on the actual bioburden level (i.e. 1–50 or 51–1000 CFU), a linear extrapolation of the appropriate SDR survival curve is made from either (log N_0 or bioburden, 0 kGy) or (log 10^{-2}–10^{-6}, 25 kGy) for 1–50 CFU and 51–1000 CFU, respectively. The AAMI TIR 27 (2001) may therefore be adopted as a formal replacement of ISO 13409 (1996) (IAEA 2004; Yusof 2005).

The sterility test results of bone allografts at the verification doses stated in Table 3 were 10 negative and 0 positive for bone grafts; thus, this experiment was successful according to ISO 11737-2 (1998). Based on these experiments, the radiation sterilization dose (RSD) at an SAL of 10^{-6} for each method was obtained. The RSD for method A1, 15.2 kGy, was obtained from Table 2b of the Code. The RSD of 25 kGy was substantiated for both method B (ISO 13409, 1996) and method C (AAMI TIR 27, 2001). If the VD experiments of methods A1 and B fail, and the experiment of method C succeeds (because of higher VD at the same bioburden number), then the RSD of 25 kGy can still be used to sterilize products. It can also be seen that a validated RSD lower than 25 kGy can be obtained by using method A1; this is beneficial to sterilize radiosensitive soft tissues such as tendons, facias, vessels, heart valves, and cartilages. The validation experiments of the RSD at an SAL of 10^{-6} are done once every 6 months or whenever needed.

It can be concluded that an RSD lower than 25 kGy for tissue allografts can be validated using method A1 of the Code, i.e. 15.2 kGy for bone allografts. Method B (ISO 13409, 1996) and method C (AAMI TIR 27, 2001) substantiate an RSD of 25 kGy. For products using 25 kGy as the sterilization dose, the probability of success on VD experiments using AAMI TIR 27 is higher than those using ISO 13409.

Documentation

The graft should be properly documented for easy tracing. All work steps are documented in a related worksheet form and signed by the technicians.

Distribution

Before distribution, the grafts are controlled by the quality control manager or chief technician. The distribution of grafts should be well documented and accompanied by a signed dispatched Bone Graft Form.

References

American Association of Tissue Banks (AATB) (2002). Standards for Tissue Banking, McLean, VA.

Association for the Advancement of Medical Instrumentation (AAMI) (2001). Sterilization of Health Care Products — Radiation Sterilization — Substantiation of 25 kGy as a Sterilization Dose — method VD_{max}, AAMI TIR 27, McLean, VA.

Basril A, Febrida A, and Nani S (2006). Validation of Ca Content and Residual Moisture Content of Radiation Sterilization of Demineralized Bone Powder Allografts, BATAN Research Tissue Bank, BATAN, Jakarta (to be published).

Basril A, Febrida A, Surtipanti S, Petrus Z, and Hilmy S (2000). The effects of gamma irradiation and demineralization process on mechanical properties of lyophilized bovine bone. *Proc 8th APASTB International Conference on Tissue Banking,* Bali, Indonesia, p. 44.

European Association of Tissue Banks (EATB) (1997). General Standards for Tissue Banking, OBIG Transplant, Vienna.

Hilmy N, Febrida A, and Basril A (2000). Validation of radiation sterilization dose for lyophilized amnion and bone grafts. *Cell Tissue Bank* **1**(2):143–147.

Hilmy N, Febrida A, and Basril A (2003). Indonesia: statistical sampling technique in validation of radiation sterilization dose of biological tissue. *Cell Tissue Bank* **4**(2):185–191.

Hilmy N, Febrida A, and Basril A (2006). Experiences in using the IAEA Code of Practice for the Radiation Sterilization of Tissue Allografts: validation and routine control. In: *Proc 14th International Meeting of Radiation Processing (IMRP) 2006*, Kuala Lumpur, Malaysia.

International Atomic Energy Agency (IAEA) (2002). International Standards for Tissue Banks, IAEA, Vienna.

International Atomic Energy Agency (IAEA) (2004). Code of Practice for the Radiation Sterilization of Tissue Allografts, IAEA, Vienna.

International Atomic Energy Agency and National University of Singapore (IAEA/NUS) (1997). Module 4: Procurement. Multimedia Distance Learning Package on Tissue Banking, Interregional Training Centre, Singapore.

International Standards Organization (ISO) (1995a). Sterilization of Health Care Products — Requirements for Validation and Routine Control — Radiation Sterilization, ISO 11137, 1995, Geneva.

International Standards Organization (ISO) (1995b). Sterilization of Medical Devices — Microbiological Methods, ISO 11737-1, 1995, Geneva.

International Standards Organization (ISO) (1996). Sterilization of Health Care Products — Radiation Sterilization — Substantiation of 25 kGy as a Sterilization Dose for Small or Infrequent Production Batches, ISO 13409, 1996, Geneva.

International Standards Organization (ISO) (1998). Sterilization of Medical Devices — Microbiological Methods — Part 2: Tests of Sterility Performed in the Validation of a Sterilization Process, ISO 11737-2, 1998, Geneva.

Kowalski JB and Tallentire A (1999). Substantiation of 25 kGy as a sterilization dose: a rational approach to establishing verification dose. *Radiat Phys Chem* **54**:55–64.

Pharmaceutical Inspection Convention and Pharmaceutical Inspection Cooperation Scheme (PIC/S) (2000). Guide to Good Manufacturing Practice (GMP) for Medicinal Products, PIC/S, Geneva.

Yusof N (2005). Is the irradiation dose of 25 kGy enough to sterilize tissue grafts? In: Nather A (ed.), *Bone Grafts and Bone Substitutes*, World Scientific, Singapore, pp. 189–212.

Chapter 17

Validation for Processing and Irradiation of Amnion Grafts

Nazly Hilmy, Basril Abbas and Febrida Anas

BATAN Research Tissue Bank (BRTB)
Center for Research and Development of Isotopes and Radiation Technology, BATAN
Jakarta 12070, Indonesia

Introduction

Tissue banking has many similarities with the pharmaceutical and medical device manufacturing industry, in particular with respect to the safety aspects. Tissues from which virulent microorganisms have been isolated are not acceptable for transplantation, unless the procedure has been validated to effectively inactivate the microorganisms without causing potentially harmful effects (AATB 2002; EATB/EAMST 1997; IAEA 2002).

The validation process is the establishment of documented evidence, which provides a high degree of assurance that a specific process will consistently produce a product meeting its predetermined specifications and quality attributes. Each process step in tissue banking should have validated standard operating procedures (SOPs), such as for the retrieval of raw materials; for methods of screening, washing, freezing, and lyophilizing; and for the radiation sterilization dose to be used. Predetermined specifications and quality attributes of biological tissues (such as amnion membranes) both before and after processing should be set up before preparing the SOPs. In general, there are three types of validations in tissue banking: validation of personnel, validation of the presterilization process, and validation of the sterilization process (IAEA 2002).

The radiation process can be used to sterilize amnion grafts in their final package. Validation of the radiation sterilization dose (RSD) can be done according to the IAEA Code of Practice (2004), and consists of three methods: method A1 or A2 (IAEA 2004), method B (ISO 13409, 1996), and method C (AAMI TIR 27, 2001). These standards are for small or infrequent production batches, namely products with an average bioburden less than 1000 colony-forming units (CFU) and manufactured in small quantities (i.e. less than 1000 product units per batch). These categories are relevant to tissue bank products. Viral contamination is excluded from all of these standards. To overcome viral contamination problems, tissues should be well screened (IAEA/NUS 1997; IAEA 2002; Hilmy *et al.* 2000).

The objective of this chapter is to describe the process validation of washing and lyophilizing amnion membranes (i.e. part of the validation of the presterilization process), as well as the amount of the radiation sterilization dose to be used as amnion grafts for clinical use at the BATAN Research Tissue Bank (BRTB).

Preparation of Amnion Membranes for Validation Process

Retrieval

Amnion membranes are retrieved aseptically in hospitals from healthy donors who are free of HIV and hepatitis B/C. They can also be obtained from vaginal delivery or caesarean section. There is no difference in the mechanical properties of both membranes; however, vaginally delivered amnion membranes have a higher microbial content compared to amnions obtained from caesarean section (Hilmy *et al.* 1987). Serological donor screening tests that consist of obligatory blood tests (e.g. HIV 1-2, VDRL, hepatitis B/C) and optional tests (e.g. CMC antibodies) are done at the hospitals, while the microbiology swab tests and bioburden determination are done at the BRTB.

The placenta is collected aseptically from the labor room or operation theatre in sterile basins, and the amnion–chorion membranes are separated from the placenta mass (Fig. 1). The membrane, which is made up of the chorion layer (the dull aspect of the amniotic membrane) and

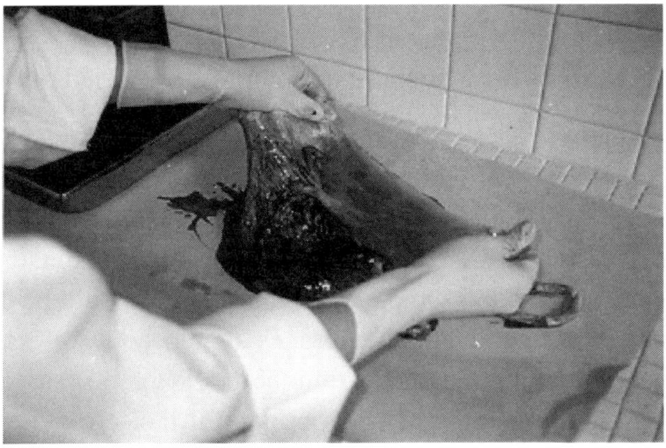

Fig. 1. Retrieval of amnion membrane from fresh placentae.

the amnion layer (the glistening layer of the amniotic membrane), is then cleaned with normal saline to remove blood and other blood products. The amnion is separated by peeling off from the chorion layer. The amnion is submerged in sterile normal saline either for storage at 4°C or for transportation. The amnion is retrieved as soon as possible, not less than 6 h after labor, to prevent microbial contamination and problems in separating the amnion from the chorion (IAEA/NUS 1997; Jerzy *et al.* 1999; IAEA 2002).

Before processing, tissues are stored in a sterile pouch/bag containing sterile saline solution at a low temperature (i.e. 4°C) to prevent microbe proliferation and proteolysis enzyme action. The pouch and the container should be labeled. Each step of work should be documented and carried out according to the SOPs (IAEA 2002).

Donor documentation should be recorded in terms of the following details:

- Name of donor and sex of child
- Name of hospital
- Time and date of delivery
- Time of amnion collection
- Type of delivery and related problems
- Screening of donor (free from HIV, hepatitis B/C)

- Donor consent

Quality control of fresh amniotic membranes is carried out as follows:

- Donor screening. Serological test results should be negative and swab test results should be free of contaminated pathogenic bacteria such as *Streptococcus* sp., *Pseudomonas* sp., *Staphylococcus* sp., coliform bacteria, and *E. coli*, which are isolated by using selective media. If pathogenic bacteria are found in the sample, then the sample should be discarded.
- Appearance of amnion. The membranes should be colorless, clear, and transparent. Meconium-stained amnion should be discarded. The processing of amnion membranes is continued if the serological and swab test results are negative.

Discarded amnion should be documented and can be used for research.

Processing

The processing steps of amnion membranes are conducted as follows:

1. Washing is done nine times, using nine bottles each containing 400 mL of sterile water, except for bottle 5 which contains 0.05% sodium hypochlorite (NaOCl) solution in sterile water (Fig. 2). The amnion is first washed and shaken well four times in 400 mL of sterile water (bottles 1–4), and then immersed in 0.05% sodium hypochlorite solution (bottle 5) for 10 min before being washed four more times in bottles

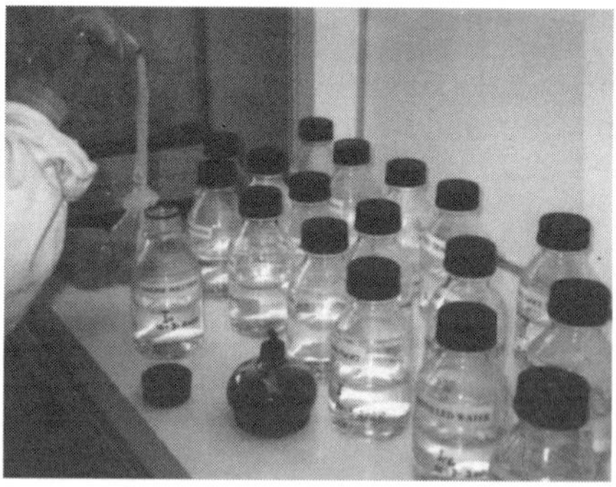

Fig. 2. Washing process of amnion membrane.

6–9. Each bottle is shaken for 10 min. The used washing water in bottle 9 is subject to control for validation (IAEA/NUS 1997; Hilmy *et al.* 2000; Hilmy *et al.* 2003).

2. The amnion is stretched and mounted on a sterile cotton gauze or polyester net with the chorion side of the amnion placed directly on the cotton gauze, and is then frozen (−70°C for 24 h for lyophilized amnion grafts, or until sterilization for frozen amnion grafts).
3. The amnion is freeze-dried/lyophilized for 5 h (validation is done by calculating the water content, i.e. less than 5%).
4. The amnion is cut into 4 cm × 4 cm (or another size) and then triple-packed in a polyethylene pouch. About 20–30 packets can be produced from one piece of amnion membrane.
5. Bioburden enumeration is done on the amnion (validation is done according to ISO 11737-1, 1995b).
6. The amnion is packaged.
7. The amnion is labeled.
8. The amnion is radiation sterilized at a dose of 25 kGy (validation is done according to the IAEA Code of Practice 2004).
9. The amnion is stored at 5°C or at room temperature.
10. The amnion is distributed.
11. The amnion is documented.

Validation of Washing Process of Amnion Membranes (Hilmy *et al.* 2002)

The aim of process validation is to validate the nine-time washing process of amnion membranes according to the IAEA/NUS module 4 (1997) by controlling the used washing water in bottle 9 with respect to the following:

- NaOCl residue
- Microbe contamination
- Red blood cell/blood particle residue
- Neutral pH

The used washing water should be free of all of these contaminations and residues.

Process validations

The 400 mL of water in bottles 7, 8, and 9 is divided as follows:

- 200 mL for microbiology examination
- 60 mL for red cell examination (microscopy examination)
- 100 mL for sodium hypochlorite residue

Microbiology examination

The technique for removing microbes from amnion membranes (i.e. bioburden enumeration) is done according to ISO 11737-1 (1995b), i.e. by using the membrane filtration method. Approximately 200 mL of washing water is filtered, and then the filter paper is incubated at 30°C in trypticase soy agar (Difco) for 2 weeks.

Red cell examination

About 60 mL of the washing water is centrifuged, and the sediments are observed for red cell residue via a microscopic examination.

Results of validation experiments (Hilmy et al. 2002)

The validation results of the washing process are shown in Table 1.

The validation process shows that the results of bottle 9 are accepted and that the predetermined specifications are fulfilled. Therefore, the nine-time washing process of amnion is accepted.

Table 1. Results of validation experiments.

Tests	No. of bottles		
	7	8	9
Residue of microbes	+	–	–
Residue of red cells	+	+	–
Residue of NaOCl	+	–	–

Validation of Lyophilizing Process of Amnion Membranes

All of the equipment used is calibrated for a period stated in the SOPs. After freezing for 24 h and then lyophilizing for 5 h, the water content of the amnion should be less than 5% (IAEA/NUS 1997; and stated in SOPs). Validation is carried out by using five amnion graft packets produced from one amnion membrane. The water content examination is done according to the methods stated in the Indonesian Pharmacopeia (1995), that is, by heating the samples up to a constant weight at 70°C.

At the BRTB, the water content results ranged between 3% and 5%. Given that these results are less than 5% (as stated in the SOPs), they are thus accepted.

Validation of Radiation Sterilization Dose of Amnion Membranes (IAEA 2004; Hilmy *et al.* 2000; Hilmy *et al.* 2002; Hilmy *et al.* 2004)

Sampling method

The radiation process can be used to sterilize amnion grafts in their final package. Validation of the radiation sterilization dose can be done according to the IAEA Code of Practice (2004), ISO 13409 (1996), and AAMI TIR 27 (2001).

According to the IAEA Code of Practice (2004), the minimum number of uniform samples for statistical sampling needed for the verification dose experiment at the selected sterility assurance level (SAL) per production batch size is 20: 10 for the bioburden determination/enumeration (ISO 11737-1, 1995b), and the remaining 10 for the verification dose (VD) experiment (IAEA 2004; ISO 11737-2, 1998). The bioburden number is used to determine the VD at an SAL of 10^{-1}. There are three methods that can be used: method A1 (IAEA 2004), method B (ISO 13409, 1996), and method C (AAMI TIR 27, 2001). If the verification dose experiment passes, then the radiation sterilization dose (RSD) at an SAL of 10^{-6} is either 25 kGy (methods B and C) or lower (method A1).

Each amnion membrane obtained from one donor can produce 20–30 packets of amnion grafts with a size of 4 cm × 4 cm. The grafts are used for ocular, dental, and other surgeries. A total of 20 packets with a sample item portion (SIP) of one that were processed according to a single processing protocol during the same processing cycle are used for this experiment: 10 packets for bioburden determination, and the other 10 for the verification dose (VD). The verification dose is determined based on the bioburden number (Table 2a of the Code).

There are two kinds of batches at tissue banks:

- Production batch — a specific quantity of cells and/or tissues that are intended to have a uniform character and quality as well as specific limits, and are produced according to a single processing protocol during the same processing cycle (i.e. precluding mixing from two or more donors)
- Irradiation batch — quantity of final products irradiated at the same cycle in a qualified facility (AATB 2002; IAEA 2002)

Validation steps

1. Determine the bioburden from 10 samples (ISO 11737-1, 1995b).
2. Determine the verification dose (VD) at an SAL of 10^{-1}. This is either based on the bioburden number (Table 2a of the Code for method A1) or calculated using a formula (for methods B and C). Ten samples are irradiated at the VD in gamma cells, followed by a sterility test according to ISO 11737-2 (1998). The results are accepted only if there is one maximum positive (Hilmy *et al.* 2004).
3. If the experiment succeeds, then the RSD to achieve an SAL of 10^{-6} is determined according to Table 2b of the Code for method A1 or is 25 kGy for methods B and C.

Method for bioburden determination

Bioburden estimation is determined according to ISO 11737-1 (1995b), using bacterial media of trypticase soy agar (Difco); while the sterility test is done according to ISO 11737-2 (1998), using trypticase soy broth (Difco). The incubation temperature and time are 30°C and 14 days, respectively. The methods stated in ISO 11737-1 (1995b) should be used to determine the bioburden for RSD validation if the IAEA Code of Practice (2004) and ISO 13409 (1996) are applied. One of these methods is to remove microbes from tissues via the shaking method for 10 min and to transfer them to a culture medium by using the membrane filtration method. Gram staining and

D_{10} value determination are then done to all of the contaminated microbe colonies. Viral contaminations are not included in the bioburden enumeration according to ISO 11737-1 (1995b). To overcome viral contamination problems, tissues should be well screened.

Morphology of microbe contamination

The morphology of the amnion membrane contaminations should be observed. At the BRTB, the morphology was found to be Gram-positive coccoid forms (98%) and Gram-positive vegetative rods (2%), with D_{10} values of 0.25–0.50 kGy. No pathogenic spore-forming Gram-negative bacteria, mold, or yeast were found in these contaminants. Based on this microbiological evaluation, all of the samples investigated met the requirement of the BRTB, and so all of the samples can be processed for allografts (Hilmy *et al.* 2000).

Validation results

As shown in Table 2, the average bioburden per sample (SIP = 1) of lyophilized amnion membranes is 55 CFU (min. 35 and max. 72 CFU), which is less than 1000 CFU; thus, method A1 of the Code (IAEA 2004) can be used to validate the RSD at an SAL of 10^{-6}. Referring to Table 2a of the Code, the VD is 4.6 kGy; if calculated using formula in methods B (ISO 13409, 1996) and C (AAMI TIR 27, 2001), the VD is 4.7 and 8.2 kGy, respectively. The Table also shows that the RSD according to method A1 is 21 kGy, which is less than the RSD of 25 kGy for the other two methods. Validation experiments of the radiation sterilization dose at an SAL of 10^{-6} are done once every 6 months or whenever needed.

According to several authors, an irradiation dose of 40 kGy can be used to eliminate HIV from fresh-frozen patella ligaments and freeze-dried bone grafts; however, such high doses (i.e. those above the currently used

Table 2. Results of validation of RSD experiment.

Method	Bioburden exp.	VD	Results	Table 2b	RSD (kGy)
A1 (IAEA 2004)	55 CFU	4.6 kGy	Success	20.2	20.2/21
B (ISO 13409, 1996)	55 CFU	4.7 kGy	Success	—	25
C (AAMI TIR 27, 2001)	55 CFU	8.2 kGy	Success	—	25

sterilization dose of 25 kGy) may evoke the degradation of important proteins and mechanical properties of the grafts, although some changes are desirable (e.g. decrease in immunogenicity of the grafts) (Hilmy *et al.* 1987; Dziedzic-Goclawska *et al.* 1991; Anderson *et al.* 1992; Fideler *et al.* 1994; Hilmy *et al.* 1994). No data has been obtained on the sensitivity of the hepatitis B virus (HBV) to radiation, but this virus is known to be resistant to heat sterilization. It has a small genome (only 3.2-kb pairs) and a double-stranded DNA; therefore, it is assumed to be resistant to radiation. Many D_{10} values of viruses exceed 5 kGy; in fact, some viruses (e.g. foot and mouth disease virus) have a D_{10} value of 13 kGy when irradiated at frozen state (Chisari and Ferrari 1997). A radiation dose of 25 kGy at an SAL of 10^{-6} can reduce the viral contamination of certain viruses, but cannot sterilize them.

Packaging of Amnion Membranes

After freeze-drying, each amnion is cut into appropriate shapes, packed into polyethylene pouches (or into other materials as stated in ISO 11137, 1995a), and sealed with a heat sealer under a laminar airflow cabinet. The packaging is done in triple layers, and then sterilized at a dose of 25 kGy.

Labeling of Amnion Membranes

The label of the products should display the following:

- Date, name and address of the tissue bank
- Graft name and code number
- Size/volume of product
- Irradiation indicator (go/no-go)
- Expiration date
- Accompanying note that states "do not use if package is damaged"

Documentation of Amnion Membranes

The graft should be documented properly for easy tracing. All steps of work are documented in a related worksheet form and signed by the technicians.

Distribution of Amnion Membranes

Before distribution, grafts are controlled by the chief technician. The distribution of grafts should be well documented and accompanied by a signed dispatched Amnion Graft Form.

Conclusions

- The nine-step washing method of amnion membranes for amnion grafts fulfills the predetermined specifications, and is thus accepted.
- ISO 11737-1 (1995b) can be used as a standard for bioburden determination.
- The IAEA Code of Practice (2004), ISO 13409 (1996), and AAMI TIR 27 (2001) can be used to validate the RSD of amnion grafts.

References

American Association of Tissue Banks (AATB) (2002). Standards for Tissue Banking, McLean, VA.

Anderson MJ, Keyak JH, and Skinner HB (1992). Compressive mechanical properties of human cancellous bone after gamma irradiation. *J Bone Joint Surg Am* **74**:747–752.

Association for the Advancement of Medical Instrumentation (AAMI) (2001). Sterilization of Health Care Products — Radiation Sterilization — Substantiation of 25 kGy as a Sterilization Dose — Method VD_{max}, AAMI TIR 27, 2001, Arlington, VA.

Chisari FV and Ferrari C (1997). Viral hepatitis. In: Nathanson N, Ahmed R, Scarano FG, Griffin DE, Holmes KV, Murphy FA, and Robinson HL (eds.), *Viral Pathogenesis*, Lippincott-Raven, Philadelphia, PA, pp.745–747.

Dziedzic-Goclawska A, Ostowski K, Stachowick W, Michalik J, and Grzesik W (1991). Effect of radiation sterilization on osteoinductive properties and the rate of remodeling of bone implants preserved by lyophilization and deep freezing. *Clin Orthop Relat Res*: 30–37.

European Association of Tissue Banks and European Association of Musculoskeletal Transplantation (EATB/EAMST) (1997). Common Standards for Musculoskeletal Tissue Banking, OBIG Transplant, Vienna.

Fideler BM, Vangsness CT, Moore T, Li Z, and Rasheed S (1994). Effects of gamma irradiation on the human immunodeficiency virus. *J Bone Joint Surg Am* **76**:1032–1035.

Hilmy N, Basril A, and Febrida A (1994). The effects of procurement, packaging materials, storage and irradiation dose on physical properties of lyophilized amnion membranes. In: *Proc IAEA Meeting of Radiation Sterilization of Tissue Grafts*, Manila, Philippines.

Hilmy N, Basril A, and Febrida A (2002). Validation of washing process of amnion membrane for amnion grafts. In: *9th APASTB Conference*, Seoul, Korea.

Hilmy N, Febrida A, and Basril A (2000). Validation of radiation sterilization dose for lyophilized amnion and bone grafts. *Cell Tissue Bank* **1**(2):143–148.

Hilmy N, Febrida A, and Basril A (2003). Indonesia: statistical sampling technique in validation of radiation sterilization dose of biological tissue. *Cell Tissue Bank* **4**(2):185–191.

Hilmy N, Febrida A, and Basril A (2004). Experiences in using IAEA Code of Practice for validation of radiation sterilization dose for tissue allografts. In: *10th APASTB Conference*, Hong Kong.

Hilmy N, Siddik S, Gentur S, and Gulardi W (1987). Physical and chemical properties of freeze dried amnion membranes sterilized by irradiation. *J Atom Indones* **13**(2):1–14.

Indonesian Pharmacopeia (1995). Ministry of Health, Jakarta, Indonesia.

International Atomic Energy Agency (IAEA) (2002). International Standards for Tissue Banks, IAEA, Vienna.

International Atomic Energy Agency (IAEA) (2004). Code of Practice for the Radiation Sterilization of Tissue Allografts, IAEA, Vienna.

International Atomic Energy Agency and National University of Singapore (IAEA/NUS) (1997). Module 4: Procurement. Multimedia Distance Learning Package on Tissue Banking, Interregional Training Centre, Singapore.

International Standards Organization (ISO) (1995a). Sterilization of Health Care Products — Requirements for Validation and Routine Control — Radiation Sterilization, ISO 11137, 1995, Geneva.

International Standards Organization (ISO) (1995b). Sterilization of Medical Devices — Microbiological Methods, ISO 11737-1, 1995, Geneva.

International Standards Organization (ISO) (1996). Sterilization of Health Care Products — Radiation Sterilization — Substantiation of 25 kGy as a Sterilization Dose for Small or Infrequent Production Batches, ISO 13409, 1996, Geneva.

International Standards Organization (ISO) (1998). Sterilization of Medical Devices — Microbiological Methods — Part 2: Tests of Sterility Performed in the Validation of a Sterilization Process, ISO 11737-2, 1998, Geneva.

Jerzy T, Isabela A, Kaminski A, and Dziedzic-Goclawska A (1999). Amnion allografts prepared in Central Tissue Bank in Warsaw. *Ann Transplant* **4**(3–4):85–90.

Chapter 18

Validating Pasteurization Cycle Time for Femoral Head

Norimah Yusof and Selamat S. Nadir

Malaysian Nuclear Agency (NM)
Bangi, 43000 Kajang, Selangor
Malaysia

Introduction

The risk of transmitting diseases through organ and tissue transplantation remains the major limitation for the availability of suitable donors. The problem was highlighted in the 1980s with the emergence of the acquired immune deficiency syndrome (AIDS), which is caused by the human immunodeficiency virus (HIV). Screening tests for the detection of antibodies to HIV are commercially available; however, the incubation period (window period) of HIV — during which the antibody markers of infection are undetectable — is long and varies (Kitchen *et al.* 1989).

Early HIV infection, i.e. before HIV antibody production, may be the most infectious period (Asselmeier *et al.* 1993). On this basis, screening of donor blood alone cannot completely prevent the transmission of the virus. Several methods are recommended for the inactivation of infectious agents in tissues during processing and preservation. Treatment with chemicals such as alcohols and sodium hypochlorite (Spire *et al.* 1984) or physical methods such as heat can be used primarily as disinfection procedures (Spire *et al.* 1985; Tjotta *et al.* 1991). The half-life of the virus has been shown to be approximately 9 days at 4°C and 24 h at 37°C (Tjotta *et al.* 1991). Gamma irradiation, which has been studied extensively as a terminal process for sterilization, can also be considered for the inactivation of viruses (Yusof 2000; Kitchen *et al.* 1989).

The use of dry heat has been widely adopted for the inactivation of HIV in lyophilized blood products (Rousell 1986), while Vajaradul (1998) has been using dry heat for viral inactivation in massive bone allografts prior to deep-freezing. Spire *et al.* (1985) reported that a 30-min heating time of HIV-1 at 56°C is sufficient to kill the virus. The advantage of pasteurization in routine bone processing procedures is twofold: to inactivate viruses in bone allografts, and to safeguard the tissue bank operators handling the tissues. Our previous work showed that pasteurization treatment at the beginning of processing could inactivate almost all microorganisms (Yusof *et al.* 1994). Therefore, wet pasteurization at 56°C–57°C is carried out during the processing of bone allografts prior to freeze-drying.

Even though the pasteurization of bone at 56°C is only for 30 min, the actual time taken for the whole process of pasteurizing bones is definitely longer, taking into account the time taken for the center part of the bone to reach the critical temperature and maintain it for 30 min. Various factors, including the size, shape, and state of the bone (either still frozen or already thawed when first immersed in water), will influence the duration of the whole process. Under the tissue banking quality system, the process must be validated to ensure that the pasteurization is complete.

This chapter describes how the authors conducted a validation trial through a series of experiments on femoral heads with the main objective being to determine the actual heating time before the innermost part of the femoral head reaches 56°C, after which time the actual pasteurization period of 30 min commences. We varied the initial temperature of water bath and sterile water in which the bone was placed. In addition, the study looked into how the heating time varies with the initial temperature of bone (i.e. frozen or thawed bone).

Pasteurization

Bone allografts obtained mainly from orthopedic surgeries were sent to the authors' tissue bank for processing only after a seronegative result occurred. They were mainly femoral heads or knee slices. For validation work, femoral heads were selected because of their size and density so that it was more

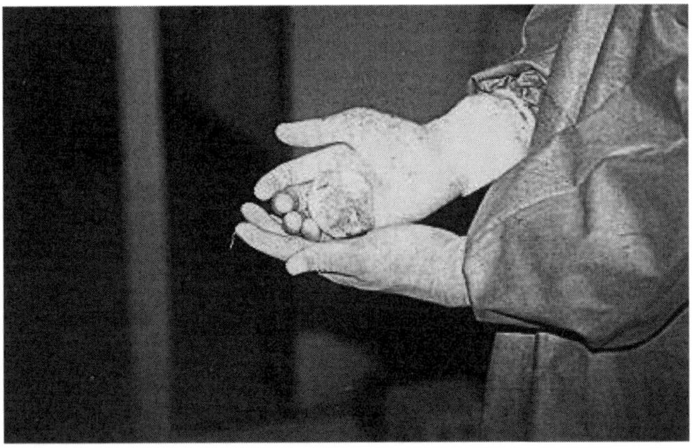

Fig. 1. Femoral head.

difficult for heat to penetrate. The femoral heads were either in frozen state (directly removed from the quarantine freezer) or thawed at room temperature (Fig. 1).

For pasteurization, each bone was immersed in sterile water in a screwed-cap bottle, which was then placed in a water bath. Initial temperatures of water bath and sterile water were varied. Increasing temperatures were monitored over time. A thermocouple thermometer (Kane-May, model KM 2013) calibrated against a mercury thermometer was inserted right in the center of the femoral head. Any gap on the bone surface was covered using plasticine. The temperature of water bath was controlled to ensure that the bone temperature was maintained at 56° C to 57°C and never exceeded 60° C, as bone proteins might be denatured at temperatures higher than 60°C. The experimental setup is illustrated in Fig. 2.

Using Preheated Water Bath at 60°C

The water in the water bath was preheated at 60° C. Bones (frozen or thawed) were immersed in bottles containing sterile water either at room temperature or at more than 50°C (by keeping the bottles in water bath before the experiment). Monitored temperatures were plotted against time, and some complete results are presented in Fig. 3. The time taken for the center point of each bone to reach 56°C was estimated from the graphs and is summarized in Table 1.

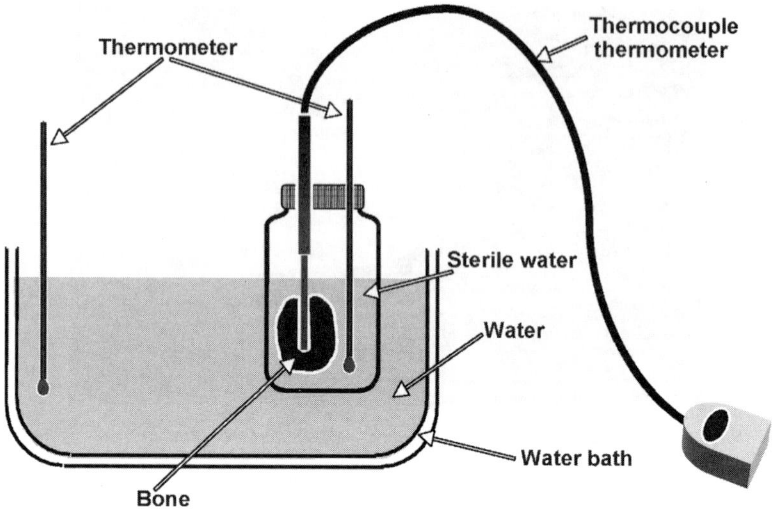

Fig. 2. Experimental setup for the validation trial of the pasteurization cycle time of femoral head.

In preheated water bath, thawed bones [Fig. 3(a)] and frozen bones [Fig. 3(b)] required almost similar heating times of about 16–22.5 min; thus, the total pasteurization cycle time would be 46–52.5 min (by adding 30 min of heating at 56°C to inactivate the virus). The heating duration was reduced to 15 min when the sterile water in the bottles was prewarmed at over 50°C in water bath before placing the bones [Fig. 3(c)]. In cases where the bones themselves were prewarmed at about 37°C before immersion, the heating time was further reduced to 9 min [Fig. 3(d)].

Using Nonpreheated Water Bath

In this case, the water in the water bath was just starting to heat up to 60°C when the bottles containing the bones were placed in sterile water. The results are presented in Fig. 4, and the heating times to reach 56°C obtained from the graphs are summarized in Table 2. The time taken for thawed femoral heads [Fig. 4(a)] to reach 56°C was approximately 23–25 min, which was slightly higher than that of those using a preheated water bath. However, for frozen bones [Fig. 4(b)], the heating time was comparably longer, i.e. more than 40 min; thus, the total pasteurization cycle time was 1.2 h.

(a) Thawed bone in sterile water at room temperature.

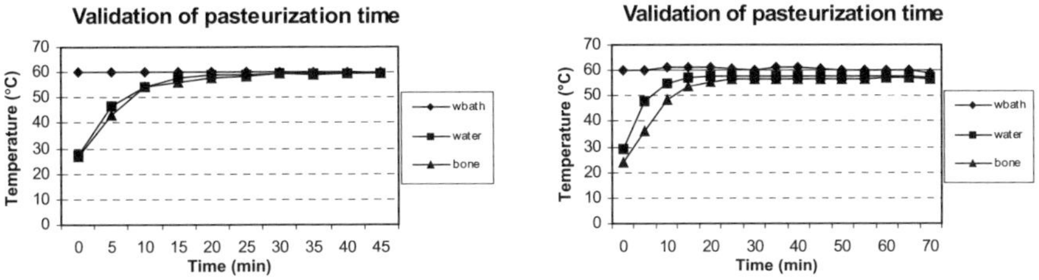

(b) Frozen bone in sterile water at room temperature.

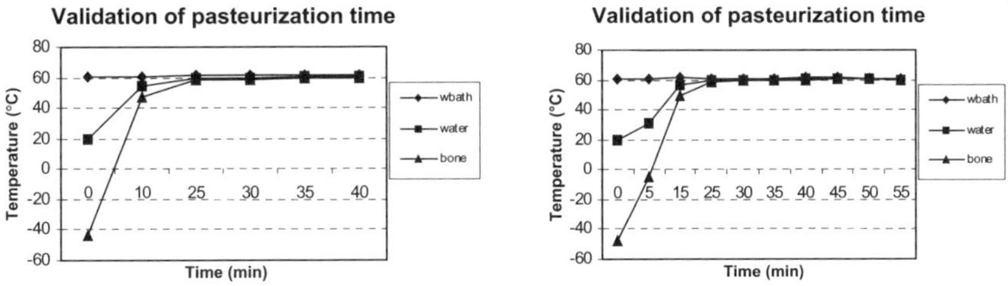

(c) Thawed bone in sterile water prewarmed at >50°C.

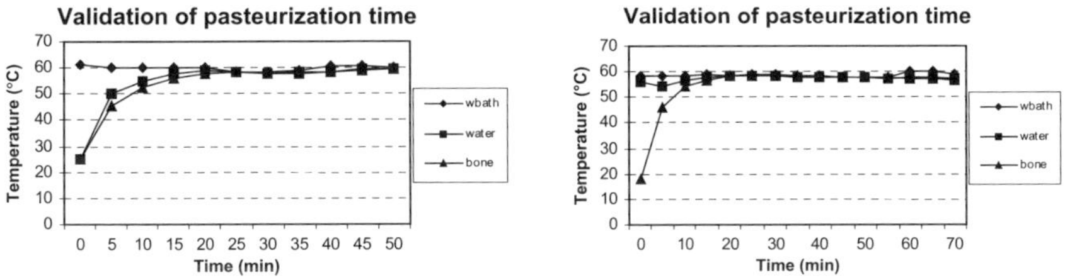

(d) Sterile water prewarmed at >50°C, and bone prewarmed at >37°C.

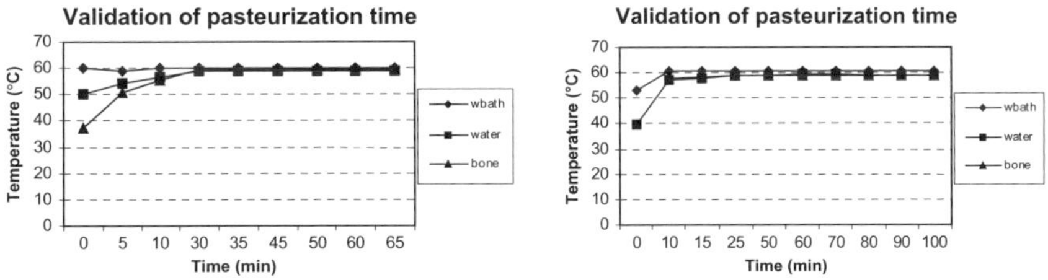

Fig. 3. Monitored temperatures of bone and sterile water in preheated water bath at 60°C.

Table 1. Determination of heating time and pasteurization cycle in preheated water bath at 60°C.

Initial temp. of water bath (°C)	Initial temp. of sterile water in bottle (°C)	Initial temp. of femoral head (°C)	Heating time for whole bone (min)	Pasteurization cycle (min)
60	29.0 (RT)	24.1 (thawed)	22.5	52.5
60	27.5 (RT)	27.8 (thawed)	16.0	46.0
61	50 (heated)	25.0 (thawed)	15.0	45.0
58	56 (heated)	17.4 (thawed)	15.5	45.5
60.1	50.2 (heated)	37.6 (prewarmed)	13.0	43.0
53	57.5 (heated)	39.4 (prewarmed)	9.0	39.0
60	27 (RT)	−40.0 (frozen)	18.0	48.0
61	28 (RT)	−47.8 (frozen)	22.5	52.5

RT: room temperature.

(a) Thawed bone in sterile water at room temperature.

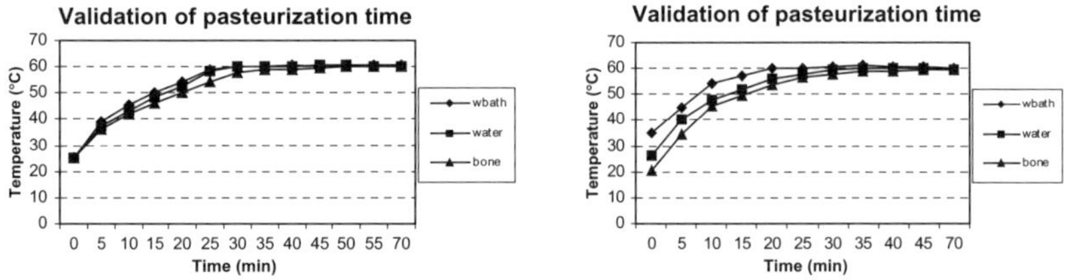

(b) Frozen bone in sterile water at room temperature.

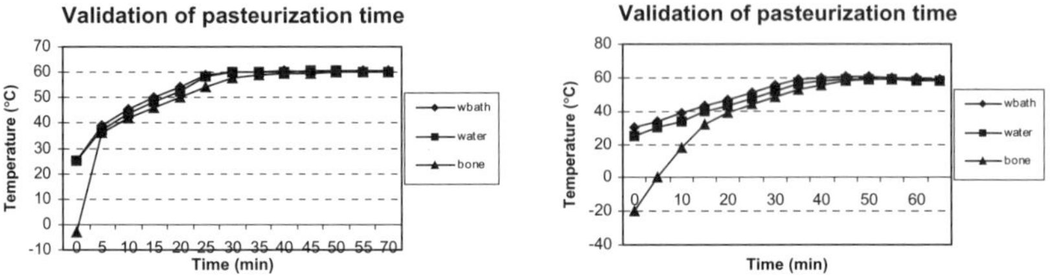

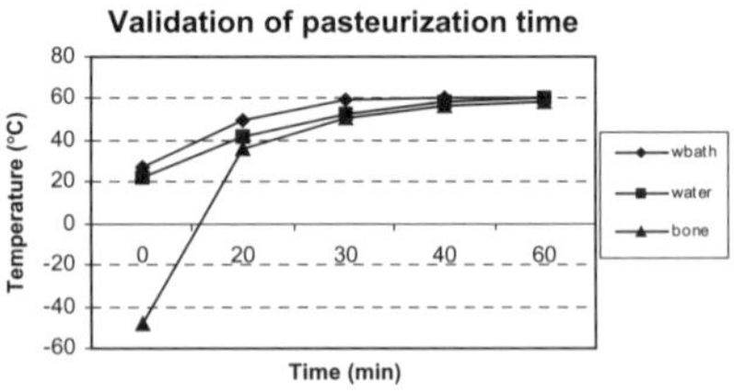

Fig. 4. Monitored temperatures of bone and sterile water in nonpreheated water bath.

Table 2. Determination of heating time and pasteurization cycle in nonpreheated water bath.

Initial temp. of water bath (°C)	Initial temp. of sterile water in bottle (°C)	Initial temp. of femoral head (°C)	Heating time for whole bone (min)	Pasteurization cycle (min)
25	25.0 (RT)	25.0 (thawed)	23.0	53.0
35	26.0 (RT)	20.4 (thawed)	25.0	55.0
27	25.0 (RT)	−48.6 (frozen)	40.0	70.0
30	25.0 (RT)	−20.1 (frozen)	41.0	71.0
28	27.0 (RT)	−15.6 (frozen)	44.5	74.5

RT: room temperature.

Validated Pasteurization Process

Based on this validation trial, the authors recommend that the water bath be preheated up to 60°C and bottles with sterile water be placed in the water bath (Fig. 5). The temperature of the sterile water must reach 58°C–59°C before placing the bone. Frozen bones are preferably thawed at room temperature so that they can be pasteurized for a minimum total time of 45 min. This includes 15 min for the heating time, allowing the center part of the bone to reach the required temperature; and a further 30 min for maintaining heating at 56°C to inactivate the HIV, as recommended in the

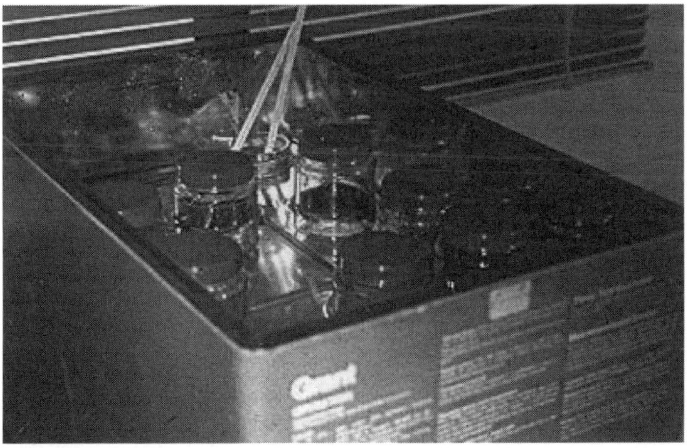

Fig. 5. Bottles with sterile water in water bath.

literature. This validated pasteurization process is included in the authors' work instructions for bone processing.

The authors later found that at least five washing steps are required after pasteurization for a complete clean-up. Washing is done using preheated water, and the bones are shaken for 30–45 min in each washing step (Fig. 6). In fact, warm water can help remove fat to a certain extent. In isolated cases where big bones have to be pasteurized, a minimum pasteurization period of 3 h — as recommended by the Clwyd and Oswestry Research Tissue Bank (1991) — is employed.

As described in chapter 15, the pasteurization process has been found to be an effective method for killing microbes. Microbiological analysis carried out on washing solutions and bones taken from different stages of bone processing showed that the pasteurization process inactivated almost all of the microbes, as no colony count was detected in the washing solutions immediately after pasteurization (Yusof *et al.* 1994). The bioburden for the processed bones was also very low.

A sufficient time of 15 min to heat up a whole femoral head has been properly validated at the authors' tissue bank; and by adding the actual pasteurization at 56°C–57°C for 30 min, a total pasteurization cycle time of 45 min for femoral heads has been verified. However, a report by Tjotta *et al.* (1991) requires reconsideration in validating the pasteurization treatment and safe handling of tissues. They heated HIV-1 samples for 30 min

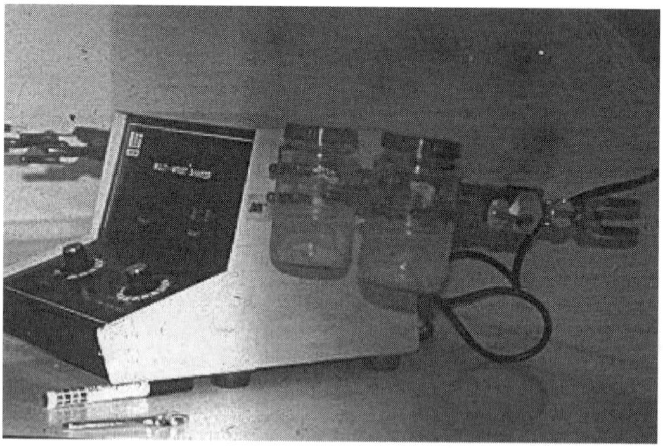

Fig. 6. Bones are shaken in preheated sterile water.

at temperatures ranging from 37°C to 64°C; despite drastic inactivation between 48°C and 56°C, a significant number of HIV particles still survived at higher temperatures. Prince (1986) reported that the pasteurization of serum at 60°C may require 10 h to sufficiently kill the virus. The use of gamma irradiation for the terminal sterilization of bone allografts provides an additional means of assuring the safety of tissues.

Conclusion

Pasteurization at 56°C for 30 min during the early stage of bone processing not only inactivates HIV and safeguards bank operators from any risk of transmissible diseases during the handling of tissues, but also effectively kills almost all of the microbes. Using a preheated water bath at 60°C, the shortest heating time of 15 min was validated for thawed bones immersed in sterile water preheated at over 50°C before pasteurization. It is recommended that the total duration of the pasteurization process for thawed femoral heads is 45 min; however, for large-sized bones, a pasteurization cycle of 3 h is required. The examples given here may be a useful guide for any tissue bank to validate its pasteurization cycle time.

References

Asselmeier MA, Caspari RB, and Bottenfields S (1993). A review of allograft processing and sterilization techniques and their role in transmission of the human immunodeficiency virus. *Am J Sports Med* **21**(2):170–175.

Clwyd and Oswestry Research Tissue Bank (1991). A Protocol for the Production of Bone Allografts.

Kitchen AD, Mann GF, Harrison AJ, and Zuckerman AJ (1989). Effect of gamma irradiation on the human immunodeficiency virus and human coagulation proteins. *Vox Sang* **56**:223–229.

Prince AM (1986). Effect of heat treatment of lyophilised blood derivatives on infectivity of human immunodeficiency. *Lancet* **1**:1280–1281.

Rousell RH (1986). Heat treatment of FVIII concentrate. *Lancet* **1**:1389.

Spire B, Barre-Sinoussi F, Montagnier L, and Chermann JC (1984). Inactivation of lymphadenopathy-associated virus by chemical disinfectants. *Lancet* **2**:899–901.

Spire B, Dormont D, Barre-Sinoussi F, Montagnier L, and Chermann JC (1985). Inactivation of lymphadenopathy-associated virus by heat, gamma rays, and ultraviolet light. *Lancet* **1**:188–189.

Tjotta E, Hungnes O, and Grindle B (1991). Survival of HIV-1 activity after disinfection, temperature and pH changes, or drying. *J Med Virol* **35**:223–227.

Vajaradul Y (1998). Personal communication.

Yusof N (2000). Gamma irradiation for sterilising tissue grafts and for viral inactivation. *Malays J Nucl Sci* **18**(1):23–35.

Yusof N, Noor Azlan MA, Selamat SN, and Lee CM (1994). Radiation sterilised freeze dried bone allograft — process validation. In: *Proc 8th Int Conf on Biomed Eng*, National University Singapore, Singapore, pp. 303–305.

Chapter 19

Radiation Sterilization Dose Establishment for Tissue Grafts — Dose Setting and Dose Validation

Norimah Yusof

Malaysian Nuclear Agency (NM),
Bangi, 43000 Kajang, Selangor
Malaysia

Introduction

Radiation sterilization has been widely used to sterilize medical products for several decades. The most common dose, 25 kGy, has been the dosage of choice for many medical product manufacturers including tissue bankers. However, given that the dose has started to have detrimental effects on the products or is insufficient to make the products sterile, they have started to ask irradiation personnel for alternative doses. According to the international radiation sterilization standard ISO 11137 (1995a), it is the manufacturers of medical products or the tissue bankers who process the tissues themselves, not the irradiation personnel, who are responsible for deciding the radiation doses used to sterilize their products. The ISO 11137, based on AAMI recommendations, clearly guides manufacturers on how to set a radiation dose that can effectively sterilize their products.

As described in several chapters in this book, the radiation dose is actually very much dependent on the microbiological quality of the products, namely the bioburden as well as the number and types of microorganisms present on or in the product. Tissue bankers must be aware by now that the dose they set is ultimately reliant on how effectively they screen, handle, and process their tissues. They must be able to identify the dose that effectively sterilizes their tissues, yet has no detrimental effects on the required clinical functions of the tissue grafts (e.g. weight bearing in the case of long bones, burn coverage in the case of amnions, or filling in the case of morselized bones).

The main challenge in deciding on the dosage is how to validate it. Validation exercises must be conducted to verify the dose, and the results of the exercise must be documented under the quality system. Since the ISO 11137 caters mainly for medical items, the International Atomic Energy Agency (IAEA) has released a Code of Practice (2004) that provides guidelines for tissue bankers in determining and validating the radiation doses used to sterilize tissues. The Code explains three methods that can be used: methods A and B are based on IAEA 11137 (1995a) and ISO/TR 13409 (1996), respectively; while method C is generated from AAMI TIR 27 (2001). Method A offers a validation exercise for setting a dose other than 25 kGy that is specific to a particular product via two approaches (methods A1 and A2), while methods B and C describe how to do substantiation for 25 kGy if the tissue banker does not intend to change the sterilization dose. The use of the Code in validation exercises will be elaborated in this chapter together with worked examples.

A revision of the ISO 11137 document was undertaken over the past 5 years based on the experience gained in applying the earlier version (Hoxey and Tallentire 2006). As a result, changes have been made to the following:

- The vocabulary of dose establishment
- The conditions that apply to the various methods of sterilization dose choice
- The frequency of and actions following sterilization dose auditing

The revised ISO 11137-2 (2006) describes methods that may be used to establish the sterilization dose in accordance with the following approaches:

1. Dose setting to obtain a product-specific dose
2. Dose substantiation to verify a preselected dose of 25 or 15 kGy

The latter, as put forward by Kowalski and Tallentire (1999), substantiates a sterilization dose using a maximal verification dose or VD_{max}. Therefore, $VD_{max}{}^{25}$ is the maximal verification dose for a given bioburden (not exceeding 1000 CFU), consistent with the attainment of a sterility assurance level (SAL) of 10^{-6} at a specified sterilization dose of 25 kGy. Method $VD_{max}{}^{15}$ is based on the same principles as method $VD_{max}{}^{25}$, but is limited to products with an average bioburden less than 1.5. Tissue bankers may consider this new VD_{max} approach, especially in choosing and substantiating a low dose of 15 kGy to sterilize soft tissues. Nevertheless, it is still necessary to quantify the bioburden and to know the radiation resistance of the natural contaminants of the product prior to sterilization. This chapter will summarize the options available.

IAEA Code of Practice

Following the successful regional and interregional program on the radiation sterilization of tissues by the IAEA from the 1990s to the early 2000s, many tissue banks — mainly in the Asia-Pacific region — are now using ionizing radiation to terminally sterilize tissues. Most tissue bankers simply use 25 kGy, believing that only a 25-kGy dose can attain a sterility assurance level (SAL) of 10^{-6}. Only recently, especially when validating the dose, have they realized that they can choose other doses. Understanding the relationship between the SAL and the tissue microbiological quality (bioburden) prior to sterilization has enabled tissue bankers to establish their own sterilization dose. By producing tissue products with a consistently low bioburden, they can in fact lower the sterilization dose. As has been described elsewhere (Yusof 2000; Yusof 2005; Yusof *et al.* 2005; Yusof *et al.* 2006), this concept is based solely on the number of microbes on/in the tissues prior to irradiation and on the types of microbes in relation to radiation resistance.

By exposing tissue to doses lower than 25 kGy, the damage due to radiation can definitely be minimized, especially in soft tissues whereby radiation doses higher than 25 kGy have been reported to affect the physical properties of the tissue (Tomford 2005; Koller 2005). The IAEA Code of Practice (2004) — which is based on several ISO and AAMI documents — offers three methods suitable for tissues, as tissues (unlike medical items) cannot be produced in large quantities and may not have the same type and distribution of microbial contaminants. All of these methods involve performing bioburden and sterility tests on product items that have received radiation doses lower than the sterilization dose. The Code provides the necessary guidance in the use of ionizing radiation to sterilize tissue allografts in order to ensure their safe clinical use.

Samples for Bioburden and Verification Dose Exercises

Tissues, unlike healthcare products, have variability in the types and levels of bioburden. Due to the limited number of tissues that can be spared for the validation exercise, some tissue banks have to be creative in acquiring enough samples for the exercise. If dummy samples are used, then they have to ensure that the microbial content of the tested samples must be similar to that in/on the finished tissue products. The nonuniformity of tissue size must also be taken into consideration in deciding on the size of tested samples or sample item portions (SIPs).

Tissues are processed according to an established and validated method. Ten packages are randomly picked from a processing/production batch (preferably from one donor) for bioburden estimation using the filtration method according to ISO 11737-1 (1995). From the author's experience, 10 packages from each of three different production batches should be taken to determine the overall average bioburden, which in turn helps to determine whether the tissues processed from several batches are of consistent quality. The results from the bioburden test are then used to obtain or calculate a verification dose. For the dose validation experiment, 10 packages of samples from the batch with the highest bioburden should be taken. The verification dose should be delivered within a $\pm 10\%$ variation, preferably using an irradiation facility (which can deliver better dose uniformity). After being exposed to the verification (substerilization) dose (at an SAL of 10^{-1}), these 10 samples are then subjected to a sterility test, which is conducted according to ISO 11737-2 (1998). The sterility test should not yield more than one positive growth. Dosimeters such as ceric/cerous and Amber Perspex dosimeters can be used to measuring the absorbed dose.

The methods are described here with some worked examples on amnions that were procured from screened mothers, treated with sodium hypochlorite during processing, and air-dried. For easy understanding, the same bioburden value was used in all of the examples with SIP $=1$ (i.e. the whole sample was used for the bioburden test).

Method A1: Establish Sterilization Dose for Tissues with Standard Distribution of Resistance (SDR)

Method A1, based on the ISO 11137 (1995a) document for medical products, allows tissue bankers to validate sterilization doses other than 25 kGy. Assuming the tissue has a microbial population of the standard distribution of resistance (SDR) for medical items, method 1 of ISO 11137 (1995a) is adopted. Ten samples are taken for average bioburden estimation. The verification dose is obtained from Table 2a of the Code at the estimated initial bioburden to achieve an SAL of 10^{-1}. The 10 samples are then exposed to that verification dose within a $\pm 10\%$ variation. If the exercise is valid (i.e. there is not more than one positive growth in the sterility test), Table 2b of the Code is referred to for the sterilization dose at an SAL of 10^{-6} and for the closest bioburden number that is equal to or greater than the estimated bioburden.

The worked example in Table 1 shows that method A1 can offer a new dose when the bioburden is less than 1000 CFU/product unit. The tested amnion with a bioburden of 7.63 CFU/amnion that passed the sterility test after being exposed to a verification dose of 2.8 kGy could now be sterilized at 17.2 kGy instead of 25 kGy.

Method A2: Establish Sterilization Dose for Tissues with a Population Different from the Standard Distribution of Resistance (SDR)

Method A2, an alternative method by calculation, can be considered if the microbial population differs from the SDR. When the distribution of microbial radiation resistance is known and different to the SDR, the verification dose is calculated using the following survival equation:

$$N = N_0 \times 10^{-(D/D_{10})}$$

It is simplified as

$$D = D_{10}\,[\log N_0 - \log N]$$

where

D_0 is the verification dose (kGy)
D_{10} is the radiation dose (kGy) required to reduce a population of microorganisms to 10% of the initial number, 90% killing, by a factor of 10, or by one log cycle

Table 1. Establishing the sterilization dose using method A1 of the IAEA Code of Practice. Sample: amnion (from screened mother, treated with sodium hypochlorite, air-dried).

Stage	Value	Comments
Stage 1		
Production batch size	10 pieces/batch	10 cm × 10 cm amnion samples, obtained from 3 processing batches (mothers)
Test sample size for bioburden determination	$3 \times 10 = 30$	Bioburden test on 3 different batches with 10 samples per batch
Test sample size for the verification dose exercise	10 10	Samples from one processing batch for exposure to verification dose required at SAL of 10^{-1} (= 1/10)
Stage 2		
Obtain samples	40*	3 batches ×10 samples for bioburden, and 10 samples for verification dose experiment
Stage 3		
SIP	1	The entire amnion is used
Average bioburden	7.63 CFU/amnion	Overall average bioburden of 3 processing batches: Batch 1: 9.3 CFU/amnion Batch 2: 6.1 CFU/amnion Batch 3: 7.5 CFU/amnion None of the bioburdens are twice the overall average bioburden, therefore 7.63 is used to establish the verification dose
Stage 4		
Verification dose calculation	2.8 kGy	Assuming that the microbial population of amnion is of SDR, the verification dose is obtained from Table 2a of the Code for bioburden of 8 and SAL of 10^{-1} (sample size of 10)

(*Continued*)

Table 1. (*Continued*)

Stage	Value	Comments
Stage 5		
Verification dose experiment	3.0 kGy delivered	The actual dose delivered to the 10 samples must be within 10% variation, i.e. 2.52–3.08 kGy. The experiment is accepted
Sterility test	No positive	The verification exercise is accepted
Stage 6		
Sterilization dose	17.2 kGy	Refer to Table 2b of the Code. The radiation dose required to achieve SAL of 10^{-6} at a bioburden of 8.0 is obtained

*Under the IAEA Code of Practice, only 10 samples are required for average bioburden estimation.

N_0 is the initial number of microorganisms
N is number of microorganisms surviving the dose D, i.e. 10^{-1}

Ten samples are exposed to the verification dose D within a $\pm 10\%$ variation. When the sterility test yields not more than 1 positive sample out of 10 samples, the sterilization dose at an SAL of 10^{-6} is calculated from the same equation given above.

The worked example in Table 2 used the same bioburden results from three processing batches (7.63 CFU) as in Table 1. When the microbial population was known and different from the SDR, the sterilization dose based on calculation (method A2) was 12.4 kGy — even lower than that obtained through method A1. The dose was validated when 10 samples exposed to a verification dose of 3.4 kGy passed the sterility test.

Method B: Substantiate 25 kGy as Sterilization Dose

Method B — which adopts ISO/TR 13409 (1996) — is used to substantiate 25 kGy as the sterilization dose, based on the average bioburden estimation from 10 samples and on the number of samples used in the verification dose

Table 2. Establishing the sterilization dose using method A2 of the IAEA Code of Practice. Sample: amnion (from screened mother, treated with sodium hypochlorite, air-dried).

Stage	Value	Comments
Stage 1		
Production batch size	10 pieces/batch	10 cm × 10 cm amnion samples, obtained from 3 processing batches (mothers)
Test sample size for bioburden determination	10	Bioburden test on 3 different batches
Test sample size for the verification dose exercise	10	Verification dose required at SAL of 10^{-1} (=1/10)
Stage 2		
Obtain samples	40	3 batches × 10 samples for bioburden, and 10 samples for verification dose experiment
Stage 3		
SIP	1	The entire amnion is used
Average bioburden	7.63 CFU	Overall average bioburden of 3 processing batches: Batch 1: 9.3 CFU/amnion Batch 2: 6.1 CFU/amnion Batch 3: 7.5 CFU/amnion
Stage 4		
Verification dose calculation	3.4 kGy	The microbial population of amnion is known and different from SDR. The most common and most resistant microbe on amnion is *Bacillus* sp., with D_{10} value of 1.8 in aerobic condition. The verification dose is calculated: $\mathrm{VD} = D_{10}\,[\log N_0 - \log N] = 1.8\,[\log 7.63 - \log 10^{-1}] = 3.39$
Stage 5		
Verification dose experiment	3.5 kGy delivered	The actual dose delivered to the 10 samples must be within 10% variation, i.e. 3.06–3.74 kGy. The experiment is accepted

(*Continued*)

Table 2. (*Continued*)

Stage	Value	Comments
Sterility test	No positive	The verification exercise is accepted
Stage 6		
Sterilization dose	12.4 kGy	The sterilization dose is calculated to achieve SAL of 10^{-6} at bioburden of 7.63: $SD = D_{10}\,[\log N_0 - \log N]$ $= 1.8\,[\log 7.63 - \log 10^{-6}]$ $= 12.39$

experiment. The verification dose at an SAL of 10^{-1} (sample size of 10) for an SDR population is estimated using the following equation:

$$\mathrm{VD} = I + [S \times \log(\text{average SIP bioburden})]$$

where

VD	is the verification dose (kGy)
I and S values	are given in Annex C in Table 3 of the Code
SIP	is the sample item portion or standardized portion of a tissue graft that is tested

The verification dose should be delivered within a ±10% variation. The sterility test on 10 samples should not yield more than one positive growth. To be able to use this method to substantiate 25 kGy, the bioburden for the whole sample (SIP = 1) must be less than 1000 CFU.

The worked example in Table 3 showed that a sterilization dose of 25 kGy was selected and substantiated. The verification dose in method B was 2.7 kGy. The author's tissue bank has proven that the selected sterilization dose is capable of achieving the specified requirements for sterility. The same amnion (bioburden of 7.63 CFU/amnion) could be sterilized at 17.2 kGy and even lower at 12.4 kGy as verified through methods A1 and A2, respectively; therefore, using a 25-kGy dose is indeed preferable over killing.

Table 3. Substantiating 25 kGy as the sterilization dose using method B of the IAEA Code of Practice. Sample: amnion (from screened mother, treated with sodium hypochlorite, air-dried).

Stage	Value	Comments
Stage 1		
Production batch size	10 pieces/batch	10 cm × 10 cm amnion samples, obtained from 3 processing batches (mothers)
Test sample size for bioburden determination	10	Bioburden test on 3 different batches
Test sample size for the verification dose exercise	10	Verification dose required at SAL of 10^{-1} (=1/10)
Stage 2		
Obtain samples	40	3 batches × 10 samples for bioburden, and 10 samples for verification dose experiment
Stage 3		
SIP	1	The entire amnion is used
Average bioburden	7.63 CFU	Overall average bioburden of 3 processing batches: Batch 1: 9.3 CFU/amnion Batch 2: 6.1 CFU/amnion Batch 3: 7.5 CFU/amnion
Stage 4		
Verification dose calculation	2.7 kGy	The verification dose is calculated using the method in ISO/TR 13409 (1996), which is only applicable to SDR: $VD/SIP = I + [S \times \log(\text{average bioburden})]$ $= 1.25 + [1.65 \times \log(7.63)]$ $= 2.71$ The I and S values are obtained from Table 3 of the code for bioburden of 1–10 and sample size of 10. The verification dose is rounded to one decimal place

(*Continued*)

Table 3. (*Continued*)

Stage	Value	Comments
Stage 5		
Verification dose experiment	2.8 kGy delivered	The actual dose delivered to the 10 samples must be within 10% variation, i.e. 2.44–2.98 kGy. The experiment is accepted
Sterility test	One positive	The verification exercise is accepted
Stage 6		
Sterilization dose	25 kGy	The use of 25 kGy as a sterilization dose (SAL of 10^{-6}) is substantiated

Method C: Substantiate 25 kGy as Sterilization Dose

Method C, based on AAMI TIR 27 (2001), is also for substantiating 25 kGy to achieve an SAL of 10^{-6}. This method allows a better chance to pass the verification dose during the validation experiment. The verification dose varies with the bioburden level for a given SAL and sample size.

Ten samples are taken for average bioburden estimation. The verification dose is calculated using the following formula:

1. For bioburden levels of 1–50 CFU per product,

$$\text{Step 1: } D_{\text{lin}} = 25\,\text{kGy}/(6 + \log N_0)$$
$$\text{Step 2: VD} = D_{\text{lin}}(\log N_0 - \log \text{SAL}_{\text{VD}})$$

2. For bioburden levels of 51–1000 CFU per product,

$$\text{Step 1: } TD_{10} = \text{Dose}_{-6}\,\text{kGy} + \text{Dose}_{-2}\,\text{kGy}$$
$$\text{Step 2: VD} = 25\,\text{kGy} - [TD_{10}(\log \text{SAL}_{\text{VD}} + 6)]$$

where

D_{lin} is the D_{10} dose for a hypothetical survival curve that is linear between the coordinates ($\log N_0$, 0 kGy) and ($\log 10^{-6}$, 25 kGy)

N_0 is the bioburden or count prior to sterilization

SAL_{VD} is the sterility assurance level at which the verification dose experiment is to be performed

TD_{10} is the hypothetical D_{10} value of a survival curve for an SDR population that is linear between log 10^{-2} and log 10^{-6} (log SAL values)

$Dose_{-6}$ and $Dose_{-2}$ are the doses corresponding to SAL values of 10^{-6} and 10^{-2}, respectively, obtained from Table B1 of ISO 11137 (1995)

The verification dose should be delivered within a $\pm 10\%$ variation. The sterility test on 10 samples should not yield more than one positive growth. Values of verification doses at an SAL of 10^{-1} for a bioburden of 0–1000 CFU are given in Table 4 of the Code. For other SAL values, the methods of calculation described above should be used.

The worked example in Table 4 indicated that method C allows the use of a higher verification dose (6.8 kGy) than would be allowed using the formula given in method B (2.7 kGy). For those tissue banks that prefer to use a sterilization dose of 25 kGy, the Code suggests that method C should be used as fewer verification dose exercises will fail.

In all of the above methods, the irradiation conditions of the samples for the verification experiment at the verification (substerilization) dose should be the same as the conditions for the sterilization of the whole batch. Where the verification dose experiment is successful, the dose required to produce an SAL of 10^{-6} for the allograft product can be obtained from Table 2b for method A1, or the sterilization dose should be calculated according to method A2. For the procedures in method B and method C, a successful verification dose experiment substantiates the use of 25 kGy as a sterilization dose. As summarized in Table 5, the verification dose for methods A1 and C were almost similar and lower than the verification dose for method A2. Therefore, validation conducted at an SAL of 10^{-1} with a verification dose of 2.7 kGy allowed the amnion to be sterilized at 25 kGy as well as at lower doses of 17.2 kGy and 12.4 kGy.

Concept of VD_{max} Approach

The revised version of ISO 11137-2 (2006) describes methods of choosing a sterilization dose and demonstrating its effectiveness over time. Method

Table 4. Establishing the sterilization dose using method C of the IAEA Code of Practice. Sample: amnion (from screened mother, treated with sodium hypochlorite, air-dried.)

Stage	Value	Comments
Stage 1		
Production batch size	10 pieces/batch	10 cm × 10 cm amnion samples, obtained from 3 processing batches (mothers)
Test sample size for bioburden determination	10	Bioburden test on 3 different batches
Test sample size for the verification dose exercise	10	Verification dose required at SAL of 10^{-1} (=1/10)
Stage 2		
Obtain samples	40	3 batches × 10 samples for bioburden, and 10 samples for verification dose experiment
Stage 3		
SIP	1	The entire amnion is used
Average bioburden	7.63 CFU	Overall average bioburden of 3 processing batches: Batch 1: 9.3 CFU/amnion Batch 2: 6.1 CFU/amnion Batch 3: 7.5 CFU/amnion
Stage 4		
Verification dose calculation	6.8 kGy	The verification dose is calculated using the method in AAMI TIR 27 (2001) for bioburden levels of 1–50 CFU with SDR: Step 1: $D_{\text{lin}} = 25\,\text{kGy}/(6 + \log N_0) = 25/(6 + \log 7.63) = 3.63$ Step 2: $\text{VD} = D_{\text{lin}} (\log N_0 - \log \text{SAL}_{\text{VD}}) = 3.63 (\log 7.63 - \log 10^{-1}) = 6.83$ Table 4 of the Code also provides the verification dose

(*Continued*)

Table 4. (*Continued*)

Stage	Value	Comments
Stage 5		
Verification dose experiment	7.1 kGy delivered	The actual dose delivered to the 10 samples must be within 10% variation, i.e. 6.12–7.48 kGy. The experiment is accepted
Sterility test	One positive	The verification exercise is accepted
Stage 6		
Sterilization dose	25 kGy	The use of 25 kGy as a sterilization dose (SAL of 10^{-6}) is substantiated

Table 5. Summary of verification dose (VD) and radiation sterilization dose for amnion with a bioburden of 7.63 CFU/product item using the methods described in the IAEA Code of Practice (2004) for validation exercise.

Method	Verification dose (VD)	Radiation sterilization dose
A1	2.8 kGy	17.2 kGy
A2	3.4 kGy	12.4 kGy
B	2.7 kGy	25 kGy
C	6.8 kGy	25 kGy

VD_{max}, which substantiates a specific preselected sterilization dose, verifies that the bioburden present on that particular product prior to sterilization is less resistant to radiation than a microbial population of maximal resistance consistent with the attainment of an SAL of 10^{-6} at the selected sterilization dose. Verification is conducted at an SAL of 10^{-1} with 10 product items. For the substantiation of a sterilization dose of 25 kGy, the method is designated $VD_{max}{}^{25}$ and is applicable to products having an average bioburden less than or equal to 1000 CFU. This is similar to methods B and C of the Code.

Method $VD_{max}{}^{15}$ is used to substantiate 15 kGy to achieve an SAL of 10^{-6}, but is limited to products with an average bioburden less than 1.5 CFU. This allows tissue banks to validate and use 15 kGy, the dose that has been recommended by several tissue standards to sterilize especially soft tissues.

The method may be adopted to substantiate 15 kGy as the sterilization dose for tissues. By lowering the sterilization dose, the damage in physical properties of tissues due to irradiation can be avoided.

For a low bioburden (e.g. lower than 10 CFU), it is permissible to pool the 10 product items to determine the batch average bioburden. VD_{max} is obtained from Table 10 of the ISO document, and the sterility test on 10 samples should not yield more than 2 samples with positive growth.

The bioburden of 7.63 CFU/amnion used in the worked examples above is obviously higher than the bioburden limit allowed by method $VD_{max}{}^{15}$. This implies that an improved process is required to produce very clean tissues with a bioburden lower than 1.5 CFU in order to substantiate 15 kGy as the sterilization dose. In applying method $VD_{max}{}^{15}$, an entire tissue product item (SIP = 1) is used.

Conclusion

The validation of a radiation sterilization dose can only be conducted if the tissues processed are of consistent quality. Tissue bankers must ensure that tissues are processed according to validated procedures and are carried out by trained staff. Good hygienic processing and preservation lowers the bioburden, thus lowering the sterilization dose. Sterilization doses lower than 25 kGy can only be determined when the bioburden is less than 1000 CFU per tissue product. For the substantiation of 25 kGy, the bioburden for the whole sample must also be less than 1000 CFU. For the substantiation of 15 kGy using method $VD_{max}{}^{15}$, tissue products must have a very low bioburden (i.e. less than 1.5 CFU). It is the responsibility of tissue bankers to ensure that the bioburden of each processing batch is consistently low after dose validation is conducted. Microbiological analysis must be in place, with bioburden being one of the product quality controls.

References

Association for the Advancement of Medical Instrumentation (AAMI) (2001). Sterilization of Health Care Products — Radiation Sterilization — Substantiation of 25 kGy as a Sterilization Dose, AAMI TIR 27, 2001, Arlington, VA.

Hoxey EV and Tallentire A (2006). Sterilisation dose establishment under the revised radiation standard (EN ISO/FDIS 11137:2005). In: *Proc 14th International Meeting of Radiation Processing (IMRP) 2006*, Kuala Lumpur, Malaysia, p. 204.

International Atomic Energy Agency (IAEA) (2004). Code of Practice for Radiation Sterilization of Tissue Allografts: Requirements for Validation and Routine Control, Project No. INT/6/052, IAEA, Vienna.

International Standards Organization (ISO) (1995a). Requirements for Validation and Routine Control — Radiation Sterilisation, ISO 11137, 1995(E), Switzerland.

International Standards Organization (ISO) (1995b). Sterilization of Medical Devices — Microbiological Methods — Part 1: Estimation of Population of Microorganisms on Products, ISO 11737-1, 1995, Geneva.

International Standards Organization (ISO) (1996). Sterilization of Health Care Products — Radiation Sterilization — Substantiation of 25 kGy as a Sterilization Dose for Small or Infrequent Product Batches, ISO/TR 13409, 1996, Geneva.

International Standards Organization (ISO) (1998). Sterilization of Medical Devices — Microbiological Methods — Part 2: Tests of Sterility Performed in the Validation of a Sterilization Process, ISO 11737-2, 1998, Geneva.

International Standards Organization (ISO) (2006). Sterilization of Health Care Products — Radiation — Part 2: Establishing the Sterilization Dose, ISO 11137-2, 2006, Geneva.

Koller J (2005). Effects of radiation on the integrity and functionality of amnion and skin grafts. In: Kennedy JF, Phillips GO, and William PA (eds.), *Sterilisation of Tissues Using Ionising Radiations*, CRC Woodhead Publishing, England, pp. 197–220.

Kowalski JB and Tallentire A (1991). Substantiation of 25 kGy as a sterilization dose: a rational approach to establishing verification dose. *Radiat Phys Chem* **54**(1):55–64.

Tomford WW (2005). Effects of gamma irradiation on bone — clinical experience. In: Kennedy JF, Phillips GO, and Williams PA (eds.), *Sterilisation of Tissues Using Ionising Radiations*, CRC Woodhead Publishing, England, pp. 133–140.

Yusof N (2000). Gamma irradiation for sterilising tissue grafts and for viral inactivation. *Malays J Nucl Sci* **18**(1):23–35.

Yusof N (2005). Is the irradiation dose of 25 kGy enough to sterilise tissue grafts? In: Nather A (ed.), *Bone Grafts and Bone Substitutes — Basic Science and Clinical Applications*, World Scientific, Singapore, pp. 189–212.

Yusof N, Abdul Rani S, Hasim M, Hassan A, Ang CY, and Muhamad Firdaus AR (2005). Bioburden estimation in relation to tissue product quality and radiation dose validation. In: Kennedy JF, Phillips GO, and Williams PA (eds.), *Sterilisation of Tissues Using Ionising Radiations*, CRC Woodhead Publishing, England, pp. 319–329.

Yusof N, Hassan A, Firdaus AR, and Suzina AH (2006). Challenges in validating the sterilisation dose for human amniotic membranes in complying with the IAEA Code of Practice. In: *Proc 14th International Meeting of Radiation Processing (IMRP) 2006*, Kuala Lumpur, Malaysia, p. 64.

Chapter 20

Quality System in Radiation Sterilization of Tissue Grafts

Nazly Hilmy

BATAN Research Tissue Bank
Center for Research and Development of Isotopes and Radiation Technology, BATAN
Jakarta 12070, Indonesia

Introduction

The radiation sterilization of tissue allografts can only be successfully achieved when tissue bank activities are carried out as described in the International Atomic Energy Agency (IAEA) International Standards for Tissue Banks (2002), which should be used as a starting point for good tissue banking practices. These Standards describe the safety and quality dimensions of human tissues for transplantation, such as quality management, processing methods, tissue sterilization, and validation. These Standards apply to all types of tissues (including corneas) and cells.

An essential step in the radiation sterilization of tissues is rigorous donor selection to eliminate specific contaminants, e.g. viruses. Full details about donor selection, tissue retrieval, general tissue banking procedures, specific processing procedures, labeling, and distribution are given in the Standards. These tissue donor selection, retrieval, processing, and preservation processes determine the characteristics of tissue allografts prior to the radiation sterilization process.

In 2004, the IAEA published the Code of Practice for the Radiation Sterilization of Tissue Allografts. The objective of the Code is to provide necessary guidance in the use of ionizing radiation to sterilize tissue allografts in order to ensure their safe clinical use. This IAEA Code adopts the principles that the International Standards Organization (ISO) has applied to the radiation sterilization of healthcare products (ISO 11137, 1995a; ISO 13409, 1996; AAMI TIR 27, 2001), with appropriate modifications for the low numbers of tissue allograft samples typically available. The Code specifies requirements for validation, process control and routine monitoring of donor selection, tissue processing and preservation, storage, and radiation sterilization of tissue allografts at the terminal stage. They apply to continuous- and batch-type gamma irradiators using the radioisotopes ^{60}Co and ^{137}Cs, electron beam accelerators, and X-rays.

A radiation sterilization dose of 25 kGy or lower, depending on the bioburden number of the products, can be determined and validated according to the Code. The Code is not applicable if viral contamination is identified. It is emphasized that human donors of the tissues must be medically and serologically screened. However, these sterilization methods may adversely affect the mechanical properties of tissues if the radiation sterilization dose is higher than 25 kGy. Following intensive studies on the effects of ionizing radiation on the chemical, physical, and biological properties of tissue allografts and their components, there are now a variety of methods and practices of radiation sterilization.

In order to reduce the risk for patients by the transplantation of tissue to an acceptable level, it is necessary to operate an effective quality management system in tissue banking, including a quality system in the radiation sterilization of allografts. Each processing step in tissue banking should have validated standard operating procedures (SOPs), such as procedures for retrieval of raw materials; methods of screening, washing, freezing, and lyophilizing; as well as experiments to determine the radiation sterilization dose to be used. Predetermined specifications and quality attributes of biological tissues both before and after processing should be set up before preparing the standard operating procedures.

The quality management system stated in the IAEA International Standards for Tissue Banks (2002) should be implemented in all tissue processing steps prior to the radiation sterilization of tissue allografts. Validation of the radiation sterilization dose can be done according to the IAEA Code of Practice (2004). This chapter discusses the quality system in the radiation sterilization of tissue allografts.

Quality Management in Tissue Banking System (IAEA 2002)

In order to reduce the risk for patients by the transplantation of tissues to an acceptable level, it is necessary to operate an effective quality management system. The system may include extensive testing of donor blood and tissue samples, but this alone does not sufficiently guarantee safety and efficacy. Therefore, the system should include other management and control measures, such as those pertaining to the procurement, processing, and supply of tissues for transplantation.

Quality requirements

Quality requirements form the basis of all quality assurance and quality control (QC) programs. It is necessary to define the quality requirements not only for the final product, but also for the starting material collected, reagents and equipment used, staff competencies, testing techniques, packaging materials, labels, and process intermediates. These quality requirements are best prescribed and quantified in written specifications that determine the quality control testing/inspection procedures performed, on the basis of which release decisions are made. The quality requirements are based on characteristics that affect both patient safety and the maintenance of the clinical effectiveness of the product.

Figure 1 shows the transplant management according to the IAEA International Standards (2002) and the IAEA Code of Practice (2004). All steps of work should be documented.

Quality management

It is recognized that quality has to be managed in organizations, and that a systematic approach is the only way to ensure that the quality of products produced and services delivered consistently meets the quality requirements. The high level of quality assurance required for the safety of critical therapeutic medical products and clinical services can only be achieved through the implementation of an effective quality management system.

The international standard for quality management is the ISO 9000 (2000) series. Specific principles incorporated into the quality system that

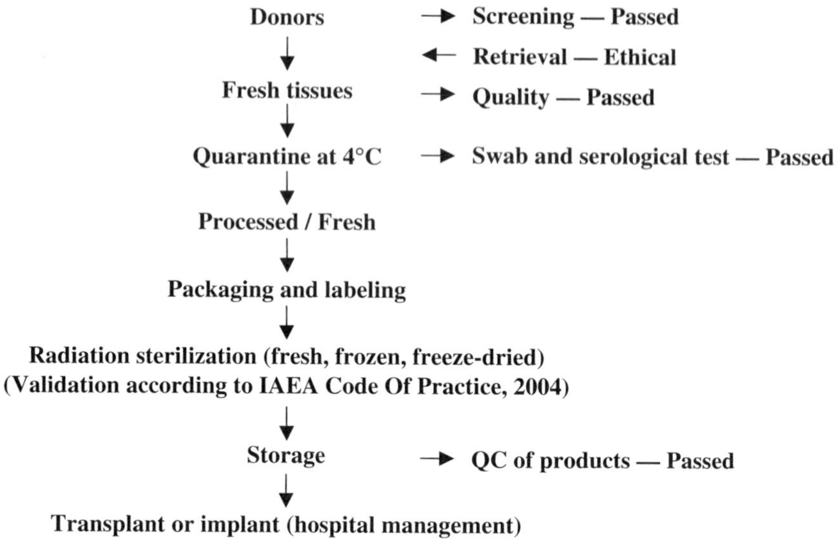

Fig. 1. Transplant management of biological tissues: from donor screening to radiation sterilization. SOPs should be followed according to the IAEA Standards. Products can be released after passing the QC evaluation.

cover the manufacture and quality control of medicines are known as Good Manufacturing Practice (GMP) (PIC/S 2000). The ISO 9000, GMP, or other applicable standards — as well as other applicable intergovernmental, national, regional, and local law or regulation — should be consulted when developing quality management for tissue banking organizations and other procurement organizations.

The basic elements of an appropriate quality management system

Organizational structure and accountability

This is necessary to achieve the quality requirements and to review the effectiveness of the arrangements for quality assurance. There should be a suitably qualified and experienced member of staff appointed to verify that the quality requirements are being met, and that there is compliance with the quality management system. The quality manager should be a designated individual who is independent of production (i.e. not directly responsible for or involved in the procurement, processing, and testing of tissue) and preferably of other responsibilities within the tissue bank.

Documentation

The objectives of thorough documentation are to define the system of information and control, to minimize the risk of misinterpretation and error inherent in oral or casually written communication, and to provide unambiguous procedures to be followed. Documents should clearly state the quality requirements, organizational structure and responsibilities, the organization's policies and standards, the management and technical procedures employed, and the records required. All of the procedures in the processing of tissue should be documented, and the documents controlled. Any correction should be clearly and legibly handwritten in permanent ink, and signed and dated by an authorized person.

The system for document control should identify the current revision status of any document and the holder of the document. Documented procedures should be established and maintained for identification, collection, filing, storage, retrieval, and maintenance of all documents.

Control of processes (SOPs)

Written instructions of standard operating procedures (SOPs) should be in place wherever it is essential that tasks be performed in a consistent way. Equipment, processes, and procedures should be validated as effective before being implemented or changed. Equipment essential to the quality of the product shall be routinely serviced and calibrated, if appropriate. The processing environment and the staff performing the processes shall meet minimum prescribed standards of cleanliness and hygiene.

The tissue bank shall maintain an SOP manual, which details in writing all aspects of these standards. The SOPs shall be utilized to ensure that all of the materials released for transplantation meet at least the minimum requirements defined by professional standards and by applicable intergovernmental, national, regional, and local law or regulation. The SOP manual should include, but should not be limited to, the following:

- Standard procedures for donor screening, consent, retrieval, processing, preservation, testing, storage, and distribution
- Quality assurance and quality control policies

- Laboratory procedures for tests performed in-house and in contracted laboratories
- Specifications for materials used including supply, reagent, storage media, and packaging materials
- Personnel and facility safety procedures
- Standard procedures for facility maintenance, cleaning, and waste disposal
- Methods for verification of the effectiveness of sterilization procedures
- Equipment maintenance, calibration, and validation procedures
- Environmental and microbiological conditions as well as the methods used for controlling, testing, and verification
- Physiological and physical test specifications for materials
- Methods for determination of shelf life, storage temperature, and expiry date of tissues
- Determination of insert and/or label text
- Policies and procedures for exceptional release of materials
- Procedures for adverse event reporting and corrective action
- Donor/recipient tracking as well as product recall policies and procedures

All SOPs, their modifications, and associated process validation studies must be reviewed and approved by either the medical or administrative director, as dictated by the content. All medically related SOPs shall be reviewed and approved by the medical director. Copies of the SOP manual shall be available to all staff, and to authorized individuals for inspection upon request. Upon implementation, all SOPs should be followed as written. SOPs shall be updated at regular intervals to reflect modifications or changes. The authorized person, depending on the content, shall approve each modification or change.

Appropriate training shall be provided to pertinent staff. Obsolete SOP manuals shall be archived for a minimum of 10 years, taking into account the shelf life of the material.

Record keeping

Records shall be confidential, accurate, complete, legible, and indelible. All donor, processing, storage, and distribution records should be maintained for 30 years or in accordance with applicable intergovernmental, national, regional, and local law.

Records shall hold all information that identifies the origins of the product and demonstrates that the product meets all of the quality requirements. Records shall show that all of the required processing steps and quality control tests have been performed correctly by trained staff, and that the product has been released for use only after the correct authorization. Records shall also demonstrate the correct handling and storage of materials, and track the final status of products (whether they are transplanted, discarded, or used for research). The use and storage of records shall be controlled.

1. Contract records
When two or more tissue banks participate in tissue procurement, processing, storage, or distribution functions, the relationships and responsibilities of each shall be documented to ensure compliance with relevant scientific and quality professional standards. Tissue banks should perform on-site audits of contract laboratories to ensure their compliance with relevant scientific and professional standards, technical manuals, and the tissue bank's own requirements.

2. Donor tracking
Each component shall be assigned one unique identifier that serves as a lot number to identify the material during all of the steps, from collection to distribution and utilization. This unique number shall link the donor to all tests, records, organs, and other material, as well as to the final packaged material. It will also be used for tracking purposes to the recipient.

Records shall include identification and evaluation of the donor; blood testing and microbiological evaluation of the donor; conditions under which the material is procured, processed, tested, and stored; and the final destination of the material. Records shall indicate the dates of and the staff members involved in each significant step of operation.

3. Inventory
A record of unprocessed, processed, quarantined, and distributed tissues shall be maintained.

4. Recipient-adverse events and noncompliances
An adverse event file shall be maintained, including any noncompliances.

5. Electronic records
If a computer record-keeping system is used, there should be a system not only to ensure the authenticity, integrity, and confidentiality of all the records, but also to retain the ability to generate true paper copies. A description of the system, its functions, and specified requirements must be documented. The system shall record the identity of persons entering or confirming critical data. Alteration to the system or program shall only be made in accordance with defined procedures. Where the release of finished batches is conducted by computerized systems, it must identify and record the person(s) releasing the batches. Alternative management systems should be available to cope with failures in computerized systems.

Methods for detecting, correcting, and preventing quality failures from recurring

Quality failures

Quality failures include in-use product deficiencies (complaints, adverse events, etc.), failures to meet quality control specifications, and noncompliance with procedures. Methods for detecting failures include quality control tests, inspections, quality audits, and staff and end-user feedback. The ability to trace, locate, quarantine, and recall materials, consumables, and products at any stage is essential to patient safety. Serious failures shall be thoroughly registered and investigated; and appropriate changes to specifications, systems, and procedures implemented to prevent further failures of a similar nature.

Audit

The tissue bank shall participate in an audit program. Quality assurance staff shall perform internal audits. Focused audits shall be conducted to monitor critical areas and when problems with quality have been identified. Regular audits shall be performed by qualified staff who do not have direct responsibility for the processes being audited.

Competency

The educational and training requirements for each member of staff shall be determined and specified. There shall be regular and formal appraisals of staff competency. Training and education shall include the requirements for quality, standards of practice, good hygiene, as well as appropriate continuing professional development. Records of training shall be maintained up to date.

Specific Processing Procedures

General

Section A — which relates to written procedures, process validation, quality control, and record management — always applies.

Rejected tissues due to donor ineligibility cannot be used for transplantation, even after processing (including sterilization or disinfection). Even if terminal sterilization or disinfection using physical or chemical agents is conducted, the procurement and processing shall be adequate to minimize the microbial content of tissues in order to ensure the effectiveness of the subsequent sterilization–disinfection process. Appropriate indicators for sterilization must be included in each sterilization batch.

Disinfectant or antibiotic immersion

If disinfectants or antibiotics are used after retrieval, the tissues shall be immersed in a disinfectant or antibiotic solution following sterility testing and before final packaging. The type of solution used shall be specified in the documentation.

Fresh tissue

Fresh allografts (e.g. small fragments of articular cartilage and skin) are aseptically procured in an operating room. Fresh tissue is usually stored refrigerated at 4°C or in accordance with written procedures. Fresh tissue shall not be used in a patient until donor blood testing has been completed according to the prescribed standards, available bacteriological results are acceptable, and donor suitability has been approved by the medical director or designee.

Frozen tissue

After aseptic procurement in the operating room, frozen tissues are placed in a −40°C (or colder) controlled environment within 24 h of procurement.

Subsequent manipulation of tissues (e.g. cleaning and cutting) shall be undertaken aseptically.

Cryopreserved tissue

A cryopreservative solution (e.g. DMSO or glycerol) is usually added to treat the tissue prior to freezing. Documentation of the concentration of cryoprotectants and nutrients or isotonic solutions in the cryopreservative solution shall be maintained.

Properly packaged specimens are frozen either by placing the specimens below −40°C or by subjecting them to control-rate freezing using a computer-assisted liquid nitrogen freezing device. If a programmed control-rate freezing method is employed, a record of the freezing profile shall be evaluated, approved, and recorded.

Freeze-dried tissue

Freeze-drying methods

Various protocols for freeze-drying tissues exist. Freeze-drying is a method for preservation, but is not a sterilization method; sterility shall be assumed by aseptic protocol or additional sterilization.

After a standardized procedure for freeze-drying has been developed, a quality control program for monitoring the performance of the freeze-dryer shall be documented. Freeze-dried tissues shall be stored at room temperature or colder.

Freeze-drying controls

Each freeze-drying cycle must be clearly documented, including the length, temperature, and vacuum pressure at each step of the cycle. Representative samples shall be tested for residual water content.

Simply dehydrated tissue

Dehydration method

The use of simple dehydration (evaporation) of tissues as a means of preservation shall be controlled in a manner similar to that of freeze-drying. Temperatures of simple dehydration shall be below 60°C.

Dehydration controls

The temperature of each dehydration cycle shall be monitored during operation. Following dehydration, representative samples shall be tested for residual moisture.

Irradiated tissue

Irradiation methods

Commercial or hospital radiation facilities are available for ionizing radiation. The minimum recommended dose for bacterial decontamination is 15 kGy. The minimum recommended dose for bacterial sterilization is 25 kGy. Viral inactivation requires a higher dose and depends on numerous factors; for this reason, no specific dose can be recommended, but shall be validated when applicable.

The used protocol shall be validated taking into account the initial bioburden, and shall be performed by facilities following good irradiation practices (see Appendix 2).

Irradiation sterilization controls

Sterilization by ionizing radiation shall be documented. The processing records include the name of the facility and the resultant dosimetry for each batch.

Selection of Potential Donor (IAEA 2002)

Donor selection to eliminate specific contaminations such as viruses is an essential step in the radiation sterilization of tissues because the contamination of viruses is not included in bioburden determination, which is carried out in the verification dose experiment to validate the radiation sterilization dose (RSD). Each virus has a specific window period, i.e. the period between the time of infection and the time the virus is detectable by screening tests. Allografts without proper processing techniques and terminal sterilization can be affected by viruses during the window period (Table 1).

Table 1. Window period (WP) of several viruses (Busch and Kleinman 2000).

Virus	Human immuno-deficiency virus (HIV)	Hepatitis C virus (HCV)	Hepatitis B virus (HBV)
WP (using FDA[a]-licensed test kit)	22 days (anti-HIV)	70 days (anti-HCV)	56 days (HBsAg)
WP (using nucleic acid test)	7–12 days	10–29 days	41–50 days

[a]Food and Drug Administration.

Donor selection

The suitability of a specific donor for tissue allograft donation is based on medical and behavioral histories, medical record reviews, physical examinations, cadaveric donor autopsy findings (if an autopsy is performed), and laboratory tests.

Donor history review

Donor evaluation includes an interview with the potential living donor or the cadaveric donor's next of kin, performed by suitably trained personnel using a questionnaire. A qualified physician shall approve donor evaluation.

Exclusion criteria

The following conditions contraindicate the use of tissues for therapeutic purposes:

- History of chronic viral hepatitis
- Presence of active viral hepatitis or jaundice of unknown etiology
- History of (or clinical evidence, suspicion, or laboratory evidence of) HIV infection
- Risk factors for HIV, HBV, and HCV, as assessed by the medical director according to existing national regulations (taking into account national epidemiology)
- Presence or suspicion of central degenerative neurological diseases of possible infectious origin, including dementia (e.g. Alzheimer's disease, Creutzfeldt–Jakob disease or familial history of Creutzfeldt–Jakob disease, multiple sclerosis)

- Use of all native human pituitary–derived hormones (e.g. growth hormone), possible history of dura mater allograft (including unspecified intracranial surgery)
- Septicemia and systemic viral disease, mycosis, or active tuberculosis at the time of procurement (in the case of other active bacterial infections, tissues may be used only if they are processed for bacterial inactivation using a validated method and after approval by the medical director)
- Presence or history of malignant disease (exceptions may include primary basal cell carcinoma of the skin, histologically proven and unmetastatic primary brain tumor)
- Significant history of connective tissue disease (e.g. systemic lupus erythematosus and rheumatoid arthritis) or any immunosuppressive treatment
- Significant exposure to a toxic substance that may be transferred in toxic doses or damage the tissue (e.g. cyanide, lead, mercury, gold)
- Presence or evidence of infection or prior irradiation at the site of donation
- Unknown cause of death (if the cause of death is unknown at the time of death, then an autopsy shall be performed to establish this cause)

Physical examination

Prior to the procurement of tissue, the donor body shall be examined for general exclusion signs and for signs of infection, trauma, or medical intervention over donor sites that can affect the quality of the donated tissue.

Cadaveric donor autopsy report

If an autopsy is performed, the results shall be reviewed by the medical director or designee before the tissue is released for distribution.

Transmissible disease blood tests

Tissues shall be tested for transmissible diseases in compliance with the laws and practices of the country concerned. In the case of living donors, applicable consent procedures for blood testing shall be followed. Tests shall be performed and found acceptable on properly identified blood samples from the donor, using recognized and (if applicable) licensed tests according to the manufacturer's instructions. Tests shall be performed by a qualified and (if applicable) licensed laboratory according to Good Laboratory Practice (GLP).

Blood for donor testing should be drawn at or within 7 days of the donation, preferably within 24 h after death. For potential tissue donors who have received blood, blood components, or plasma volume expanders within 48 h prior to death, a pretransfusion blood sample shall be tested if there is an expected hemodilution of more than 50% (based on calculation algorithm).

The living donor or the cadaveric donor's next of kin or physician shall be notified in accordance with state laws of confirmed positive results having clinical significance. Confirmed positive donor infectious disease tests shall be reported to the local/national health authorities, when required.

A sample of donor serum shall be securely sealed and stored frozen in a proper manner until 5 years after the expiration date of the tissue or according to applicable intergovernmental, national, regional, and local law or regulation.

1. Blood tests

Minimum blood tests include the following:

- Human immunodeficiency virus 1/2 antibody (HIV-1/2 Ab) test
- Hepatitis B virus surface antigen (HBsAg) test
- Hepatitis C virus antibody (HCV Ab) test
- Syphilis test — nonspecific (e.g. VDRL) or preferably specific (e.g. TPHA)

Optional blood tests may be necessary for compliance with applicable intergovernmental, national, regional, and local law or regulation and/or to screen for endemic diseases:

- Hepatitis B core antibody (HBcAb) test — should be negative for tissue validation, although confirmation cascade can be entered if the HBcAb test is positive and the HBsAg test is negative. If antibodies against the surface antigen (HBsAb) are found, then the donor can be considered to have recovered from an infection and the tissue can be used for transplantation.
- Antigen test for HIV (p24 antigen) or HCV, or validated molecular biology test for HIV and HCV (e.g. PCR) — performed by an experienced laboratory

- HTLV-1 antibody test — depending on the prevalence in some regions
- Cytomegalovirus (CMV), Epstein–Barr virus (EBV), and toxoplasmosis antibody tests — for immunosuppressed patients
- Alanine aminotransferase (ALT) test — for living donors (in addition to the general testing requirements, testing living donors of tissue for ALT is recommended)

2. Living donor retesting
Retesting of living donors for HIV and HCV at 180 days is recommended. If another method of increasing safety rather than retesting (antigen testing, molecular biology testing, or viral inactivation method) is used and allowed by applicable regulation, it must be documented and validated.

3. Exclusion criteria
Positive results for HIV, hepatitis, and HTLV-1 are general reasons for exclusion. However, in specific life-threatening situations for the recipient (e.g. related HPC donation), positive results for hepatitis are no reason for exclusion in accordance with applicable regulations. In these situations, tissues with a higher risk for the recipient may be offered as long as full information is given to the recipient or (if it is not possible) to his/her relatives.

Bacteriological studies of donor and tissues

Representative samples of each retrieved tissue have to be cultured for bacteria if the tissues are to be aseptically processed without terminal sterilization. Samples shall be taken prior to exposure of the tissue to antibiotic-containing solution. The culture technique shall allow for the growth of both aerobic and anaerobic bacteria as well as fungi. Results shall be documented in the donor record.

If procurement is performed on a cadaver donor, blood cultures may be useful in evaluating the state of the cadaver and interpreting the cultures performed on the grafts themselves. They shall be reviewed by the medical director or designee.

If bacteriological testing of tissue samples obtained at the time of donation reveals a growth of low-virulence microorganisms, which are commonly considered nonpathogenic, the tissue may not be distributed without being further processed in a way that effectively decontaminates the tissue.

Tissue from which high-virulence microorganisms have been isolated are not acceptable for transplantation, unless the procedure has been validated to effectively inactivate the organisms without harmful potential effects (taking into account possible endotoxins).

Nonmicrobiological tests

Nonmicrobiological tests depend upon the tissues and cells to be transplanted. Hematopoietic progenitor cell donor selection requires the following as a minimum:

- ABO blood group and rhesus group
- Human leukocyte antigen (HLA) typing
- Whole blood cell count

Age criteria

Donor age criteria for each type of tissue shall be established and recorded by the tissue bank.

Cadaver donor retrieval time limits

Tissues shall be retrieved as soon after death as is practically possible. Specific time limits vary with each tissue obtained, and shall be determined by the medical director. Usually, the procurement of tissues should be completed within 12 h after death (or circulatory arrest if also an organ donor). If the body has been refrigerated within 4–6 h of death, procurement should preferably start within 24 h and no later than 48 h.

Quality Control (Hilmy 2005)

Quality control (QC) is part of the quality management system. It is concerned with sampling, specifications, and testing — as well as organizational, documentation, and release procedures — to ensure that the necessary and relevant tests are carried out, and that the products are not released for use until their quality has been judged satisfactory. QC is not only confined to laboratory operations, but must also be involved in all decisions that may concern the quality of products. The independence of QC personnel from production is considered fundamental to the satisfactory operation of QC.

Adequate trained resources must be available to ensure that all QC arrangements are effectively and reliably carried out. QC personnel should have access to all of the steps of production for sampling and investigation. The QC department as a whole also has other duties, such as to establish, validate, and implement all QC procedures; keep the reference samples of materials and products; ensure the correct labeling of containers of materials and products; ensure the monitoring of product stability; and participate in the investigation of complaints related to product quality.

Tests and procedures shall be performed to measure, assay, or monitor the processing, preservation, and storage methods as well as the equipment and reagents for compliance with established tolerance limits. The results of all such tests shall be recorded (PIC/S 2000). Several QC procedures that should be set up according to the American Association of Tissue Banks (AATB) are as follows:

- Environmental monitoring — including temperature, relative humidity, air quality, contamination control, and cleanliness in the processing room
- Equipment maintenance, calibration, and monitoring — should be carried out regularly, at least once a year
- Tolerance limits — i.e. the limits defining a range of acceptable values for each testing procedure that, when exceeded, require the implementation of corrective action
- In-process control monitoring — including final or intermediate sterilization
- Reagent and supply monitoring — including raw materials for allografts (e.g. quality of biological tissues after procurement)
- Laboratory performance monitoring

In small tissue banks with limited trained resources available, problems in implementing the QC program exist. In addition to the QC personnel, these tissue banks also face problems in the limited number of samples available for testing and evaluation.

The roles of the QC manager in tissue banking include (but are not limited to) the following:

- To ensure that the processed tissue grafts are reliable for clinical use
- To check all documents
- To evaluate all QC tests

Bacteria, yeast, fungi, and viruses can contaminate the tissues during procurement, processing, and storage, or directly from the donor's blood. Therefore, several steps should be taken to minimize the risk of infectious disease transmission by using allografts, e.g. serological screening of donors, processes such as demineralization and freeze-drying, pasteurization, sterilization by irradiation, as well as implementation of quality management system and Good Manufacturing Practice (GMP) in all steps of tissue banking activities. In order to prevent cross-contamination, the AATB (2002), the European Association of Tissue Banks (EATB 1995), the IAEA International Standards (2002), and the Therapeutic Goods Administration (TGA 2000) have prohibited the comingling of tissues from more than one donor during procurement/retrieval, processing, preservation, or storage. Tissue banks must prepare, validate, and follow written procedures (SOP manual) designed to prevent the transmission of infectious diseases during tissue processing.

The steps of activities in tissue banking that need to be controlled for quality are procurement; processing; preservation; storage; accuracy and reliability of the tissue bank's equipment and operational procedures; control of material; as well as the monitoring of supplies, equipment, and facilities (von Versen and Monig 2000; EATB 1995; AATB 2002).

Implementation of QC in tissue banking

Procurement

Procurement refers to the removal, acquisition, recovery, harvesting, and collection activities of donor cells and/or tissue. They are conducted by specially trained personnel in a clean room, and are procured from accepted donors. All of the activities should follow the written SOP manual, including environment control in the procurement area.

Before procurement, documentation on donor criteria as stated in the SOP manual should be evaluated (e.g. documentation on disease-transmitting agents HBsAg, HIV-1/2 Ab, HCV Ab). All procedures on disease-transmitting agents should be validated for suitable sensitivity and specificity. Surface swab tests for culturing contaminated microbes are done for each individually recovered or packaged tissue intended for transplantation, while a preprocessing culture shall be obtained prior to the exposure of cells and/or tissue to antibiotics, disinfectants, or sterilizing agents; and then the results shall be documented in the donor record. Cells and/or tissue contaminated with anaerobic spore-forming organisms shall be discarded, unless they can be processed in a manner that will eliminate the contaminant via a validated process (e.g. final sterilization by irradiation).

Methods of sampling tissues for culture, depending on the condition at each tissue bank, can be chosen from the following methods (Martinez 2002; ISO 11737-1, 1995b):

- Bone surface swab
- Medullary canal swab
- Bone segment immersion
- Complete bone wash or immersion

The wrapping materials for tissues after procurement should be sterilized, and the temperature during transportation from the procurement area to the tissue bank should be controlled. Each package should be labeled and coded (PIC/S 2000; EATB 1995; AATB 2002; IAEA 2002).

Quarantine

The tissues should be kept in a specified place at a specified temperature in accordance with the SOP manual until the swab test results and donor criteria are obtained. If the results are accepted, then the tissues can be processed. According to von Versen and Monig (2000), there are several quarantine steps:

1. Waiting for serological test and swab test results
2. Serological and swab test passed; waiting for preparation/processing
3. Processing finished; waiting for freeze-drying
4. Freeze-drying and packaging finished; waiting for final sterilization
5. Sterilization finished; waiting for sterile control or dosimetry release
6. Sterile control accepted; release for clinical application

Processing

Processing is defined as any activity other than procurement, donor screening, donor testing, storage, labeling, packaging, and distribution that is performed on cells and/or tissue-based products. It includes (but is not limited to) preparation such as the cutting and washing processes, as well as preservation for storage and/or removal from storage (e.g. from the freezing, lyophilization, or dehydration process) to assure the quality and/or sterility of cells and tissue.

The main criteria for an orthopedic allograft are the retention of strength, retention of biologic factors, and reduction of risk of disease transmission. The first two should not be affected by processing, while processing should eliminate the risk of disease transmission.

Several processing factors that might affect the graft's integrity and function are as follows:

1. Residue of processing reagents, such as water and chemicals, could have an adverse effect on allograft function and integrity. Therefore, procedures that use and remove the processing materials at a limited amount without affecting allograft function and integrity should be set up.
2. The physical and mechanical properties of grafts may be reduced due to processing steps such as lyophilization, freezing, heating, and sterilization.

   QC programs for monitoring the performance of lyophilizers/dehydrators should be documented. Either one representative sample for each type of dried tissue or duplicate cortical bone samples from each drier run shall be tested for residual moisture and residual reagents used during the processing.

   Tolerance limits should be fixed; for example, the tolerance limit for the moisture content of lyophilized samples is 5% ± 2% (i.e. minimum of 3% and maximum of 7%). If the tissue bank produces demineralized bones, the calcium content of the products should be controlled.

Mechanical devices used for processing activities (including storage) shall be subjected to no less than annual calibration in accordance with national standards. All critical procedures such as sterilization should be validated for their effectiveness according to the standards.

The validation of methods used for viral or bacterial removal/inactivation (such as pasteurization) should not be conducted in the production facilities so as not to put the routine manufacture at any risk of contamination with the viruses/bacteria used for validation (PIC/S 2000; EATB 1995; AATB 2002; IAEA 2002; TGA 2000).

The SOPs for the washing process should, whenever possible, be validated. More specifically, this means validating the washing of amnion membranes, other soft tissues, and bones to evaluate the residue of blood as well as the residue of chemical reagents and contaminating microbes (Hilmy *et al.* 2002).

Final prepackaging

All cells and/or tissue to be released for human transplantation shall have representative microbiological cultures obtained and the results documented in the donor record, unless dosimeter release has occurred by validated processes according to terminal tissue sterilization by irradiation. Dosimeter release is defined as the release of cells and/or tissues based on dosimetry instead of sterility control.

Microbiological testing of processed cells and/or tissue shall be performed on each donor lot. Skin samples shall be cultured for the presence of fast-growing fungal organisms (AATB 2002). Skin shall not be used for transplantation if any of the following is noted at final culture:

- *Staphylococcus aureus*
- *Streptococcus pyogenes*
- *Enterococcus* sp.
- Gram-negative organism
- *Clostridia* sp.
- Fungi (yeast or mold)

Samples taken for testing should be representative of the whole batch.

Packaging materials

The criteria of packaging materials used must be controlled for their suitability for the proposed purpose in accordance with national/international requirements. Certification should be obtained to show that the packaging material is suitable for storage over the desired period (e.g. expiration date) at room temperature and for certain sterilization processes (e.g. irradiation), not permeable to bacteria (von Versen and Monig 2000).

If cells and/or tissues to be shipped require specific environmental conditions other than ambient temperature, QC monitoring of shipping packaging must be performed according to the SOP manual in order to verify the maintenance of the required environmental conditions. These QC checks shall be documented (AATB 2002).

Retention samples

Where possible, samples of individual donors should be stored to facilitate any necessary look-back procedures.

Control of nonconformity products

It must be ensured that faulty allografts do not end up back in processing by mistake.

Control before product release for clinical application

The QC department should control all documents related to product quality, including (but not limited to) packaging, expiration date, and labeling. It should also ensure that all tests related to QC have been completed before product release.

Personnel

All personnel involved in the QC program must be trained in their specific responsibilities. To this end, training plans are created and documented. Although the number of staff involved in tissue banking is small, there should be separate people responsible for production and quality control.

Laboratory for quality control

QC laboratory premises and equipment should meet the requirements of standard use, including calibration of the instruments and maintenance of the equipment. Analytical methods according to the SOP manual should be validated.

Special attention should be given to the quality of laboratory reagents and culture media, which should be prepared in accordance with written procedures. Laboratory reagents intended for prolonged use should be marked with the preparation date and the signature of the person who prepared them. The expiry date of unstable reagents and culture media should be indicated on the label, together with specific storage conditions.

Contract analysis may be accepted, but this should be stated in the quality control record. Written sampling procedures should be prepared to ensure that the critical manufacturing steps from procurement to final product meet customer requirements and standards.

QC documentation entails the following (TGA 2000; OECD 1998):

- Product specifications
- Sampling procedures
- Testing procedures and records
- Data from environmental monitoring
- Validation records of test methods
- Records of calibration of instruments and maintenance of equipment

Validation of Radiation Sterilization Dose According to the IAEA Code of Practice (2004) (see chapter 19; Hilmy *et al.* 2006)

The validation process is the establishment of documented evidence, which provides a high degree of assurance that a specific process will consistently produce a product meeting its predetermined specifications and quality attributes. Although international standards — e.g. ISO 11137 (1995a), ISO 13409 (1996), ISO 11737-2 (1998), and AAMI TIR 27 (2001) — have been established for the radiation sterilization of healthcare products (including medical devices, medicinal products, and *in vitro* diagnostic products), not all of them can be applied for the validation of the radiation sterilization dose (RSD) of tissue allografts. Problems in using ISO 11137 (1995a) and ISO 11737-2 (1998) for tissue allografts are limited numbers of uniform products per production batch size, and whether these low numbers of samples can be used for sterilization dose-setting purposes.

A tissue allograft is a graft transplanted between two different individuals of the same species. They are not commercially produced products involving a large number of samples. The size and type of products vary from long bones and cancellous chips to bone powders, cartilages, tendons, ligaments, heart valves, vessels, fascias, skin, and amnions. Compared to healthcare products, the variability in types and levels of bioburden is much greater in tissue allografts; therefore, the number of bioburden per production batch cannot be treated equally. Bioburden is defined as the total number of viable contaminant microbes (bacteria, yeast, and mold) on packaged products before sterilization, excluding viral contamination (ISO 11137, 1995). Frozen samples cannot be considered as part of the same production batch as lyophilized/freeze-dried samples because of different processing and irradiation temperatures.

One of the major differences between tissue allografts and other health-care products is the possibility of viral contamination in tissues obtained from a donor, thus transmitting the virus from donor to recipient. Most of those contaminated viruses can be eliminated by strict donor screening. Viral screening on donors is done according to the IAEA International Standards for Tissue Banks (2002), and includes screening for HIV, hepatitis B virus, hepatitis C virus, and pathogenic bacteria.

According to the IAEA Code of Practice (2004), validation of the processes prior to radiation sterilization includes the following:

- Qualification of tissue bank facilities
- Qualification of tissue donors
- Qualification of tissue processing and preservation
- Certification procedures to review and approve documentation of the above three qualifications
- Maintenance of validation
- Process specification

Implementation of the qualifications can be done according to the IAEA Standards (2002).

The aim of using radiation sterilization as the terminal sterilization for tissue allografts is to minimize the risk of disease transmission from donor to recipient by eliminating contaminant bacteria and viruses (Hilmy and Lina 2001). Several tissue bank standards, such as the AATB (2002) and EATB (1995), recommend 15 kGy as the minimum dose for bacterial decontamination and 25 kGy as the minimum dose for bacterial sterilization; all of these doses should be validated.

ISO 13409 (1996) has been successfully used to validate an RSD of 25 kGy for tissue allografts produced from one cadaver donor, but this standard cannot be used to validate an RSD lower than 25 kGy (Hilmy *et al.* 2000; Hilmy *et al.* 2003). The RSD can be lower than 25 kGy if the bioburden can be reduced by strictly applying Good Manufacturing Practices (PIC/S 2000) and Quality Management System (ISO 9000, 2000) in each processing step. The lower RSD will protect the radiosensitive polymeric and valuable biological materials (growth factors) of tissues from degradation (Hilmy 2005; Yusof 2005).

According to the IAEA Code of Practice (2004), there are four methods that can be used to determine the RSD: method A1, a modification of method 1 of ISO 11137 (1995a); method A2, based on knowledge of the different proportions of contaminated microbes and their respected D_{10} values; method B, for substantiation of 25 kGy as the RSD (ISO 13409, 1996); and method C, for substantiation of 25 kGy as the RSD (AAMI TIR 27, 2001). Depending on the bioburden level of the product, method A1 can be applied to validate an RSD lower than 25 kGy at sterility assurance level (SAL) values between 10^{-2} and 10^{-1} of Table 1 of ISO 11137 (1995a). It can be found for bioburden levels up to 1000 CFU per allograft product. The SAL values correspond to a relatively small sample size of 10–100. It should be noted that for this method, low bioburden levels combined with low sample numbers will give rise to an increased probability of failure of the validation dose (VD) experiment. In the event of VD experiment failure for method A1, methods B and C may decrease the risk and the RSD would be 25 kGy. The amount of RSD depends on the number of bioburden to be used for determinating the VD.

The radiation process can be used to sterilize amnion grafts in their final package. Validation of the radiation sterilization dose (RSD) can be done according to the IAEA Code of Practice (2004), which lists three methods: method A1 or A2 (IAEA Code 2004), method B (ISO 13409, 1996), and method C (AAMI TIR 27, 2001). These standards are for small or infrequent production batches, namely products with an average bioburden less than 1000 CFU and manufactured in small quantities (i.e. less than 1000 product units per batch). These categories are relevant to the tissue bank products. Viral contaminations are excluded from all of these standards. To overcome viral contamination problems, tissues should be well screened (IAEA/NUS 1997; IAEA 2002; Hilmy *et al.* 2000).

Experiences in using the IAEA Code of Practice (2004) to determine the radiation sterilization dose have been presented by Hilmy *et al.* (2006). In October 2006, ISO 13409 (1996) was replaced by AAMI TIR 27 (2001) and ISO 11137 (1995a) was replaced by a new version of ISO 11137 (2006).

Labeling

Tissue container labeling

Tissue containers shall be labeled so as to identify, as a minimum, the following:

- The human nature of the contents
- Product description
- Name and address of the tissue bank
- Tissue identification number
- Expiration date
- Amount of tissue in the container expressed as volume, weight, dimension, or a combination of these as needed, for an accurate description of the contents
- Sterilization by irradiation accompanied by "go/no-go" indicator
- Batch number, if applicable
- Recommended storage conditions

Package insert

All tissues shall be accompanied by a document describing the nature of the tissue as well as the processing methods and instructions for proper storage and reconstitution, when appropriate. Specific instructions shall be enclosed with tissues that require special handling.

Accompanying documentation requirements

Accompanying documentation shall contain all of the information described for container labeling and the following additional information:

- Origin of tissue (country of procurement)
- The nature and results of biological tests performed on the donor using appropriate and licensed tests
- Processing methods used and the results of sterility tests or inactivation controls
- Special instructions indicated by the particular tissue for storage or implantation (tissue that is to be reconstituted at or prior to the time of use shall include information on the conditions under which such tissue shall be stored and reconstituted prior to implantation)

- Indications and contraindications for use of tissue, when necessary
- Statement that each tissue shall only be used for a single patient

References

American Association of Tissue Banks (AATB) (2002). Standards for Tissue Banking, AATB, McLean, VA.

Association for the Advancement of Medical Instrumentation (AAMI) (2001). Sterilization of Health Care Products — Radiation Sterilization — Substantiation of 25 kGy as a Sterilization Dose — Method V_{Dmax}, AAMI TIR 27, 2001, McLean, VA.

Busch MP and Kleinman SH (2000). Nuclear acid amplification testing and disease transmission. *Transfusion* **40**:143–146.

European Association of Tissue Banks (EATB) (1995). General Standards for Tissue Banking, OBIG Transplant, Vienna.

Hilmy N (2005). Quality control issue in tissue banking. In: Nather A (ed.), *Bone Grafts and Bone Substitutes*, World Scientific, Singapore, pp. 173–187.

Hilmy N, Febrida A, and Basril A (2000). Validation of radiation sterilization dose for lyophilized amnion and bone graft. *Cell Tissue Bank* **1**(2):143–148.

Hilmy N, Febrida A, and Basril A (2002), Validation of washing process of amnion membranes for amnion grafts. In: *9th International Conference on Tissue Banking*, (APASTB), Seoul, Korea (to be published).

Hilmy N, Febrida A, and Basril A (2003). Indonesia: statistical sampling technique in validation of radiation sterilization dose of biological tissue. *Cell Tissue Bank* **4**(2):185–191.

Hilmy N, Febrida A, and Basril A (2006). Experiences in using the IAEA Code of Practice for the Radiation Sterilization of Tissue Allografts: Validation and Routine Control. In: *Proc 14th International Meeting of Radiation Processing (IMRP) 2006*, Kuala Lumpur, Malaysia.

Hilmy N and Lina M (2001). Effects of ionizing radiation on viruses, proteins and prions. In: Phillips GO, Strong DM, von Versen R, and Nather A (eds.), *Advances in Tissue Banking*, Vol. 5, World Scientific, Singapore, pp. 358–375.

International Atomic Energy Agency (IAEA) (2002). International Standards for Tissue Banks, IAEA, Vienna.

International Atomic Energy Agency (IAEA) (2004). Code of Practice for the Radiation Sterilization of Tissue Allografts, IAEA, Vienna.

International Atomic Energy Agency and National University of Singapore (IAEA/NUS) (1997). Module 4: Procurement. Multimedia Distance Learning Package on Tissue Banking, Interregional Training Centre, Singapore.

International Standards Organization (ISO) (1995a). Sterilization of Health Care Products — Requirements for Validation and Routine Control — Radiation Sterilization, ISO 11137, 1995, Geneva.

International Standards Organization (ISO) (1995b). Sterilization of Medical Devices — Microbiological Methods — Part 1: Determination of a Population of Microorganisms on Products, ISO 11737-1, 1995, Geneva.

International Standards Organization (ISO) (1996). Sterilization of Health Care Products — Radiation Sterilization — Substantiation of 25 kGy as a Sterilization Dose for Small or Infrequent Production Batches, ISO 13409, 1996, Geneva.

International Standards Organization (ISO) (1998). Sterilization of Medical Devices — Microbiological Methods — Part 2: Tests of Sterility Performed in the Validation of a Sterilization Process, ISO 11737-2, 1998, Geneva.

International Standards Organization (ISO) (2000). Quality Management Systems — Requirements, ISO 9000, 2000, Geneva.

International Standards Organization (ISO) (2006). Sterilization of Health Care Products — Requirements for Validation and Routine Control — Radiation Sterilization, ISO 11137, 2006, Geneva.

Martinez O (2002). Microbiologic screening of cadaver donors and tissues for transplantation. In: *AATB Conference*, Boston, MA.

Organization for Economic Cooperation and Development (OECD) (1998). Principles of Good Laboratory Practice, OECD, Paris.

Pharmaceutical Inspection Convention and Pharmaceutical Inspection Cooperation Scheme (PIC/S) (2000). Guide to Good Manufacturing Practice for Medicinal Products, PIC/S, Geneva.

Therapeutic Goods Administration (TGA) (2000). Australian Code of Good Manufacturing Practice — Human Blood and Tissues, TGA, Woden, ACT, Australia.

von Versen R and Monig HJ (2000). Quality management systems in tissue banking. In: Phillips GO, Strong DM, von Versen R, and Nather A (eds.), *Advances in Tissue Banking*, Vol. 4, World Scientific, Singapore, pp. 1–24.

Yusof N (2005). Is the irradiation dose of 25 kGy enough to sterilize tissue grafts? In: Nather A (ed.), *Bone Grafts and Bone Substitutes*, World Scientific, Singapore, pp. 189–212.

PART V.

CLINICAL APPLICATIONS OF IRRADIATED BONE GRAFTS

Chapter 21

Clinical Applications of Gamma-Irradiated Deep-Frozen and Lyophilized Bone Allografts — The NUH Tissue Bank Experience

Aziz Nather*, Kamarul Ariffin Khalid† and Zameer Aziz*

**NUH Tissue Bank*
Department of Orthopaedic Surgery
Yong Loo Lin School of Medicine
National University of Singapore
Singapore

†Department of Orthopaedics, Traumatology and Rehabilitation
Kulliyah of Medicine
International Islamic University Malaysia
Malaysia

Introduction

Gamma-irradiated deep-frozen (−80°C) large cortical bone allografts as well as gamma-irradiated morselized, freeze-dried, corticocancellous or cancellous bone strips/chips remain an important option for filling large and small bone defects in orthopedic surgery. Autografts are the preferred option, but there are limitations to using autografts, including the size, shape, and quantity of bone needed for the reconstruction as well as the complications from harvesting autografts from iliac crest (e.g. persistent donor site pain, hematoma formation, donor site infection) (Montgomery *et al.* 1990). Thus, there is a need for a good tissue bank that processes bone allografts of high quality by conforming to standards comparable to those of the American Association of Tissue Banks (AATB) and the European Association of Tissue Banks (EATB).

In Singapore, the NUH Tissue Bank — which follows the IAEA/Asia-Pacific Association of Surgical Tissue Banking Standards comparable to those of the AATB and EATB — is the national musculoskeletal tissue bank providing bone and soft tissue allografts to all hospitals in the country. Gamma irradiation at a dosage of 25 kGy is used as the final end-sterilization step in its processing techniques. Femoral heads and morselized lyophilized bones are irradiated in a gamma chamber in the Department of Nuclear Medicine, Singapore General Hospital. The long bones are gamma irradiated in a cobalt-60 plant at the Malaysian Nuclear Agency (NM) in Bangi by Dr Norimah Yusof (Nather and Thambiah 1996).

The bank requires informed consent from all recipients before the tissues are distributed to surgeons. Patients are informed that the products are not free of disease transmission. The risk of HIV transmission for deep-frozen bones is about 1 in 1 000 000 compared to 1 in 250 000 for blood transfusions. The risk is zero for lyophilized bone allografts. There is no risk of hepatitis C transmission, since a 25-kGy dose of gamma irradiation inactivates the hepatitis C virus.

The bank also provides a catalog of available products and instructions on how the grafts should be prepared and used. When new surgeons use them for the first time, the director joins the surgery team to make sure that the surgeon prepares the grafts adequately and uses them appropriately.

Preparation of Gamma-Irradiated Deep-Frozen Large Bone Allografts

The femur or tibia in its "triple wrap" (Nather 2000a) must be thawed at least 1 h before the start of the operation. A separate donor team and a separate donor trolley are needed to prepare the allografts adequately. The outer layer (plastic) is opened and the bone, wrapped in inner (plastic) and middle (linen) layers, is passed by the circulating nurse to the donor team. The bone is soaked in a large basin containing 1–2 L of normal saline with 1 g of ampicillin and 1 g of cloxacillin. The donor team starts preparing the graft by completely removing all soft tissues (including muscles and periosteum) off the bone. For intercalary grafts, the end of the bones are then osteotomized with an oscillating saw and the medullary contents meticulously removed using a manual intramedullary reamer. All blood and bone marrow must be removed. Next, the bone is mechanically flushed with normal saline using jet lavage to make sure that all soft tissues, marrow, and blood have been completely removed, as the latter are immunogenic. The cleaned bone that has been cut to its required dimensions is then soaked in a new basin containing new normal saline with 1 g of ampicillin and 1 g of cloxacillin.

Preparation of Gamma-Irradiated Deep-Frozen Femoral Heads for Spinal Fusion

The circulating nurse opens the outer jar of the "double jar technique" (Nather 2000a) to pass the inner jar to the donor team. The team opens the inner jar and soaks the femoral head in a kidney dish of saline containing antibiotics (ampicillin and cloxacillin). After thawing, all of the cartilage is meticulously removed from the head. The head is then cut into about four small pieces, which are jet lavaged with saline to remove all soft tissues, marrow, and blood. The bone pieces are then passed through a bone mill to produce smaller pieces. These are mixed with autografts to provide a 50% mix (50% allografts and 50% autografts) that is ready to be placed on the prepared raw spinal bed for spinal fusion.

Preparation of Gamma-Irradiated Lyophilized Bone Allografts

The outer layer of the vacuum-packed graft is removed by the circulating nurse and passed to the donor team. The donor team removes the pieces of bone from the inner layer. The bones are reconstituted in a small amount of saline containing antibiotics (ampicillin and cloxacillin) 5 to 10 min before their use.

Selecting the Appropriate Allografts

Gamma-irradiated, deep-frozen cortical allografts must be used for the reconstruction of large cortical bone defects, especially in the lower limbs where functional weight-bearing is required immediately after the surgery. Nather *et al.* (2004) showed that gamma-irradiated deep-frozen allografts exhibited 64% maximum torque strength of normal bone strength in adult rabbits *in vivo* at 24 weeks. Care must therefore be taken by the surgeon by using the strongest implant for the reconstruction, i.e. fluted interlocking nails rather than plating where possible to prevent the allograft from fracturing.

In contrast, gamma-irradiated lyophilized cortical allografts were significantly weaker than deep-frozen allografts, with only 12% maximum torque strength at 6 months (one fifth of the strength of deep-frozen allografts) (Nather *et al.* 2004). Irradiated, lyophilized bone allografts can only be used as "fillers" for filling bone defects and not for structural functions requiring weight loading. Clinical applications include filling bone cysts, elevating calcaneal fractures, elevating bumper fractures, etc.

By using the correct allografts for the various applications and by using high-quality bone grafts, the incidence of complications can be minimized.

Clinical Applications

Between October 1988 and December 2005, a total of 854 bone and soft tissue transplantations were performed using allografts procured and processed by the NUH Tissue Bank (Nather 2004). Of these, 238 were of soft tissue allograft transplantations. As the NUH Tissue Bank protocol does not gamma irradiate soft tissue allografts, these were excluded from the following study.

As shown in Table 1, a total of 616 gamma-irradiated musculoskeletal bone transplantations were performed during the abovementioned period. Of these, 184 were performed for spinal surgery, 123 for hip surgery, 75 for malignant bone lesions, 28 for benign bone lesions, and 88 for bone trauma. These transplantations were carried out at the National University Hospital, Tan Tock Seng Hospital, Singapore General Hospital, Alexandra Hospital, Kandang Kerbau Women's and Children's Hospital, Changi General Hospital, and private hospitals in Singapore (Mt. Elizabeth Hospital, Mt. Alvernia Hospital, and Gleneagles Hospital).

Spinal surgery

Deep-frozen femoral head allografts were used for posterior spinal fusion in 132 cases. Indications included degenerative stenosis, degenerative spondylolisthesis, burst fractures, idiopathic scoliosis, congenital scoliosis, and secondary cord compression. Pure autografts were used for facet joint fusions. The bulk of the decorticated and freshened spinal fusion bed was then packed with allografts and used as a 50% mix with autografts (Nather 2000b). Figure 1 shows a posterior spinal fusion using allografts for a burst

Table 1. The number of gamma-irradiated bone transplantations performed.

Indication	No. of cases
Spine surgery	
— Posterior spinal fusion	132
— Anterior spinal fusion	52
Hip surgery	
— Revision total hip replacement	113
— Primary total hip replacement	10
Knee surgery	
— Revision total knee replacement	10
— Knee arthrodesis	6
Malignant bone lesion	
— Massive bone reconstruction	57
— Curettage and bone grafting	18
Benign bone lesion	28
Trauma	
— Calcaneal fracture	20
— Tibial condyle fracture	18
— Periprosthetic fracture	25
— Other fractures	25
Other bone lesions (including maxillofacial lesion)	102
Total	616

fracture at lumbar 3 vertebra. Of the 132 cases, 9 (6.8%) encountered complications: 2 with deep infections, 2 with superficial infections, and 5 with pseudoarthroses with implant failure (Nather 2004).

Anterior spinal fusions using allografts with lyophilized femoral cortical rings were performed in 52 cases. Indications included burst fractures, osteoporotic burst fractures, and secondary spinal cord compression. Figure 2 shows a case of anterior reconstruction for metastasis to the spine secondary to renal cell carcinoma at lumbar 2 vertebra. No infection was seen in all 52 cases. However, one case developed persistent serous discharge from the thoracic wound following reconstruction for a burst fracture of the first lumbar vertebra. The discharge settled after 2 weeks (Nather 2004).

Hip surgery

Gamma-irradiated lyophilized cortical or corticocancellous allografts were used in 123 cases, of which 113 were for revision total hip replacement.

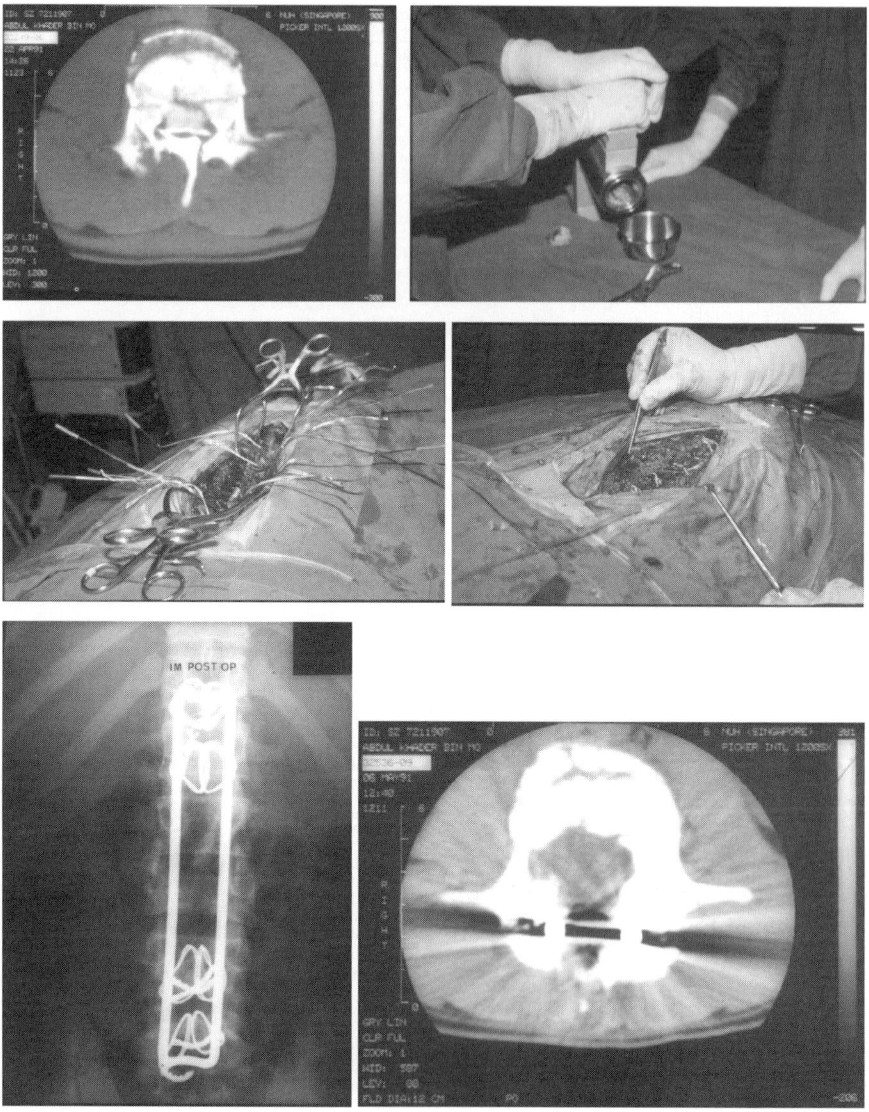

Fig. 1. A posterior spinal fusion using femoral head allografts for a burst fracture at lumbar 3 vertebra.

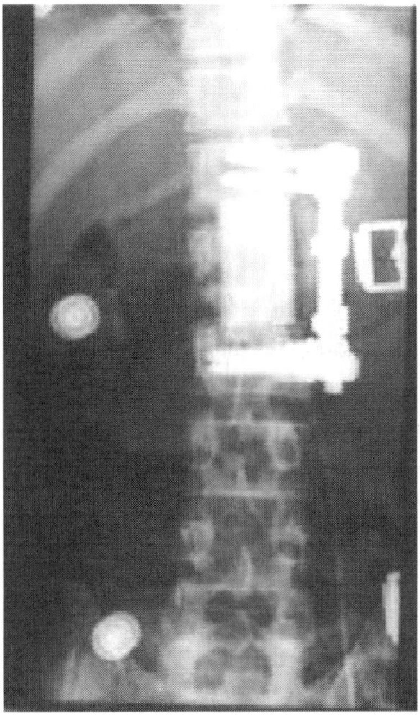

Fig. 2. A case of anterior reconstruction for metastasis to the spine secondary to renal cell carcinoma at lumbar 2 vertebra, using a lyophilized femoral cortical ring and Kaneda instrumentation.

Figure 3 shows a cortical onlay strut allograft being used for revision total hip surgery. No complications were encountered with hip surgery.

Malignant bone lesions

Out of 57 cases of massive bone reconstruction for limb salvage surgery, 6 (10.5%) complications were encountered. These included two with non-salvagable deep infections requiring above-knee amputations, and four superficial infections that were successfully treated (Nather 2004).

Benign bone lesions

Curettage and bone grafting were performed in 28 cases. Figure 4 shows allografts being used for a simple bone cyst.

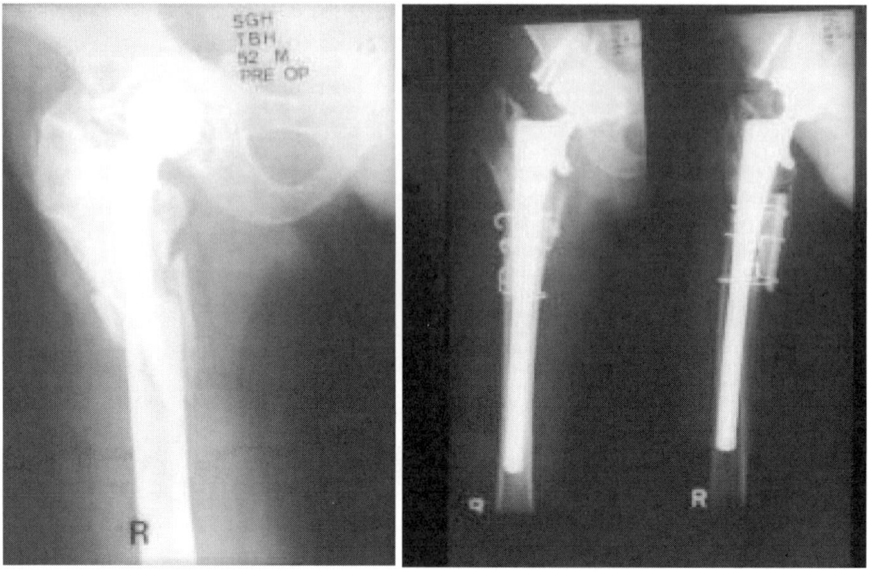

Fig. 3. A cortical onlay strut allograft being used for revision total hip surgery.

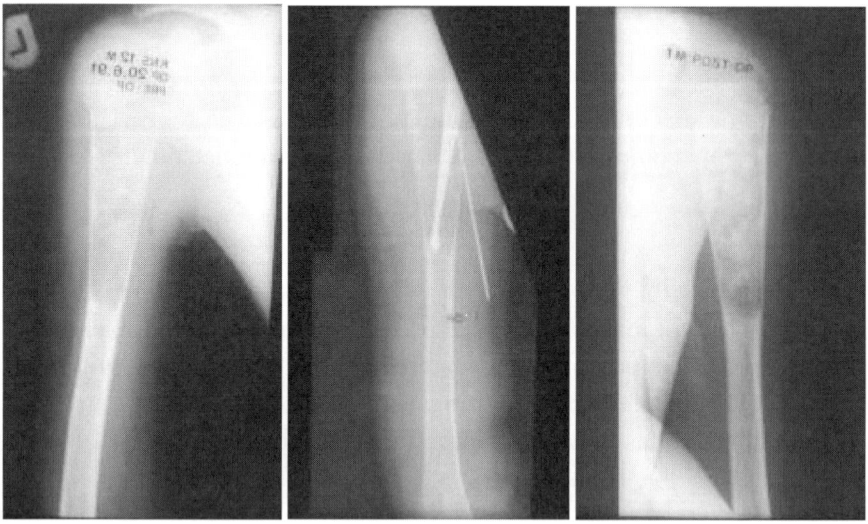

Fig. 4. Femoral head allografts being used for a simple bone cyst.

Trauma surgery

Gamma-irradiated lyophilized corticocancellous allografts were commonly used to elevate depressed calcaneal fractures. Figures 5 and 6 show their use in depressed tibial condyle fractures and depressed calcaneal fractures, respectively.

Complications from gamma-irradiated bone allografts

Complications were encountered in 19 (3.1%) of the 616 gamma-irradiated bone allografts transplanted — a good outcome. A higher (10.5%) complication rate was found with massive bone reconstruction for tumors in the limbs. This is expected for major surgery, where the complication rate (even without using gamma-irradiated allografts) is in the range of 10%–20%.

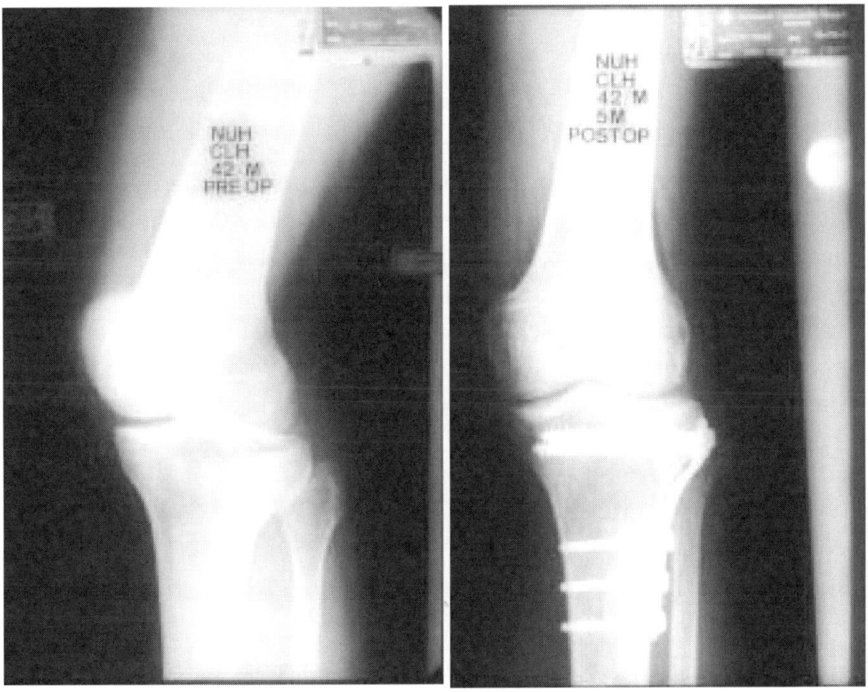

Fig. 5. The use of lyophilized corticocancellous allografts in depressed tibial condyle fractures.

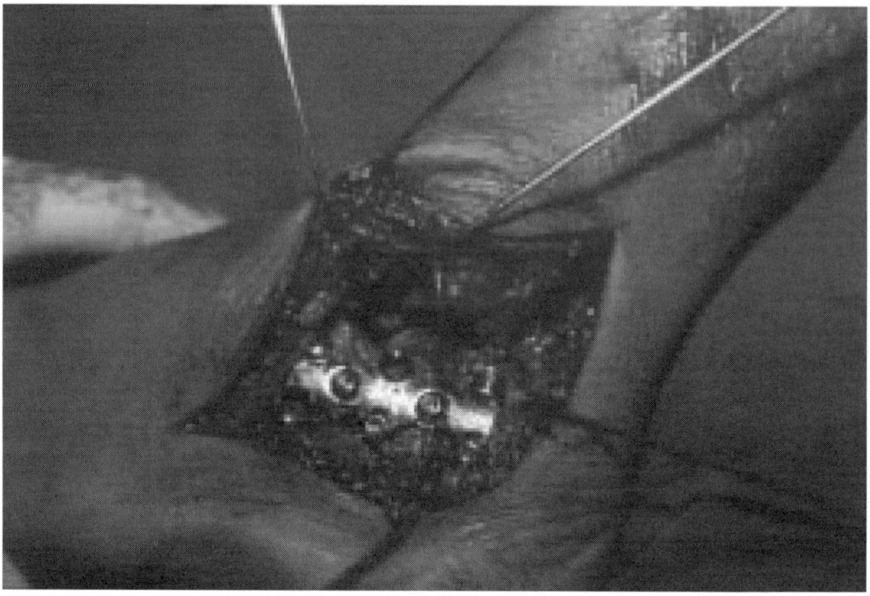

Fig. 6. The use of corticocancellous allografts in depressed calcaneal fractures.

Conclusion

Gamma-irradiated bone allografts, both deep-frozen and freeze-dried, have a definite role to play in orthopedic surgery. To reduce the number of complications, a tissue bank providing high-quality tissue allografts as well as experience in choosing the correct allografts for each indication are needed. The technical expertise of the surgeon performing the transplantation is also important. The indications for the use of such grafts are diverse, ranging from spine surgery, hip surgery, knee surgery, and trauma surgery to many other conditions in orthopedic surgery.

References

Montgomery DM, Aronson DD, Lee CL, and LaMont RL (1990). Posterior spinal fusion: allograft versus autograft bone. *J Spinal Dis* **3**:370–375.

Nather A (2000a). Procurement systems and availability. In: Phillips GO (ed.), *Radiation and Tissue Banking*, World Scientific, Singapore, pp. 263–288.

Nather A (2000b). Use of allografts in spinal surgery in Singapore. In: Phillips GO, von Versen R, and Nather A (eds.), *Advances in Tissue Banking*, Vol. 4, World Scientific, Singapore, pp. 149–167.

Nather A (2004). Musculoskeletal tissue banking in Singapore: 15 years of experience (1988–2003). *J Orthop Surg* **12**:184–190.

Nather A and Thambiah J (1996). Allografts for spinal surgery. In: Czitrom AA and Winkler H (eds.), *Orthopaedic Allograft Surgery*, Springer-Verlag, Wien, pp. 203–210.

Nather A, Thambyah A, and Goh JCH (2004). Biomechanical strength of deep-frozen versus lyophilized large cortical allografts. *Clin Biomech* **19**:526–533.

Chapter 22

Use of Freeze-Dried Irradiated Bones in Orthopedic Surgery

Ferdiansyah

Biomaterial Center – "Dr Soetomo" Tissue Bank
Department of Orthopaedics and Traumatology
Dr Soetomo General Hospital
Airlangga University School of Medicine, Surabaya
Indonesia

Introduction

The development of tissue banks in Indonesia began in around 1990. In 1986, the National Nuclear Energy Agency (BATAN) set up the country's first tissue bank in Jakarta, BATAN Research Tissue Bank (BRTB), and carried out research on the preservation of fresh amnion or fetal membranes by lyophilization and then by sterilization via gamma irradiation. In 1992, Dr Soetomo General Hospital, Surabaya, set up a bone bank producing frozen bones sterilized by ethylene oxide. In 2000, it was renamed the Biomaterial Center – "Dr Soetomo" Tissue Bank and started producing a variety of radiation-sterilized tissues, including fresh-frozen and freeze-dried bone, fresh-frozen and freeze-dried amniotic membrane, fresh-frozen and freeze-dried tendon, and fresh-frozen and freeze-dried fascia. There are currently five tissue banks in Indonesia: Dr Jamil Hospital, Padang; Sitanala Leprosy Hospital, Tangerang; Prof Dr Soeharso Orthopaedic Hospital, Solo; Dr Soetomo Tissue Bank; and BRTB.

Bone tissues can be sourced from both cadaveric and living donors. However, cadaveric donors are still limited in number because of cultural, religious, and ethical problems. Although the Indonesian Council of Ulamas

(MUI) issued guidance or fatwa on the recovery and transplantation of tissues, problems in obtaining donors still exist. The Biomaterial Center – "Dr Soetomo" Tissue Bank is developing a donation system for obtaining tissues; at present, it has secured donor candidates. Living donors are still the main source of bones, usually from orthopedic surgical procedures (head of femur bone from osteotomization) and primary traumatic amputations of the limb.

Before tissue banks were set up in Indonesia, orthopedic surgeons used commercial allograft or bone substitute products; unfortunately, the price was too high for most Indonesian people. This condition became a challenge for orthopedic surgeons and other scientists to develop tissue banks in Indonesia. However, following the development of tissue banks and campaigns by tissue bankers, the demand for both fresh-frozen and freeze-dried allografts has been high in recent years.

Procurement, Processing, and Radiation Sterilization

Procurement and processing

Bone from a living donor is taken from the hospital after the patient has signed the consent form and been screened (medical history, physical examination, and laboratory tests) by tissue bank staff. At the Dr Soetomo Tissue Bank, cadaveric bones are procured in sterile condition in the surgical room of the Forensic Department by tissue bank staff, and are then placed in a quarantine freezer in the tissue bank while waiting for the screening (laboratory) results.

Freeze-drying or lyophilization is the process of removing water from frozen samples via sublimation, i.e. the conversion of substances such as water from solid (crystalline) state to vapor state. The objective of freeze-drying is to obtain a chemically stable product at room temperature and to preserve the properties of the tissue, so that the tissue can be kept easily at room temperature and then distributed to the user after being sterilized. The freeze-drying procedure is usually divided into three stages: freezing of the tissue, primary drying by sublimation of the ice, and finally secondary drying by application of heat (IAEA/NUS 1997). The final product must not have a residual moisture content more than 7% of the dry weight. The method to determine the residual moisture is by gravimetry: after freeze-drying, the dried tissue is weighed daily on an analytical balance at 70°C until no further changes in weight are detected.

Packaging is done by wrapping the product in three layers of polyethylene plastic film in a laminar outflow cabinet and then sealing it in a vacuum sealer machine.

Radiation sterilization

At the BRTB, all freeze-dried tissue products (including bone grafts) are sterilized with gamma ray radiation using a radiation sterilization dose of 25 kGy (2.5 Mrad).

Properties of Freeze-Dried Bone

Biomechanical properties

Freeze-dried bone grafts are weaker than deep-frozen grafts. A comparison of the compression strength of freeze-dried gamma-irradiated dowel grafts from the iliac crest with identical dowel grafts obtained from fresh cadavers after reconstitution with normal saline showed that the compression strength of the former was only 50% of normal strength after 5 min of reconstitution and only 20% of normal strength after 8 min (Nather *et al.* 1987). Other research showed that the compressive strength of the bone is not modified after being freeze-dried (Bright and Burchardt 1983; Pelker *et al.* 1983), but freeze-dried cortical bone produces a significant deleterious reduction in the torsional strength of the long bone (Pelker *et al.* 1983) and in bending (Triantaphyllou *et al.* 1975). The combination of freeze-drying and irradiation causes an even more pronounced effect for compression, bending, and torsional strength, with the decrease varying from 10% to 70% (Komender 1976; Bright and Burchardt 1983; Pelker *et al.* 1983; Triantaphyllou *et al.* 1975). Consequently, freeze-dried bone grafts are rarely used as structural bone grafts; instead, they are mostly used as morselized bones to pack the cavities or gaps in the bone.

Biological properties

The biology of bone grafts and their substitutes can be appreciated from an understanding of the bone formation process as follows:

- Osteogenesis — the cellular elements within a donor graft that enable transplant survival and synthesization of the new bone at the recipient site.

- Osteoinduction — new bone realized through the active recruitment of host mesenchymal stem cells from the surrounding tissue that differentiate into bone-forming osteoblasts. This process is facilitated by the presence of growth factors within the graft, principally bone morphogenetic proteins (BMPs).
- Osteoconduction — the facilitation of blood-vessel incursion and new-bone formation into a defined passive trellis structure.

Freeze-dried bone grafts have osteoinductive, but not osteoconductive, properties. On the other hand, demineralized bone grafts have both osteoinductive and osteoconductive properties (Urist 1994; IAEA/NUS 1997; Delloye 1999; Strong and MacKenzie 1993; Reddi 2001; Yim 1999).

The sources of antigen in bone include noncellular antigens of the extracellular matrix (e.g. collagen together with noncollagenous proteins) as well as cells expressing the major histocompatibility antigens. The primary cause of the host immune response in bone allograft transplantation is the bone marrow cells, especially leukocytes. The reduction or removal of such cells by processing, freezing, freeze-drying, or irradiation reduces these cellular elements and thus lowers the likelihood of an immune response (IAEA/NUS 1997; Strong and MacKenzie 1993).

The comparative properties of bone grafts are shown in Table 1.

Table 1. Comparative properties of bone grafts (AAOS 2002).

Bone graft	Structural strength	Osteoconduction	Osteoinduction	Osteogenesis
Autograft				
• Cancellous	No	+++	+++	+++
• Cortical	+++	++	++	++
Cancellous allograft				
• Frozen	No	++	+	No
• Freeze-dried	No	++	+	No
Cortical allograft				
• Frozen	+++	+	No	No
• Freeze-dried	+	+	No	No
Demineralized freeze-dried allograft	No	+	++	No

Types of bone grafts

There are many types of bone products produced by tissue banks in Indonesia to fulfill the demand from surgeons. These include the following:

1. Human bone
   (a) Freeze-dried tissue
      i. Calvarial bone (bicortical)
      ii. Costae
      iii. Ilium (tricortical and bicortical)
      iv. Cortical strut graft (fibula and costae)
      v. Cortical chip
      vi. Cancellous chip
      vii. Bone powder
   (b) Demineralized tissue
      i. Cortical chip and powder
      ii. Cancellous chip and powder
2. Bovine bone
   (a) Cancellous chip
   (b) Bone powder
   (c) Eyeball

Clinical Application

Several indications for using freeze-dried bone allografts are to promote nonunion healing, promote spinal fusion, fill cavities after curettage of benign bone tumors, etc.

In tumor surgery, after curettage or resection of benign bone tumors (e.g. enchondroma, giant cell tumor, aneurysmal bone cyst, osteoblastoma, fibrous dysplasia, nonossifying fibroma), reconstruction can be done with freeze-dried bone allografts. In this case, allografts are mainly used to fill up cavities and maintain structural support (Gitelis and McDonald 1998; Wilkins 2002).

The Biomaterial Center – "Dr Soetomo" Tissue Bank serves about 42 hospitals in Indonesia (Fig. 1). Like other tissue banks in Indonesia, the center faces problems in donor supply, and so it also produces freeze-dried bovine bones as a bone substitute. The production of freeze-dried bovine

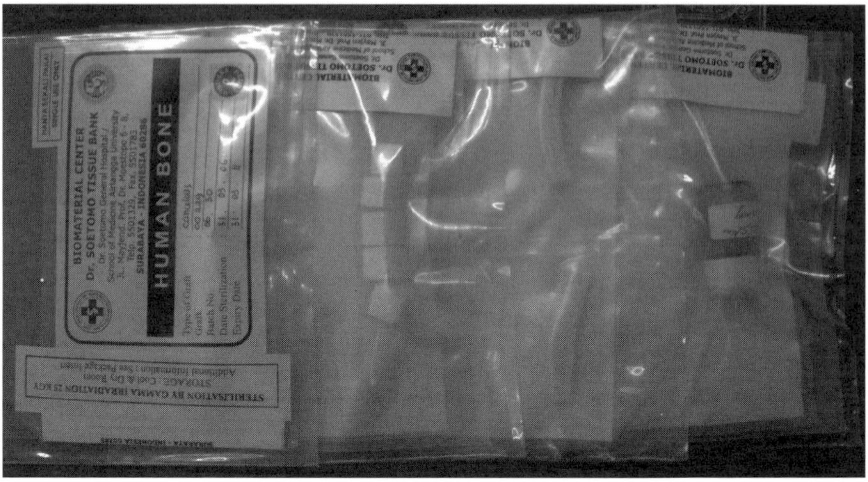

Fig. 1. Freeze-dried allografts packed with three layers of polyethylene plastic and sterilized by gamma ray irradiation at 25 kGy (Biomaterial Center, Dr Soetomo General Hospital, Surabaya, Indonesia).

bones is greater than that of freeze-dried human bones. The distribution of freeze-dried bone grafts for clinical application at Dr Soetomo General Hospital from 2002 to 2005 is shown in Table 2.

To achieve optimum results in bone tumor management, the window for curettage should be as large as possible so that the surgeon can see the full cavity. After removing the tumor tissue from the bone, intraoperative

Table 2. Distribution of freeze-dried human bone grafts for clinical application at Dr Soetomo General Hospital from 2002 to 2005.

	Cases	No. of cases
Benign bone tumors	Giant cell tumor	15
	Aneurysmal bone cyst	7
	Osteoblastoma	3
	Simple bone cyst	4
	Fibrous dysplasia	3
Trauma	Bone graft in fracture	67
	Delayed healing/Nonunion	29
Spinal fusion		4
Wedge osteotomy (valgus/ varus) around knee		11
Total		143

adjuvant therapy — e.g. hydrogen peroxide (H_2O_2), phenol, liquid nitrogen, or thermal treatment — is needed to eliminate the rest of the tumor tissue. Then, the freeze-dried bone allograft is ready to be packed into the cavities (Figs. 2 and 3).

In spine surgery, the main purpose of freeze-dried bone allografts is to achieve a bony fusion between segments of vertebra. The indications include scoliosis, trauma, degenerative disease, and tumor. Spinal fusion can be performed with or without instrumentation (Fig. 4).

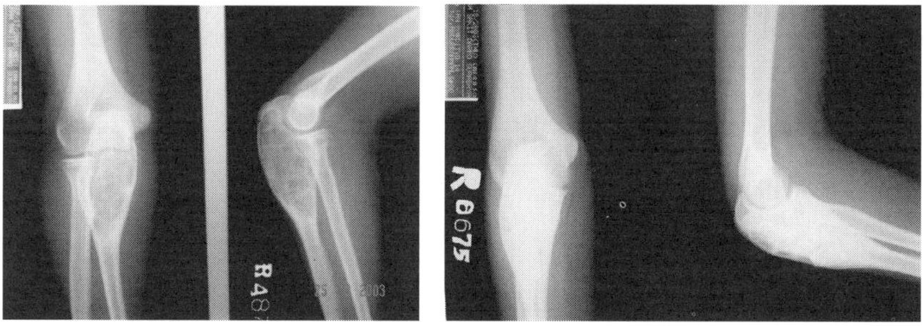

Fig. 2. X-rays of a 15-year-old boy suffering from osteoblastoma who underwent curettage and had the cavities packed with freeze-dried bone allografts. Left: preoperative X-ray; right: X-ray 1 year after curettage and bone graft surgery.

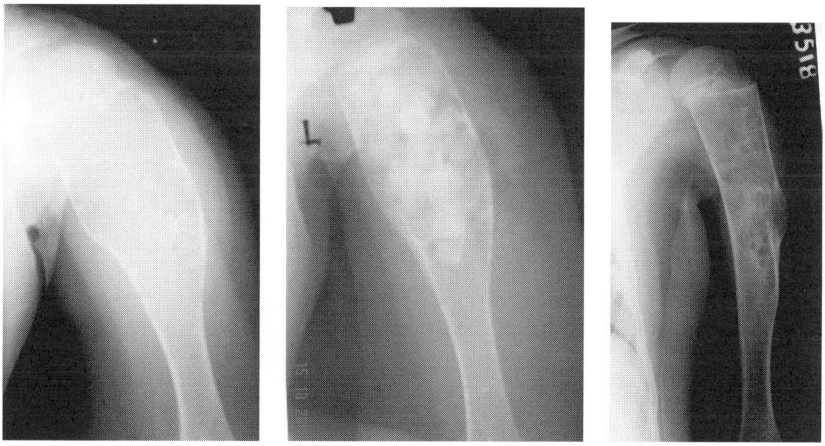

Fig. 3. X-rays of an 8-year-old boy suffering from simple bone cyst who underwent curettage and had the cavities packed with freeze-dried bone allografts. Left: preoperative X-ray; middle: immediate postoperative X-ray; right: 2-year postoperative X-ray.

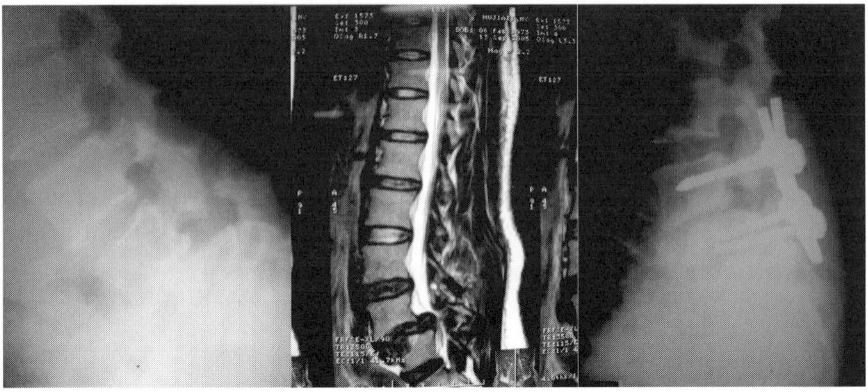

Fig. 4. X-rays of a 50-year-old woman suffering from canal stenosis (caused by spondylolisthesis vertebrae L5–S1) who underwent decompression, posterior stabilization, posterolateral fusion *in situ*, and then bone grafting with a mix of freeze-dried allograft and autograft from ilium.

Freeze-dried bone allografts can also be used for hip and knee surgery, nonunion, fractures, congenital anomaly, as well as oral maxillofacial and plastic reconstructive surgery (Figs. 5–7).

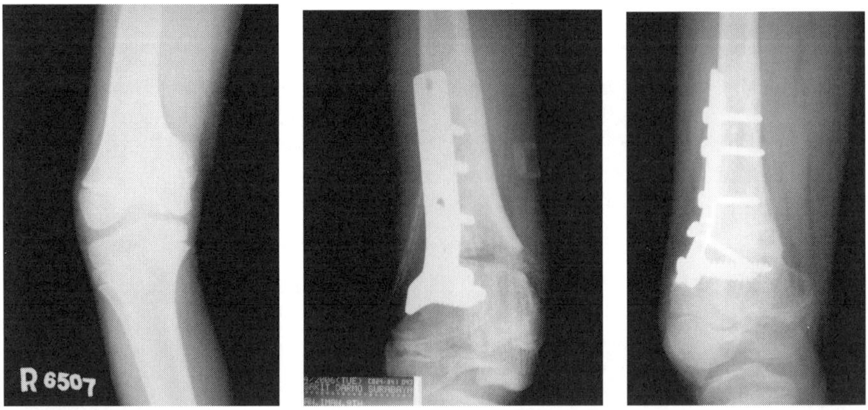

Fig. 5. X-rays of a 12-year-old boy suffering from varus deformity in his right knee (caused by disturbance of medial epiphyseal growth plate of distal right femur) who underwent valgus osteotomy of distal femur and then had freeze-dried bone allograft packed into the open wedge of the bone. Left: preoperative X-ray; middle: X-ray immediately after surgery; right: X-ray 6 months after surgery.

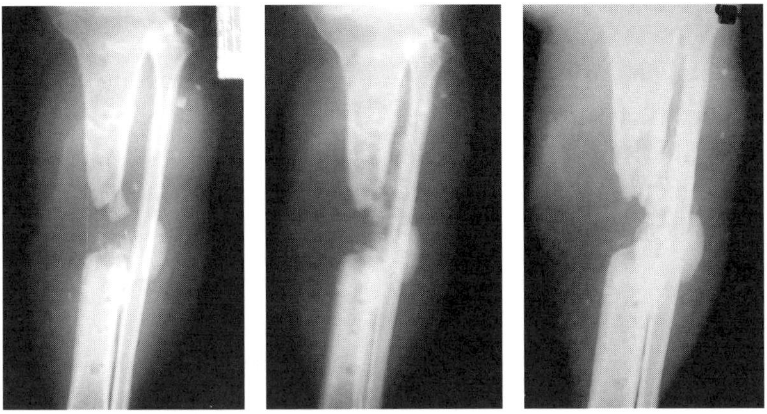

Fig. 6. X-rays of a 32-year-old man suffering from open fracture grade 3 and loose bone who underwent debridement and external fixation. After the infection subsided, he was given central bone grafting with a mix of freeze-dried bone and autograft from ilium. Left: preoperative X-ray; middle: X-ray 3 months after surgery; right: X-ray 8 months after surgery.

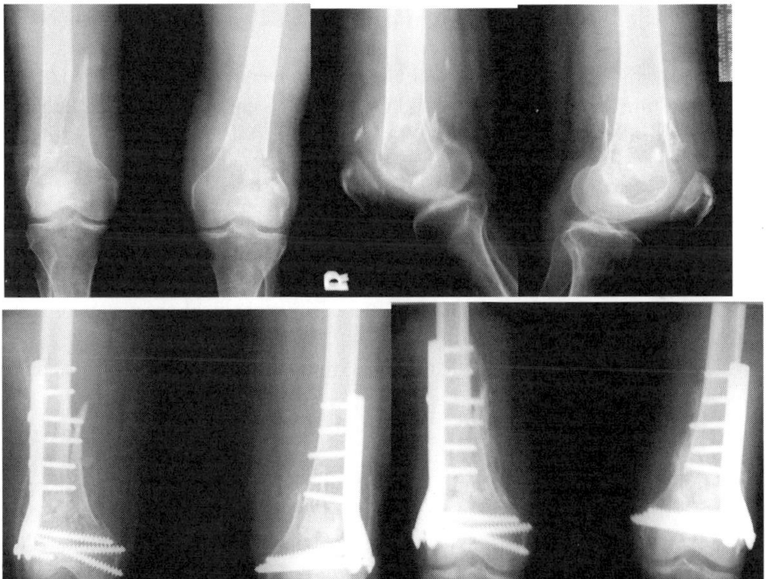

Fig. 7. X-rays of a 75-year-old woman suffering from pathologic fracture (porotic bone) of both supracondylar femurs with underlying thalassemia disease who underwent internal fixation and freeze-dried bone grafting. Top row: preoperative X-rays; below left: immediate postoperative X-ray; below right: X-ray 6 months after surgery.

Conclusion

The success rate of the application of freeze-dried allografts depends on several factors. In the author's experience, the application of freeze-dried allografts after curettage of benign bone tumors gives a satisfactory result. However, there are (sometimes recurrent) problems in applications on aggressive bone tumors such as giant cell tumor and aneurysmal bone cyst.

References

American Academy of Orthopaedic Surgeons (AAOS) (2002). Bone graft substitutes: fact, fiction and application. In: 69th Annual Meeting, AAOS, Dallas, TX.

Bright R and Burchardt H (1983). The biomechanical properties of preserved bone grafts. In: Friedlander G, Mankin H, and Sell K (eds.), *Osteochondral Allografts: Biology, Banking, and Clinical Applications*, Little Brown & Co, Boston, MA, pp. 223–232.

Delloye C (1999). The use of freeze-dried mineralised and demineralised bone. In: Phillips GO, Strong DM, von Versen R, and Nather A (eds.), *Advances in Tissue Banking*, Vol. 3, World Scientific, Singapore, pp. 45–66.

Gitelis S and McDonald DJ (1998). Adjuvant agents and filling materials. In: Simon MA and Springfield D (eds.), *Surgery for Bone and Soft Tissue Tumors*, Lippincot–Raven, Philadelphia, PA, pp. 159–166.

International Atomic Energy Agency and National University of Singapore (IAEA/NUS) (1997). Multimedia Distance Learning Package on Tissue Banking, Interregional Training Centre, Singapore.

Komender A (1976). Influence of preservation on some mechanical properties of human Haversian bone. *Mater Med Pol* **8**:13–17.

Nather A, Goh JCH, and Vajaradul Y (1987). Comparison of biomechanical strength of lyophilized versus fresh frozen Cloward's cadaveric homografts. In: *Proc 4th International Biomedical Engineering Symposium*, Singapore, pp. 31–35.

Pelker R, Friedlander G, and Markham T (1983). Biomechanical properties of bone allografts. *Clin Orthop* **174**:54–57.

Reddi AH (2001). Bone morphogenetic proteins: from basic science to clinical applications. *J Bone Joint Surg Am* **83**:1–7.

Strong M and MacKenzie A (1993). Freeze drying of tissues. In: Tomford W (ed.), *Musculoskeletal Tissue Banking*, Raven Press, New York, pp. 181–208.

Triantaphyllou N, Sotiopoulos E, and Triantaphyllou J (1975). The mechanical properties of the lyophilised and irradiated bone grafts. *Acta Orthop Belg* **5**(41 Suppl):35–44.

Urist MR (1994). The search for and discovery of bone morphogenetic protein (BMP). In: Urist MR, O'Connor B, and Burwell R (eds.), *Bone Grafts, Derivatives and Substitutes*, Butterworth-Heinzmann, Oxford, England, pp. 315–362.

Wilkins RM (2002). Treatment of benign bone tumors. In: Menendez LR (ed.), *Orthopaedic Knowledge Update: Musculoskeletal Tumors*, 1st ed., AAOS, Rosemont, IL, pp. 77–86.

Yim CJ (1999). Biology of demineralised bone and its clinical use. In: Phillips GO, Strong DM, von Versen R, and Nather A (eds.), *Advances in Tissue Banking*, Vol. 3, World Scientific, Singapore, pp. 87–112.

PART VI.

CLINICAL APPLICATIONS OF IRRADIATED AMNION GRAFTS

Chapter 23

The Use of Irradiated Amnion Grafts in Wound Healing

Menkher Manjas*, Petrus Tarusaraya† and Nazly Hilmy‡

**M. Djamil Hospital Tissue Bank*
Department of Surgery, Faculty of Medicine
Andalas University, Padang, Indonesia

†Sitinala Leprosy Hospital
Tangerang, Indonesia

‡BATAN Research Tissue Bank
Center for Research and Development of Isotopes
and Radiation Technology
BATAN, Jakarta 12070, Indonesia

Introduction

Amnion is a collagen-rich, thin, transparent, and tough membrane lining the chorion laeve and placenta that produces amniotic fluid during the earliest fetal period. It is the innermost layer of fetal membranes. Its function is to protect the fetus from unwanted material during intrauterine development.

The amnion membrane consists of a thick basement membrane and an avascular stroma, with a thickness of 0.02–0.5 mm. Basement membrane contains type IV and type VII collagen, laminin-1, laminin-5, fibronectin, allantoin, lysozyme, transferine, progesterone, and several kinds of growth factors. The collagen IV and VII subchain is identical to that of conjunctiva and laminins, which facilitate corneal epithelial cell adhesion and play an important role in ophthalmic surgery. Avascular stroma contains growth factors and anti-inflammatory proteins, and acts as a natural inhibitor to various proteases (Kamardi *et al.* 1993; Panakova and Koller 1997; Koller and Panakova 1998). The angiogenetic capability of amnion membrane stimulates neovascularization and induces the development of new blood vessels. Allantoin, lysozyme, transferine, and progesterone play an important part in the ulcer-healing mechanism, which has bacteriostatic and bactericidal effects (Rao and Chandra 1981; Nursal 1993). According to Gruss and Jirsch (1978), allantoin serves as an antibody generator, while a high concentration of lysozyme constitutes an enzyme that has bacteriostatic and bacteriolytic effects; in addition, progesterone is bacteriostatic in nature against Gram-positive bacteria.

In all of the amnion layers, there is no identifiable structure of blood vessels, lymphatic vessels, or nervous tissues. From an immunological point of view, amnion is a suitable transplant material because it does not express HLA-A, B, or DR antigens; thus, rejection does not occur (Farazdaghi *et al.* 2001).

Amnion membrane promotes wound healing, adheres tightly to the wound surface, is soft and easy to shape to conform to the wound surface, has satisfactory adhesive properties, has good elasticity and sufficient transparency (allowing wound control without secondary redressing), increases mobility and diminishes pain, prepares skin defects for closure, and stimulates neovascularization. Therefore, the amnion membrane can be used as a wound covering as well as for ulcer healing (Hilmy *et al.* 1987; Hilmy *et al.* 1994; Menkher and Helfial Helmi 2001).

Fresh amnion membranes have been used as a biological dressing since 1913 (Stern 1913), and they have been used in ophthalmology surgery since 1940 (De Roth 1940). Since 1989, preserved amnion grafts (i.e. lyophilized radiation-sterilized/ALS-radiated amnions and air-dried radiation-sterilized/AAS-radiated amnions) produced by several tissue banks in Indonesia — such as the BATAN Research Tissue Bank, M. Djamil Hospital Tissue Bank, Soetomo Hospital Tissue Bank, and Sitanala Hospital Tissue Bank — have been applied as a wound dressing for burn wounds, open wounds, postsurgical wounds, and diabetic and leprosy ulcers. Preserved amnion grafts can be kept at room temperature for up to more than 2 years. ALS-radiated amnion grafts are used in ophthalmic and dental surgeries, while AAS-radiated grafts are mostly used to dress all kinds of wounds.

In 2002, these tissue banks produced more than 8000 pieces of amnion grafts per year, and used them as a dressing for all kinds of wounds and ulcers as well as for ophthalmology and maxillofacial surgeries in more than 50 hospitals in Indonesia. The healing time of the wound using amnion membranes is reduced to about 50% of the healing time using conventional wound dressing (Hilmy *et al.* 1987; Thalut 1993; Tarusaraya and Hilmy 1998). Indira *et al.* (2000) observed that there is no difference in healing time between using fresh-frozen amnion and lyophilized, ALS-radiated amnion for ophthalmologic surgery.

This chapter describes the application of amnion grafts as a wound dressing for leprosy ulcer, burn wound, diabetic ulcer, and postsurgical wound (including post–skin graft surgery).

Types and Benefits of Amnion Grafts

The procurement, processing, packaging, and radiation sterilization of amnion membranes to be used as amnion grafts are described in chapter 17.

Types of amnion grafts

The types of amnion grafts used for clinical application can be divided as follows:

1. Viable/fresh (hypothermical preservation) amnion
   - (a) Short-term storage in saline or combined with antibiotics and then stored at 4°C in refrigerator (can be stored for up to 14 days)
   - (b) Long-term storage by freezing at –85°C in dimethyl sulphoxide (DMSO) or antibiotic solution
   - (c) Long-term storage by cryopreservation at –70°C
   - (d) Glycerolization (amnion in 85% glycerol) or other methods
2. Processed and sterilized amnion
   - (a) Sterilization of freeze-dried, air-dried, oven-dried, or frozen grafts by radiation or other methods

Benefits of amnion membrane

The healing-promoting effects of amnion as a dressing are based mostly on its chemical and biomechanical properties, which include the following:

- Antibacterial and angiogenetic effects
- Acceleration and protection of epithelization and granulation, as well as stimulation of neovascularization

- Ability to reduce pain
- Scarless healing
- No rejection or immunological reaction
- Tight adherence to the wound surface and increase in mobility
- Elasticity, translucence, semipermeability, and biodegradability (Matthews 1981; Panakova and Koller 1997; Koller 2001; Menkher and Helfial Helmi 2001)

Application of ALS-Radiated and AAS-Radiated Amnions on Several Kinds of Wounds and Ulcers as well as for Dressing onto Postsurgical Wounds in Indonesia

Some applications of amnion graft as a skin defect dressing for several kinds of wounds are as follows:

- Post–skin grafting at donor site (Hanafiah 1989)
- Shallow, clean second-degree burn and postburn deformity (Quinby *et al.* 1982; Brown 1986; Thalut 1993; Nursal 1993; Sjaifuddin Noer 2001)
- Chronic ulcerative defects (Troensagaard-Hansen 1950; Ward *et al.* 1989; Henky 2004)
- Leprosy wound/ulcer (Tarusaraya and Halim 1994; Tarusaraya and Hilmy 1998; Bari and Begum 1999)
- Wound covering after cesarean section (Menkher and Helfial Helmi 2001)
- Postcircumcision (Menkher *et al.* 2001)
- Clean open wound in daily operation (Hanafiah 1989)

Other applications of amnion grafts in surgical operation include the following:

- Vaginal reconstruction (Dhall 1984; Nisolle and Donnez 1992; Paraton 2001)
- As a molding for demineralized bone powder (it is biodegradable and compatible with oral tissues because both are ectodermal in origin)
- Eye surgical operation for conjunctival surface reconstruction and corneal defects, e.g. pterygium removal, tumor removal, and symblepharon lysis (Indira *et al.* 2000; Djiwatmo 2001; Getry Sukmawati 2005)

Suggestions before clinical application of amnion grafts include the following:

- Immerse graft in sterile saline for about 5 min before use, except for ophthalmology surgery.
- The amnion side of the defect is more effective than the chorion side for clinical use as a wound dressing (Thalut 1993).
- The chorion side of the defect is more effective than the amnion side for clinical application on eye surgery (Indira *et al.* 2000; Getry Sukmawati 2005).

Leprosy ulcer

The application of amnion as a dressing for leprosy ulcer was first practiced using fresh amnion membrane (Sabella 1913), and the latest publication was by Bari and Begum (1999). During 1997–1998, the Sintanala Hospital in Tangerang, Indonesia, observed and cured the leprosy wounds of 85 patients aged 12–60 years (65 male and 20 female patients) using AAS-radiated amnion as a dressing. The types of wounds were reactions (38 cases) or simple ulcers (60 cases). The wounds were located on the legs (52 cases) and arms (33 cases), with an average wound width of 0.5–36 cm^2. The area to be covered with AAS-radiated amnion was first debrided and cleansed; the grafts were then regularly replaced every 3–4 days until complete healing was achieved (Fig. 1) (Tarusaraya and Hilmy 1998).

The types of dressings used were AAS-radiated amnion and zinc oxide (ZnO) ointment. The following parameters were observed:

- Interaction of age and dressing type on the length of healing (days) (Table 1)
- Interaction of dressing and type of wound on the length of healing (Table 2)
- Effects of location of wound on the length of healing using amnion dressing

It was found that the healing time of the wound for younger patients took longer compared to older patients. This was probably caused by the movements of the younger patients, since most of the wounds were located on the leg. The condition was the same for both dressing types. The healing

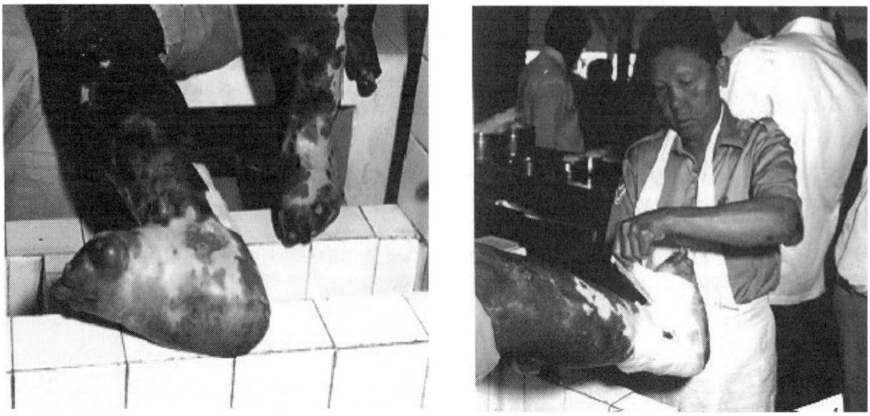

Fig. 1. Application of AAS-radiated amnion onto leprosy wound at Sitanala Hospital in Tangerang, Indonesia. The wound healing time was reduced to 50% of the healing time using conventional dressing (Tarusaraya and Hilmy 1998).

Table 1. Interaction of age and dressing type on length of wound healing (days).

Age (year)	Amnion membrane	ZnO ointment
<20	39.8 + 15.6	80.2 + 15.6
20–40	23.8 + 9.12	52.1 + 9.1
>40	27.5 + 11.6	60.1 + 11.6

Table 2. Interaction of dressing and type of wound on length of healing (days).

Type of wound	Amnion membrane	ZnO ointment
Reaction	21.3 + 13.6	63.0 + 6.2
Simple ulcer	39.4 + 4.6	82.6 + 4.6

time of the wound using amnion membrane as a dressing was about 50% shorter than that of ZnO ointment for all ages.

It was also found that both kinds of wounds — reaction and simple ulcer — could be cured using AAS-radiated amnion, and that the healing time depended on the type of wound. Tarusaraya and Halim (1994) also described the speed of the healing time of leprosy wound using several kinds of dressing on simple plantar ulcers as follows:

- ZnO ointment: 0.14 ± 0.10 cm^2/day
- Magnesium sulphate glycerine acriflavin (MSGA) mixture: 0.10 ± 0.06 cm^2/day
- Sterile amnion (AAS radiation): 0.29 ± 0.22 cm^2/day

Therefore, the application of amniotic membrane as a leprosy wound dressing was found to have several benefits: the average healing time by using amnion was about 50% shorter than that for conventional dressing, and the application of amnion provided more comfort to the patient. No difference in healing time was observed between using AAS-radiated amnion and preserved amnion (85% glycerol).

Burn wound

The use of ALS-radiated and AAS-radiated amnions began in Djamil Hospital in early 1990. They provide the following advantages, especially for second-degree burn wounds:

- Covers all surfaces of burn wounds
- Reduces pain
- Prevents further infection
- Reduces evaporation of wound, and stimulates epithelization and granulation
- Easy to procure, and has a lower price (Koller 2001; Menkher and Helfial Helmi 2001)

Thalut (1993) carried out a comparison study on the use of AAS-radiated amnion membranes and medicated antibiotic dressing as a burn wound covering for 39 patients with second- and third-degree burn wounds caused by fire, electricity, or hot water. The parameters applied were formation time of epithelization and granulation tissues as well as angiogenetic effect of the wound. The results showed that the epithelization formation time of tissue was faster with AAS-radiated amnion than with antibiotic dressing, i.e. from an average of 7 days when using antibiotic dressing to an average of 5 days when using AAS-radiated amnion. The granulation formation time also decreased from an average of 8 days to 6.5 days, respectively.

A comparison study on the angiogenetic effect (which induces epithelization and granulation) using amniotic membrane and antibiotic dressing was also conducted, with the parameter as the calculation of the total number of neovascularization profiles (30 samples for each kind of dressing). The total number of neovascularization profiles for AAS-radiated amnion was twice that of antibiotic dressing. The wound healing time using AAS-radiated amnion was about 45% shorter than that for antibiotic wound dressing (Thalut 1993). The same results were also obtained by Koller and Panakova (1998).

From 2000 to 2003, there were 63 hospitalized patients with cases of second- and third-degree burn wounds at Dr M. Djamil Hospital, Padang, Indonesia. Of these, 48 (76.3%) were men and 44 (70.9%) were over 50 years old. All of the wounds were treated with AAS-radiated amnion as a wound covering. The average healing time of the wounds was 21–26 days, and no complications or rejections were reported. Similar results were also described by Sjaifuddin Noer (2001) from Dr Soetomo Hospital, Surabaya, Indonesia, where AAS-radiated amnion has been successfully used for clinical application as a biological skin substitute and skin covering since 2000.

Diabetic ulcer

At least 15% of diabetic patients worldwide have foot ulcers and 40%–70% of these cases require amputation (Amstrong and Lavery 1998). The incidence is estimated to double by 2025. The cost rate of local management of diabetic ulcers in Indonesia is relatively high, estimated at US$15 per ulcer per day.

From 1997 to 2000, there were 37 hospitalized cases of diabetic ulcer at Dr M. Djamil Hospital, Padang, Indonesia, of which 23 (62.3%) were women and 18 (50.9%) were over 50 years old. All of the wounds were covered using ALS-radiated amnion. A total of 34 (92%) wounds were located on the leg, with an average width of 2–18 cm^2. The average healing time was 21–26 days (Dona 1996).

In 2004, a comparison study on 11 patients with grade 2 diabetic ulcer (according to the Wagner classification) using ALS-radiated amnion (group 1) and conventional medicated bandage (group 2) as a wound covering was conducted. The parameters observed were histopathology examination and length of wound healing. The results showed that diabetic ulcers using ALS-radiated amnion gave a higher histopathology grade than

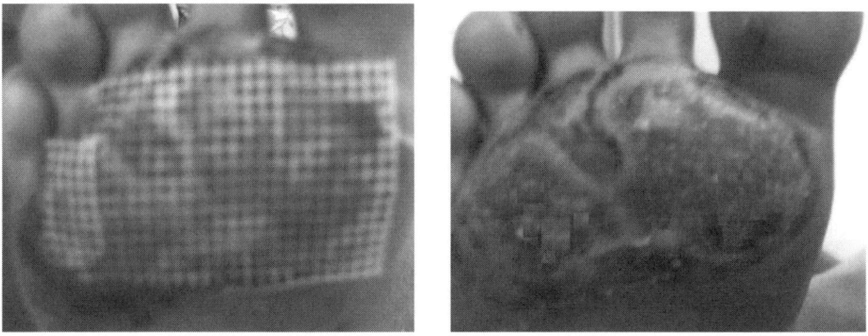

Fig. 2. Application of ALS-radiated amnion as a wound covering for diabetic foot ulcer at Djamil Hospital, Padang, Indonesia. The wound is covered with ALS-radiated amnion, and then heals without scarring after about 15 days.

those using conventional bandage. Based on the research findings, it was observed that ALS-radiated amnion stimulated an increase in cell number from replacement tissues microscopically (Table 3). The average healing time of all the wounds was 25.36 ± 4.843 days (i.e. 20–32 days), while the wound healing time for group 1 was 19.56 ± 2.035 days and for group 2 (control group) 27.18 ± 2.897 days (Fig. 2) (Henky 2004).

These studies prove that the healing time of ulcers using ALS-radiated amnion as a dressing is faster compared to using conventional sterile bandage. This is because of the response of the substance released by the amniotic membrane used.

Histological healing of skin ulcers can be detected by the increase in granulation tissues, epithelial cells, neovascularization, lymphocyte cells, and polymorphonuclear cells, as indicated in Table 3 (Bose 1979; Gruss and

Table 3. The average rate of parameters of the histological examination between the two groups (group 1 and group 2).

Histopathology description	Group 1 $N = 11$	Group 2 $N = 11$	t-test (p)
Granulation tissue	16.73 ± 3.197	4.18 ± 2.786	0.000
Epithelial cell	10.73 ± 2.328	3.82 ± 1.662	0.000
Neovascularization	8.64 ± 2.420	2.73 ± 2.054	0.000
Lymphocyte cell	11.73 ± 3.197	8.73 ± 1.954	0.015
Polymorphonuclear cell	10.45 ± 2.423	7.73 ± 1.902	0.008

Jirsch 1978). Therefore, to find out the biomolecular mechanism and the substance found in the ALS-radiated amnion, which stimulates the growth of healing cells/tissues on the ulcer, further research is required.

Post–wound surgery

There are several types of post–wound surgery in which amnion can be applied as a wound dressing, such as postcesarean operation, post–skin grafting, postcircumcision, and clean wound in daily operation. From 1998 to 2002, a total of 250 wounds were closed with AAS-radiated amnion at the Dr M. Djamil Hospital; these included 58 cases of cesarian operation, 64 cases of circumcision, and clean wound operation.

Postcesarean operation

The wound is usually covered with medicated gauze, and then abdominal strapping is applied for 3–4 days. Sometimes, the wound heals by secondary healing and leaves a scar in the abdominal wall, making it unpleasant for women. In a study by Menkher and Helfial Helmi (2001), the procedural operation was done with a Pfannenstiel incision. Abdominal strapping was used for flabby abdominal skin. Radiation-sterilized lyophilized amnion membranes (ALS radiation) produced by the Dr M. Djamil Hospital Tissue Bank were used. The size of the amnion depended on the length of the wound, but was mostly 5 cm × 20 cm. Evaluations of all the cases were followed for up to 8 days.

The results showed that this technique, which is not technically difficult, is good in achieving the best results of wound healing. Both of the operation types, whether emergency or elective, dirty or clean, gave the same results for wound healing. No complications such as severe wound infection, secondary closing of wound, wound dehiscence, allergic reaction, or bad appearance of wound were found. Therefore, the conclusion or recommendation was that amnion should be used as a wound covering for postcesarean section (Menkher and Helfial Helmi 2001).

Wound covering after circumcision

The aim of using AAS-radiated amnion here is to achieve good wound healing that is free of infection and pain, and that allows earlier use of underpants than usual.

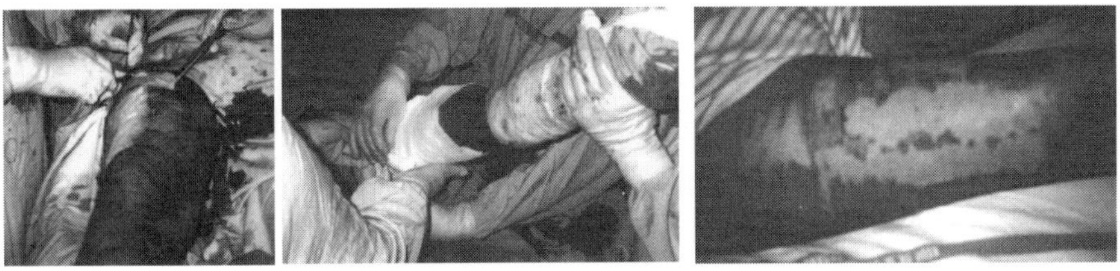

Fig. 3. Application of AAS-radiated amnion as a wound covering for skin defects at the donor site at Djamil Hospital, Padang. The wound is covered with AAS-radiated amnion and then bandaged, and heals without scarring faster than treatment using medicated covering.

In a study by Menkher *et al.* (2001), dorsal circumcision was performed on 165 boys aged 6–10 years. For 58 (35.15%) boys, the surgery was done at Djamil Hospital; while for 107 (64.85%) boys, the surgery was carried out outside of the hospital (e.g. at health centers or during mass dorsal circumcision). After suturing the wound, amnion was used as a wound covering (including covering the glans penis to protect it from external irritation). Without using any gauze or bandage, the patient was allowed for early mobilization. Antibiotics were given as a prophylactic.

For all 165 operations, the duration of wound healing was less than 6 days. There was no difference in the duration of wound healing between surgeries performed inside and outside the hospital ($P > 0.05$) (Menkher *et al.* 2001).

Post–skin grafting

The application of AAS-radiated amnion as a wound covering for skin defects at the donor site is shown in Fig. 3. The average wound healing time without scarring using AAS-radiated amnion was found to be 9 days; and using medicated dressing, 11 days (Hanafiah 1989).

From these studies, it can be concluded that AAS-radiated amnion dressing provides better results than original wound dressing, especially in terms of the rate of infection, rate of wound healing, and rate of complications.

Conclusion

Since ALS-radiated and AAS-radiated amnion can be widely used on several kinds of wounds (dirty and clean wounds, fresh and old wounds, several types of ulcers, as well as postoperative wounds), one can conclude that biological dressing is applicable for all types of wounds and gives better results than nonbiological dressing. To find out the biomolecular mechanism and the substance found in the ALS-radiated amnion, which stimulates the growth of healing cells/tissues on ulcers, further research is required.

References

Armstrong DG and Lavery LA (1998). Diabetic foot ulcers: prevention, diagnosis and classification. *Am Fam Physician* **57**:1325–1332.

Bari MM and Begum R (1999). Use of radiation-sterilised amniotic membrane grafts as temporary biological dressings for the treatment of leprotic ulcer. In: Phillips GO, Kearney JN, Strong DM, von Versen R, and Nather A (eds.), *Advances in Tissue Banking*, Vol. 3, World Scientific, Singapore, pp. 477–483.

Bose B (1979). Burn wound dressing with human amniotic membranes. *Ann R Coll Surg Engl* **61**:444–447.

Brown AS (1986). Biological dressing and skin substitute. *Clin Plast Surg* **13**:69–74.

De Roth A (1940). Plastic repair of conjunctival defects with fetal membrane. *Arch Ophthalmol* **23**:522–525.

Dhall K (1984). Amnion graft for treatment of congenital absence of the vagina. *Br J Obstet Gynaecol* **91**:279–282.

Djiwatmo (2001). Amnion membrane transplantation. In: *1st Indonesian Tissue Bank Scientific Meeting and Workshop on Biomaterial Application*, Surabaya, Indonesia, pp. 69–75.

Dona A (1996). Diabetic foot of NIDDM patient in the internal medicine department, Dr M. Djamil Hospital, 1990–1994. *Acta Med Indones* **27**:1341–1346.

Farazdaghi M, Adler J, and Farazdaghi SM (2001). Electron microscopy of human amniotic membrane. In: Phillips GO, Strong DM, von Versen R, and Nather A (eds.), *Advances in Tissue Banking: The Scientific Basis of Tissue Transplantation*, Vol. 5, World Scientific, Singapore, pp. 149–171.

Getry Sukmawati IS (2005). Multilayered amniotic membrane transplantation for the treatment of corneal epithelial defects and ulcers. Department of Ophthalmology, Faculty of Medicine, Andalas University/M. Djamil Hospital, Padang, Indonesia (to be published).

Gruss JS and Jirsch DW (1978). Human amniotic membrane: a versatile wound dressing. *Can Med Assoc J* **118**:1237–1246.

Hanafiah D (1989). Clinical studies on application of sterile lyophilization amniochorion membrane on open wound. In: *RCA Meeting on Radiation and Nuclear Technology for Sterilized and Clinical Quality Control of Tissue Graft*, Bangkok, Thailand.

Henky J (2004). The use of freeze dried radiation sterilized amniotic membrane as wound covering for diabetic ulcer. Faculty of Medicine, Andalas University, Padang, Indonesia.

Hilmy N, Basril A, and Febrida A (1994). The effects of procurement, packaging materials, storage and irradiation dose on physical properties of lyophilized amnion membranes. In: *Proc IAEA Meeting of Radiation Sterilization of Tissue Grafts*, Manila, Philippines.

Hilmy N, Siddik S, Gentur S, and Gulardi W (1987). Physical and chemical properties of freeze dried amnion membranes sterilized by irradiation. *J Atom Indones* **13**(2):1–14.

Indira S, Laksmi T, and Bambang S (2000). Freeze dried and fresh amniotic membranes with limbal stem cell transplantation in severe conjunctival tumor and corneal defect. In: *8th International APASTB Conference on Tissue Banking*, Bali, Indonesia, p. 98.

Kamardi T, Nursal H, and Nazly H (1993). Clinical studies on application of sterile irradiated freeze-dried amniochorion membranes on burn wound treatment. In: *Seminar on Wound Treatment*, Padang, Indonesia, pp. 5–24.

Koller J (2001). Healing of skin and amnion grafts. In: Phillips GO, Strong DM, von Versen R, and Nather A (eds.), *Advances in Tissue Banking: The Scientific Basis of Tissue Transplantation*, Vol. 5, World Scientific, Singapore, pp. 398–417.

Koller J and Panakova E (1998). Experiences in the use of foetal membranes for the treatment of burns and other skin defects. In: Phillips GO, Strong DM, von Versen R, and Nather A (eds.), *Advances in Tissue Banking*, Vol. 2, World Scientific, Singapore, pp. 353–359.

Matthews RN (1981). Wound healing using amniotic membrane. *Br J Plast Surg* **34**:76–78.

Menkher M and Helfial Helmi H (2001). Using amniotic membrane as wound covering after cesarian section operation. In: *Proc Scientific Meeting Research and Development on Application of Isotopes and Radiation*, BATAN, Jakarta, Indonesia, pp. 169–173.

Menkher M, Ismal, and Doddy E (2001). Experience of using amniotic membrane after circumcision. In: *Proc Scientific Meeting Research and Development on Application of Isotopes and Radiation*, BATAN, Jakarta, Indonesia, pp. 165–168.

Nisolle M and Donnez J (1992). Vaginoplasty using amniotic membranes in cases of vaginal agenesis or after vaginectomy. *J Gynecol Surg* **8**:25–30.

Nursal H (1993). The angioneogenic effect and decrease population of bacteria by amniotic membrane conservation for burn wound in Dr M. Djamil Hospital. In: *Seminar on Wound Treatment*, Padang, Indonesia, pp. 25–32.

Panakova E and Koller J (1997). Utilisation of foetal membrane in the treatment of burn and other skin defect. In: Phillips GO, von Versen R, Strong MD, and Nather A (eds.), *Advances in Tissue Banking*, Vol. 1, World Scientific, Singapore, pp. 165–173.

Paraton H (2001). Management of vaginal agenesis. In: *1st Indonesian Tissue Bank Scientific Meeting and Workshop on Biomaterial Application*, Surabaya, Indonesia, pp. 77–83.

Quinby Jr WC, Hoover HC, Scheflan M, Philemon TW, Sumner AS, and Conrado CB (1982). Clinical trials of amniotic membranes in burn wound care. *Plast Reconstr Surg* **70**:711–716.

Rao VT and Chandra SV (1981). Use of dry human bovine amnion as a biological dressing. *Arch Surg* **119**:891–896.

Sabella N (1913). Use of foetal membranes in skin grafting. *Med Rec NY* **83**:478–480.

Sjaifuddin Noer M (2001). Clinical applications of biomaterial for plastic surgery. In: *1st Indonesian Tissue Bank Scientific Meeting and Workshop on Biomaterial Application*, Surabaya, Indonesia, pp. 57–64.

Stern W (1913). The grafting of preserved amniotic membrane to burned and ulcerated skin surface substituting skin grafts. *JAMA* **1**:973–974.

Tarusaraya P and Halim PW (1994). Comparison study using amnion membrane, ZnO ointment, and magnesium sulphate glycerine acriflavin on ulcus plantar of leprosy patients. *Madjalah Kedokt Indones* **44**.

Tarusaraya P and Hilmy N (1998). Comparison study using freeze dried amnion membrane and ZnO ointment as wound covering for leprosy ulcer. In: *7th International APASTB Conference on Tissue Banking*, Kuala Lumpur, Malaysia.

Thalut K (1993). Personal communication.

Troensagaard-Hansen E (1950). Amniotic grafts in chronic ulceration. *Lancet* **1**:859–860.

Ward DJ, Bennett JP, Burgos H, and Fabre J (1989). The healing of chronic venous leg ulcers with prepared human amnion. *Br J Plast Surg* **42**:463–467.

Chapter 24

Amnion for Treatment of Burns

Hasim Mohamad

School of Medical Science
University of Science, Malaysia
Malaysia

Department of Surgery
Hospital Raja Perempuan Zainab II
Kota Bharu
Malaysia

Introduction

Amniotic membranes have been found to be effective as a temporary dressing in the management of partial-thickness burns, with clinical benefits for both the nursing staff and patients (e.g. low treatment cost). As a temporary dressing, the amniotic membrane flakes off from the healed burn wound surface with time.

Amniotic membranes are procured from the placentae of mothers who have been antenatally screened for communicable or infectious diseases (Figs. 1 and 2). Membranes from placentae with intrapartum complications are discarded. Processing of the membrane involves thorough washing with normal saline, soaking in 0.05% sodium hypochlorite solution for 30 min to 1 h, shaking several times with normal saline, drying, packing, and lastly gamma radiation at 25 kGy or lower according to the bioburden.

The ideal burn wound cover is autologous skin; however, the supply of this material may be inadequate for extensive burns. Therefore, the search for alternative biological dressings that can mimic autologous skin has been ongoing for several years now. Various substances (e.g. allograft and xenograft skins) have been used in an attempt to obtain burn wound closure, with minimal success. Problems in the availability and immunological

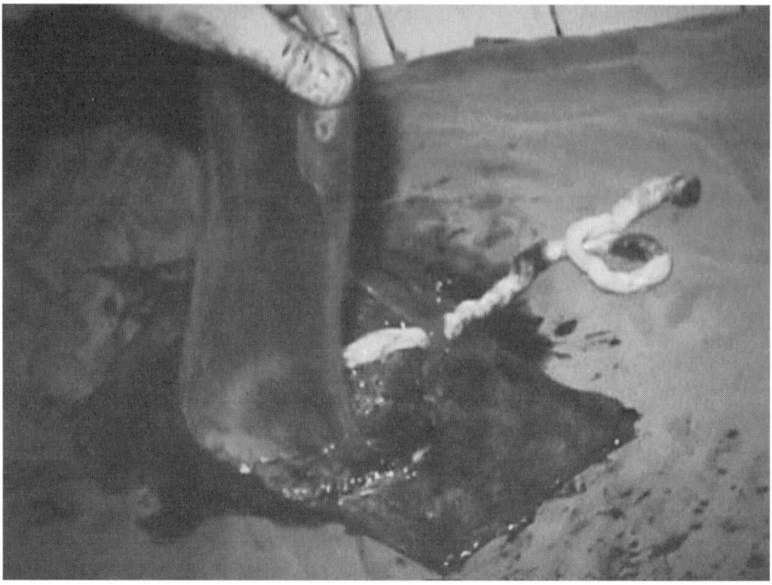

Fig. 1. Harvesting amniotic membrane from the placenta.

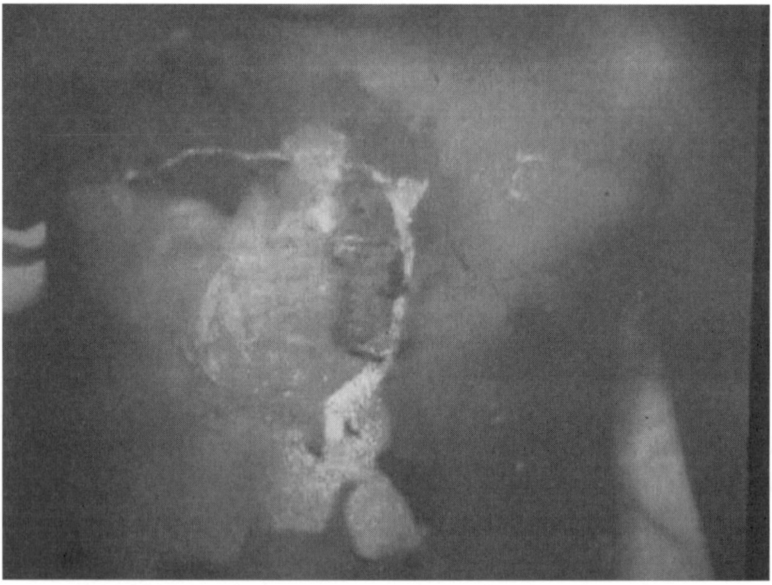

Fig. 2. Amniotic membrane without a layer of gauze.

rejection of both allograft and xenograft skin have led to further research on artificial skin for burn wound coverage. Until permanent repair with autologous skin can be instituted, temporary biological burn wound dressings are life-saving and essential, especially for extensive burns.

Amniotic membranes, which were previously discarded from hospital labor rooms, have now been found to be useful as an alternative to autologous skin for temporary wound dressings on burns, scalds, chronic ulcers, dermal injuries, and contaminated wounds. Amniotic membrane is a versatile and effective biological dressing for both superficial and deep superficial burn wounds. Clinical trials have confirmed these findings.

Amniotic membranes are histologically quite similar to skin and are made up of two layers: the amnion and the chorion. The amnion is the inner layer, which is smooth and glistening, and is composed of cuboidal cells. Its outer surface consists of mesenchymal connective tissue. The chorion is external to the mesenchymal tissue and is composed of transitional epithelial cells. The amniotic membrane has no blood vessels, nerves, or lymphatic channels. Although it is in intimate contact with the recipient burn wound, there is no occurrence of neovascularization because there are no blood vessels in the amnion that can be connected with the recipient vessels. The amniotic membrane is also nonantigenic, and so it does not show immunological reaction. Fresh amniotic membrane is purported to possess angiogenic as well as bacteriostatic effects. Both of these properties seem to remain intact in spite of sterilization by radiation, thus helping to prolong the shelf life of the membrane; however, these properties have not been experimentally confirmed.

Amniotic membrane was first reported to be used in the treatment of burn patients by Sabella in 1913. Since then, only a few reports of the use of amniotic membranes for burn wound coverage have been found in medical literature, but its other applications include treatment of leg ulcers, skin loss in Stevens–Johnson syndrome, pelvic and vaginal surgery, and otolaryngologic as well as head and neck surgery.

Methods of Preparing Radiated Amniotic Membrane

Air-drying method

Fresh amniotic membranes are obtained from mothers during delivery. Mothers must be seronegative for infectious diseases and have no history

Table 1. Procurement of amniotic membrane: maternal selection.

Inclusion	
	Clean elective cesarean section
	Uncomplicated spontaneous vaginal delivery
Exclusion	
	Prolonged rupture of membrane
	Endometritis
	Chorioamnionitis
	Meconium staining
	Drug abuse
	Positive for VDRL/TPHA
	Seropositive for hepatitis/AIDS
	Septicemia
	Toxemia of pregnancy

of premature rupture of amniotic membranes, endometritis, or meconium staining (Table 1).

According to the aseptic technique, the membrane is separated from the placenta, placed in a plastic pack containing normal saline, and appropriately labeled. This pack can be frozen and thawed for later processing or can be immediately processed. Processing of the membrane begins by dipping the fresh amniotic membrane in 0.05% sodium hypochlorite solution for 30 min to 1 h, and then washing it repeatedly with tap water until it is completely clear of blood particles and resembles a thin plastic film. After cutting the thin film to the required size (usually 10 cm × 10 cm), it is air-dried in a laminar flow cabinet or alternatively in a freeze dryer. The procedure is completed by packing the dried membrane in sterile plastic packs inside a laminar flow cabinet and then sealing it off.

Figure 3 shows the sequence of events in the preparation of amniotic membrane for packing, after which it is sterilized using cobalt-60 (Co-60) gamma radiation at 25 kGy as soon as possible. The dried, sterilized amniotic membranes are then ready for clinical use.

Freeze-drying technique

Fresh amniotic membrane is washed thoroughly with tap water to remove excess blood, and then is immersed in saline and shaken three times for 15 min each to remove amniotic fluid. If necessary, the membrane is spread over a clean flat surface and rubbed gently with sterile cotton gauze. The washed

Wash with clean water
↓
Separate chorion from amnion
↓
Wash with distilled water at pasteurization temperature of 58°C in shaking water bath for 30 min
↓
Treat with 0.5% sodium hypochlorite for 30 min
↓
Clean amnion in distilled water using multi-wrist shaker for 30 min, repeated 3 times
↓
Spread amnion for drying in laminar airflow cabinet (mount on gauze or plain dryer overnight)

or

Freeze-dry in Lyovac machine
↓
Double-pack in polyethylene bag
↓
Heat-seal
↓
Label
↓
Sterilize (gamma irradiation)

Fig. 3. Summary of amnion processing.

membrane is then stretched across over a sterile cotton gauze and freeze-dried at 40°C. Freeze-dried membrane is similarly packed and sterilized as for air-dried membrane.

Results of Clinical Applications of Radiated Amniotic Membrane

Partial-thickness burns or scalds

According to the aseptic technique, the recipient wound is thoroughly and gently cleansed with normal saline to remove all debris and dead skin. The radiated amniotic membranes are then applied with the glistening side against the wound surface, and are allowed to remain in place until they separate spontaneously. All air bubbles and excess fluid should be smoothed out

Table 2. Summary of clinical application of radiated amniotic membrane.

1.	The wound is cleansed with normal saline.
2.	Amniotic membrane is applied over the burn wound.
3.	The dressing is then covered with a thick gauze or bandage, if necessary.
4.	If there are no complications, the burn wound is inspected on the fourth or fifth day.
5.	Membrane that is stuck to the burn wound surface should be left alone, and the edge of the amnion that has peeled off should be trimmed using scissors.

to ensure good contact. However, the membranes can be changed whenever necessary, especially if the wound does not "take".

Usually, the membranes immediately adhere to the wound upon application and desiccate, thus helping to prevent excessive loss of fluids and electrolytes. If there is any sign of infection, the patient is febrile, or there is fluid or pus collection below the membrane, then the burn wound needs to be thoroughly and gently washed and redressed. The use of antibiotic cream is not necessary and not advisable. Systemic antibiotics are given only when indicated. It is not necessary to apply another dressing overlying the membrane, although light gauze dressing is sometimes applied to ensure that the amniotic membrane is in place (e.g. on the patient's back). After application of the membrane, the recipient wound will epithelize below the membrane; and within a week or so, the desiccated membrane will flake off, resulting in a shiny wound scar (Table 2).

Full-thickness defects

Radiated amniotic membrane may be similarly used for application on full-thickness skin defects. However, in this case, frequent changing of radiated membranes is necessary as the membrane may occasionally dissolve. Its main role here is to prevent infection or contamination from the environment. After wound granulation has taken place, skin grafting is indicated.

Discussion on the Clinical Use of Amniotic Membrane as Burn Wound Dressing

Radiated amniotic membranes, being thin film dressings, are easy to use clinically. They are also easy to apply onto the burn surface because of their good conformability. Radiated amnions adhere firmly to the wound, and become dry membranes covering and protecting the wound from contamination and infection. Amniotic membranes are not rejected by the host immune system; thus, they not only provide excellent protection from infection and trauma to the underlying fresh-growing epithelium, but also stimulate ideal conditions for epithelial growth. No neovascularization takes place on the overlying amnions, and the dry membranes spontaneously peel off after wound healing occurs. There is no need for regrafting of the recipient wound if it is due to partial-thickness burns or scalds; but in cases of full-thickness burn, autologous grafting is necessary once granulation tissues have formed. Table 3 summarizes the properties that contribute to the amnion as an ideal biological dressing.

Clinically, immediate coverage of open burn wounds is necessary to ensure a satisfactory outcome. In fact, it is the most important determining factor for patient recovery. For example, superficial partial-thickness lesions may be contaminated or infected and may progress to full-thickness lesions, resulting in unwanted scars or disabilities. In order to achieve an acceptable clinical outcome, autograft skin should ideally be used, but several biological dressings have been developed in the past few decades to overcome the shortage of autografts. Immediate coverage of open wounds has the following advantages:

- Prevents burn wounds from contamination and infection
- Prevents loss of fluid and electrolytes
- Prepares the wound for definite closure at a later date when autograft is available

Table 3. Physical properties of amnion that satisfy the criteria as an ideal biological dressing.

1.	Effective barrier: reduces heat, fluid, and protein loss
2.	Good adherence and durability: reduces contamination
3.	Bacteriostatic effect: reduces incidence of infection and septicemia
4.	Analgesic effect: reduces pain and analgesic usage
5.	Nonantigenic effect: has no immunological effect on patients
6.	Lightweight and elastic material: conforms easily to the body surface or contours
7.	Good acceptability by patients: allows early mobilization of patients

Allograft (cadaveric) skin satisfies the requirements, but has the disadvantage of developing rejection. Consequently, frequent removal and replacement after about 5 days from the time of application is necessary — hence, the need for a constant supply (skin bank) of donors, both living and dead. Reports of successful use of allograft skin have been reported in medical literature. Likewise, xenograft (mainly porcine) skin has been successfully used in the treatment of burn wounds. It has more favorable characteristics compared to cadaveric or other animal tissues, but it is not always socially or religiously acceptable. It is also expensive to procure and process. Artificial skin has recently been manufactured, but clinical use is limited given its exorbitant cost.

Therefore, amniotic membrane is a good alternative to other biological dressings, being easily available at little cost. The successful use of both wet and dry amnion membranes has been sporadically reported in medical literature. Robson *et al.* (1972) showed in a comparative study that amniotic membranes were found to be equal to isografts and superior to both allograft and xenograft skin in reducing bacterial levels in full-thickness skin defects in rats. Upon application, amniotic membrane alleviates pain; this has a tremendous impact, especially on children. Studies have also shown that it inhibits infection. This antibacterial property is believed to be caused by the lysozyme and progesterone present in the amniotic fluid. Moreover, its adherence to the wound surface prevents the accumulation of fluid and pus on the granulation tissues. Radiation of the amniotic membrane does not seem to cause any physical damage or damage to its antibacterial property. The advantages of radiated amniotic membrane are listed in Table 4.

Table 4. Advantages of radiated amniotic membrane.

1.	Easy to procure and process: ease of storage and long shelf life
2.	Cheap and cost-effective: monetary and hospital stay savings
3.	Reduces the contamination and infection rate
4.	Reduces the need for intensive nursing care
5.	Potential for use even in general surgical or burn wards
6.	Potential for peripheral or district hospital usage
7.	Wide availability of good-quality amnion, especially in hospitals with a high number of deliveries

The Way Ahead

Carefully selected and procured radiated amniotic membrane, with its long shelf life, definitely plays an important role in burn wound treatment. Its clinical usage as a burn wound dressing has been proven beyond doubt, especially for superficial and deep partial burn dressings. It is particularly useful in the management of burns in the young, as it alleviates pain. Clinically, its single application without any need for redressing the burn wound makes it popular among the nursing staff because of time constraints, unlike the use of silver sulfadiazine which requires frequent changes of dressings. The following Figs. 4–7 show patients who have benefited from using amniotic membranes.

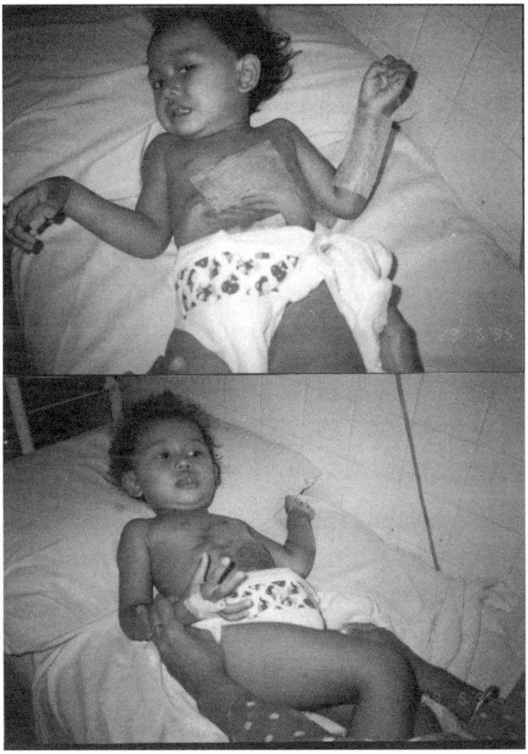

Fig. 4. Burn wound before (above) and after (below) amniotic membrane application.

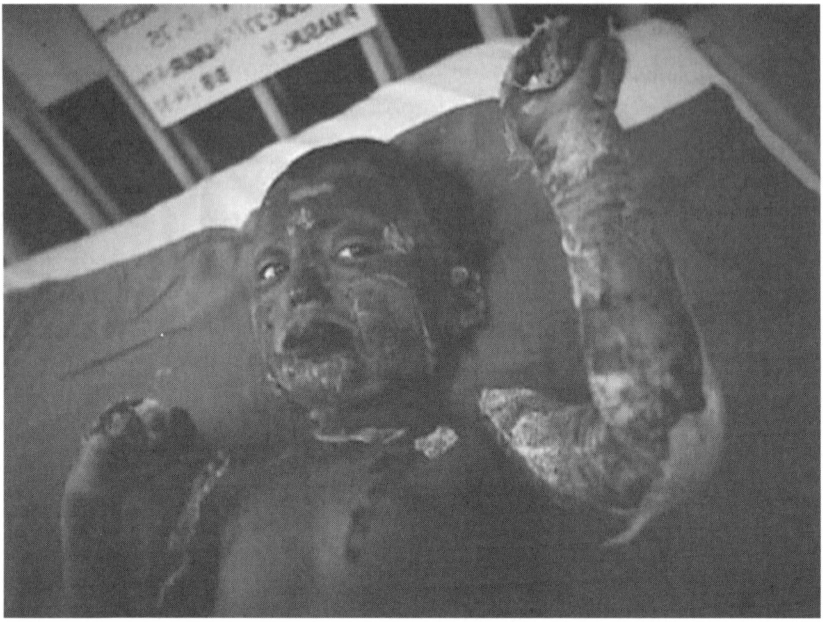

Fig. 5. Clinical application of amniotic membrane as a versatile dressing. Patient looks comfortable and pain-free.

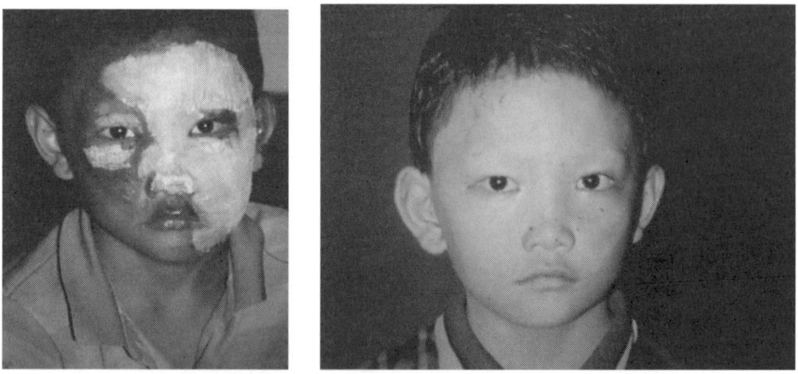

(a) (b)

Fig. 6. Application of amniotic membrane on facial burn wound. (a) Membrane on facial burn wound. (b) Healed wound.

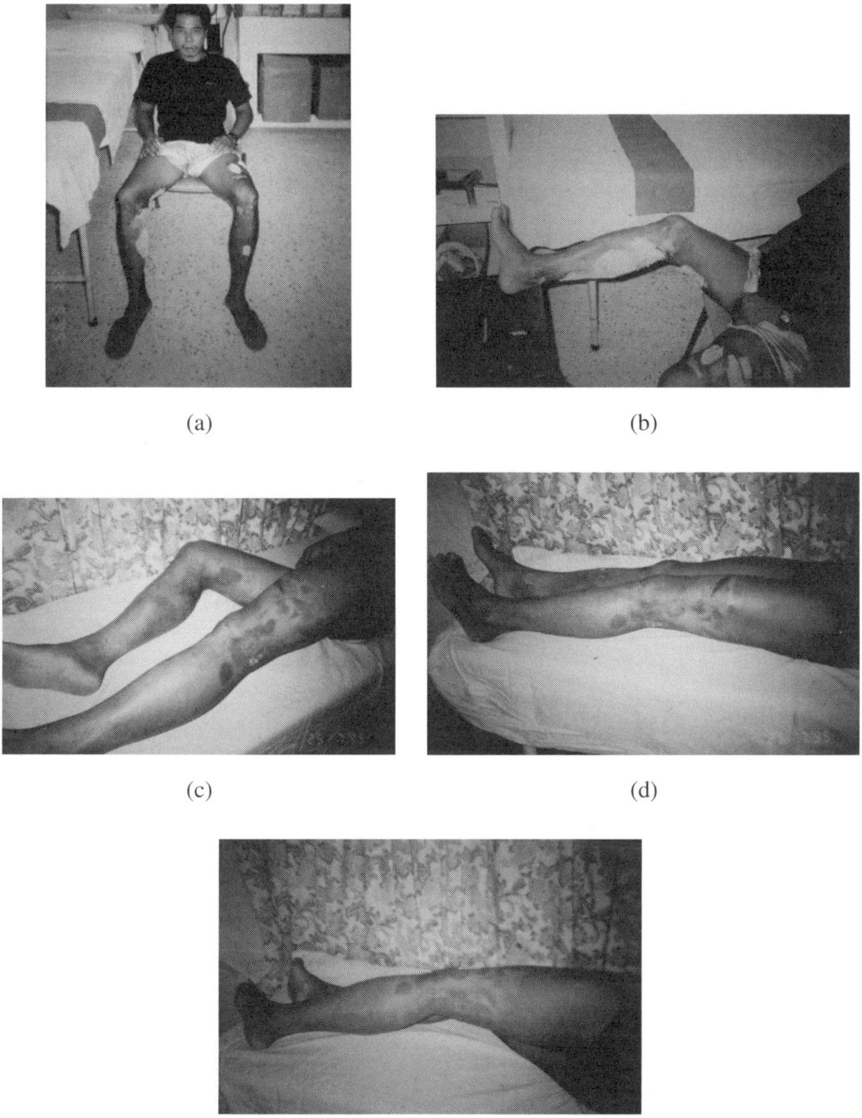

(a) (b) (c) (d) (e)

Fig. 7. Application of amniotic membrane on bilateral leg burn. (a) Patient with bilateral leg burn. (b) Application of membrane. (c) Healed wound after 1 month. (d) Lateral view of healed wound; no obvious hypertrophic scar. (e) Another view of healed wound: posterior aspect of the knee.

Acknowledgments

The author would like to thank the International Atomic Energy Agency (Grant No. MAL/7/003) and the Malaysian Intensification of Research in Priority Areas (IRPA Grant No. 323/0501/4210), as well as Mrs Radzina Ismail for typing the manuscript.

Reference

Robson MC, Samburg JL, and Krizek TJ (1972). Quantitative comparison of biologic dressings. *Surg Forum* **23**:503–507.

Chapter 25

Use of Freeze-Dried Irradiated Amnion in Ophthalmologic Practices

Nazly Hilmy*, Paramita Pandansari*, Getry Sukmawati Ibrahim†, S. Indira‡, S. Bambang‡, Radiah Sunarti‡ and Susi Heryati‡

**BATAN Research Tissue Bank (BRTB)*
Center for Research and Development of Isotopes and Radiation Technology
BATAN, Jakarta 12070
Indonesia

†Department of Ophthalmology, Faculty of Medicine
Andalas University/M. Djamil Hospital, Padang
Indonesia

‡Cicendo Eye Hospital, Faculty of Medicine
Padjajaran University, Bandung
Indonesia

Introduction

Amnion membrane was first used in ophthalmology in 1940 by De Roth, who reported partial success in the treatment of conjunctival epithelial defects after symblepharon using fresh amnion membrane. In 1946, Lavery as well as Sorsby and Symons found that both patients with lime burn of the conjunctiva with corneal involvement and patients with caustic burns could be successfully treated using amniotic membrane. Fresh amnion membranes were used in all of these studies.

In 1986, Prasad *et al.* reintroduced amnions for ocular surface reconstruction, i.e. for the treatment of Stevens–Johnson syndrome. Subsequently, Lee and Tseng (1997), Prabhasawat *et al.* (1997), Kruse *et al.* (1999), Komolsuradej *et al.* (2001), and Tseng (2005) used single- and multi-layered amnion for persistent corneal epithelial defects, severe ulceration of the cornea and sclera, and corneal perforations. Various authors have also reported beneficial effects of human amnion membrane transplantation on the ever-expanding ocular indications. All of the works used frozen or fresh amnion membranes.

Since 1999, radiation-sterilized freeze-dried amnion membranes with less than 5% water content have been used for ophthalmology surgeries (e.g. for ocular surface reconstruction, severe conjunctival tumors and corneal ulcers, corneal perforation, pterygium) in several hospitals and eye centers in Indonesia, with promising results. Some benefits of freeze-dried amnion allografts are as follows:

- Can be kept for up to 2 years at room temperature (expiration date for the BATAN Research Tissue Bank's products)
- Easy for transportation
- Easy for storage
- Sterilized by irradiation at room temperature

Prabhasawat *et al.* (1997) described some benefits of using amnion grafts for ophthalmologic practices:

- Heals all types of epithelial defects
- Reduces inflammation and scarring
- Promotes epithelial healing
- Decreases irritation as well as painful bullous and band keratopathies
- Prevents graft rejection
- Solves tissue defect problems, especially for conjuntiva
- Offers perfect grafts for conjuntival tumors
- Serves as an adjunct to limbal transplantation
- Enables antifibroblastic cell migration–promoting activities

In addition, the amniotic membrane produces various growth factors such as basic fibroblast growth factor, hepatocyte growth factor, and transforming growth factor β, which stimulate epithelization (Tseng 2005).

This chapter describes several experiences in using radiation-sterilized freeze-dried amnion membrane allografts in ophthalmologic practices.

Preparation of Radiation-Sterilized Freeze-Dried Amniotic Membranes (see chapter 17)

The processing steps of amnion membranes after screening are as follows:

1. Amniotic membranes procured from the placenta of healthy mothers must be individually washed and processed. The washing process is

done nine times, using nine bottles each containing 400 mL of sterile water, except for bottle 5 which contains 0.05% sodium hypochlorite (NaOCl) solution in sterile water. The amnion is washed and shaken well four times in 400 mL of sterile water (bottles 1–4), immersed in 0.05% sodium hypochlorite solution (bottle 5) for 10 min, and then washed again four times in bottles 6–9. Each bottle is shaken for 10 min. The used washing water in bottle 9 is subject to control for validation (IAEA/NUS 1997; Hilmy *et al.* 2000; Hilmy *et al.* 2003).

2. The amnion is stretched and mounted on a sterile cotton gauze or polyester net with the epithelial side of the amnion placed directly on the cotton gauze, and is then frozen (−70°C for 24 h for lyophilized amnion grafts, or until sterilization for frozen amnion grafts).
3. The amnion is freeze-dried/lyophilized for 5 h (validation is done by calculating the water content, i.e. less than 5%).
4. The amnion is cut into 4 cm × 4 cm or another size.
5. Bioburden enumeration is done on the amnion (validation is done according to ISO 11737-1, 1995).
6. The amnion is triple-packed in a polyethylene pouch with a thickness of 0.1 mm.
7. The amnion is labeled.
8. The amnion is radiation-sterilized at a dose of 25 kGy (validation is done according to the IAEA Code of Practice 2004).
9. The amnion is stored at 5°C or at room temperature (24°C), protected from direct sunlight.

Experiences in Ophthalmologic Practices Using Freeze-Dried Amnion Grafts

Freeze-dried amniotic membrane transplantation in corneal ulcer management (Sunarti and Heryati 2006)

The basement membrane facilitates the migration of epithelial cells, reinforces the adhesion of basal epithelial cells, promotes epithelial differentiation, and prevents epithelial apoptosis. The amnion membrane transplanted as a basement membrane acts as a new healthy substrate that is suitable for proper epithelization. Corneal ulcers are serious and urgent clinical problems that can threaten patient vision. Lee and Tseng (1997) reported that amniotic membrane transplantation may be considered as an alternative substrate for treating persistent corneal epithelial defects. Amniotic membrane transplantations were performed when corneal ulcers persisted or became worse after medication was given for a period of time, or when patients presented either with impending corneal perforation or after corneal perforation had developed.

Sunarti and Heryati (2006) have carried out a study to determine the efficacy of radiation-sterilized freeze-dried amniotic membrane transplantation in promoting wound healing in severe corneal ulcers. Freeze-dried radiation-sterilized amniotic membranes produced by the BATAN Research Tissue Bank were used in this case.

Method and surgical technique

A retrospective study on amnion membrane transplantation was performed on 18 eyes from 18 patients with corneal ulcer from January 2004 to December 2004 at Cicendo Eye Hospital, Indonesia. Of these, 16 were men and 2 were women, with an age range of 8–68 years old. Transplantation was performed under general anesthesia. Eleven (61.12%) ulcers were located centrally in the cornea, 4 (22.22%) were located peripherally, and 3 (16.66%) were located midcentrally. In the preoperative condition, 9 (50%) ulcers were perforated, 6 (33.33%) were with descemetocele, 2 (11.11%) had reached the profound stroma, and 1 was found with corneal melting.

The base of the ulcer was carefully debrided before amnion transplantation. Amnion membranes were trimmed to fit the ulcer's size, followed by placement of the amnion with stromal side down layer by layer to fill up the ulcer. Upon reaching the ulcer surface, amniotic membranes were cut into a bigger size than the ulcer and sutured with continuous 10-0 nylon suture. The top layer was sutured by 10-0 nylon suture. A bandage contact lens was applied on top of the membrane until the epithelial defect was healed. Topical medications after surgery were continued. Assessment of the surgical outcome was determined by inflammation signs, the healing time of the area covered by the membrane, and recovered visual acuity. All of the patients were examined on postoperative day 1, and every week thereafter until 1 month. All of the operations were performed after obtaining informed consent.

Clinical results and discussions

Laboratory results indicated that KOH-positive reactions were found in 7 patients, Gram-positive cocci in 4, Gram-negative rods in 3, Gram-negative diplococci in 2, and a combination of Gram-positive cocci and Gram-negative rods in the others. According to Jones' criteria, all of the ulcers were categorized as severe ulcers.

Preoperative visual acuity was categorized as poor in 14 (77.78%) patients, while the rest of the patients were categorized as having good preoperative visual acuity. Postoperatively, poor visual acuity was found in 11 (61.11%) patients and good visual acuity in 5 (27.78%). This meant that a decrease in visual acuity was found in 5, improvement in visual acuity in 5, and stable visual acuity in 6. Of the 18 eyes, 11 (61.11%) showed corneal re-epithelization and decreased inflammation, 3 (16.67%) showed worsening corneal defect, 1 (5.55%) developed endophthalmitis, and 2 (11.12%) developed corneal staphyloma (one eye underwent evisceration, and corneal ulcer persisted in the other eye after complete resolution of transplantation). Two patients did not return for follow-up.

The goal of amniotic membrane transplantation was to seal the perforation or act as a bandage in order to avoid perforation, promote corneal tissue healing, and reduce inflammation. It was observed that amniotic membrane transplantation gave an excellent result for two cases of peripheral corneal ulcers that were caused by Gram-negative diplococci, both in terms of corneal re-epithelization and visual acuity recovery. Compared to purely bacterial ulcers, KOH-positive ulcers received less benefit from the amniotic membrane transplantation procedure; however, success was found in three cases, thus this procedure could still be considered as an alternative therapy. Visual acuity was not an accurate parameter for this kind of surgical procedure, since there were many factors affecting the visual outcome after resolution of corneal ulcers, including the position of the corneal scar. The best visual acuity recovery was found in peripheral ulcers. Failure of epithelization may have been caused by imperfect surgical skill or bad ulcer condition. It was concluded that radiation-sterilized freeze-dried amniotic membranes can be considered as an alternative procedure in treating corneal ulcers to promote corneal wound healing.

Multilayered amniotic membrane transplantation (MAMT) and tarsorrhaphy for the treatment of corneal epithelial defects and ulcers (Getry Sukmawati Ibrahim 2006)

Twenty-two eyes (from 17 patients) with corneal epithelial defects and ulcers were studied from July 2005 to November 2005. The patients consisted of 13 males and 4 females, with cases as follows: 1 patient (2 eyes) suffered from corneal epithelial defects due to complications of Stevens–Johnson syndrome, 2 patients (4 eyes) suffered from limbal stem cell deficiency caused by alkali burns, and 14 patients (16 eyes) suffered from severe corneal ulcers with hypopyon.

Thirteen eyes were treated with multilayered amniotic membrane transplantation and tarsorrhaphy; 1 patient (1 eye) with Mooren's ulcer was treated via multilayered amniotic membrane transplantation and partial bare sclera. Two patients (4 eyes) presented with corneal ulcers in Graves' hyperthyroidism, and 1 patient (1 eye) was unconscious due to a head injury. Other patients included 1 eye with severe corneal ulcer caused by *Neisseria gonorrhoeeae,* 1 eye with absolute glaucoma, 2 eyes with neurotrophic corneal ulcers caused by herpes simplex virus, and 3 patients with corneal ulcers caused by bacteria and fungi. All of the patients had been treated with eye drops, eye ointment, or systemic medicine, depending on the etiology of the disease, with either slow results or no success. All of the operations were performed after obtaining informed consent.

Surgical technique

The epithelial defect and/or the base of the stromal ulcer was debrided with a microsponge, and the poorly adherent epithelium surrounding the defect or ulcer was removed. Radiation-sterilized freeze-dried amniotic membranes produced by the Djamil Hospital Tissue Bank were used in this work. The amnion graft was peeled from its holding gauze with the epithelial side up, and was placed on the defect or stromal ulcer layer by layer for filling-in, grafting, or patching, depending on the type of lesion. The entire surface of the cornea and surrounding conjunctiva was covered with two or three layers of amniotic membrane, and sutured with interrupted 10-0 nylon or 8-0 silk on the conjunctiva at eight positions (Fig. 1). The eye was then closed and patched. On the first and second day after operation, eye drops were carefully instilled through small opened palpebral fissure (<1 mm) to avoid

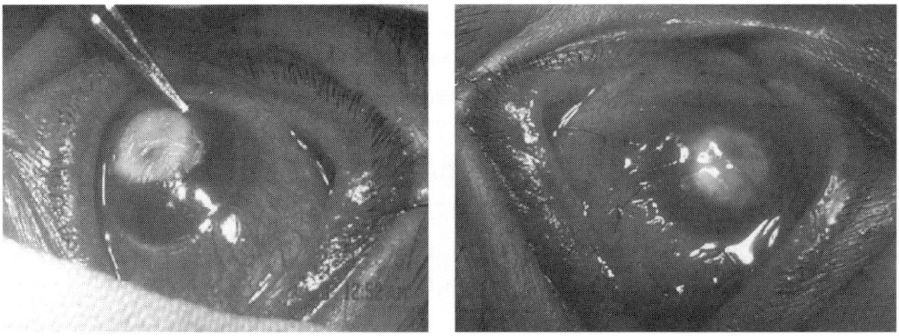

Fig. 1. The surgical technique of radiation-sterilized freeze-dried multilayered amniotic membrane transplantation carried out at the M. Djamil Hospital, Padang, Indonesia. The freeze-dried amnion was peeled from the gauze with the epithelial side up, and was placed on the defect or stromal ulcer layer by layer for filling-in, grafting, or patching on the ulcer. The entire surface of the cornea and surrounding conjunctiva was then covered with two or three layers of amniotic membrane, and sutured with interrupted 10-0 nylon or 8-0 silk on the conjunctiva at eight positions.

damage or rupture to the amniotic membrane. On the third day, the eye was inspected to see the healing process to the ulcer and epithelialization using sterile flourescein staining. The sutures were removed after 1–2 weeks.

Clinical results

The clinical results of the study showed that on the third day after multi-layered amniotic membrane transplantation, most of the cases showed corneal epithelializations. The mean time of the beginning of epithelializations was 3.9 ± 1.09 days (between 3 and 7 days). The mean time of complete epithelializations was 11.10 ± 4.95 days (between 4 and 21 days), and the median time for complete epithelializations was 15 days. Fourteen (64%) eyes acquired improved visual acuity, 6 (27%) experienced no worsening of visual acuity, and 2 (9%) could not be evaluated (i.e. one eye with absolute glaucoma and one eye from an unconscious patient due to severe head injury).

Most of the ulcerated eyes were of a severe and deep type with hypopyon. Four eyes suffered chemical and thermal burns, and two eyes had corneal erosion as a complication of Stevens–Johnson syndrome. No postoperative complications directly associated with the amnion (e.g. superinfection, new appearance of descemetocele, perforation, graft rejection) were found.

However, in one case, some hypopyons were still present, although they slowly disappeared within several days after MAMT.

It was concluded that MAMT appears to be a safe and effective method to restore a stable corneal epithelium for corneal epithelial defects, as well as an adequate base for initiating the filling of large corneal ulcers. Amnion was temporarily fixed/stabilized on the corneal surface by suturing it to the conjunctiva, and the eye was closed and patched (pressure bandage) without bandage contact lens for 3 days. No failures or complications were detected in this limited study.

Freeze-dried and fresh amniotic membranes with limbal stem cell transplantation in severe conjunctival tumors and corneal defects (Indira **et al.** *2000)*

The limbus is a junctional zone that separates the cornea and the conjunctiva into two distinctively different tissues. The limbal stem cell is the basal layer of limbal epithelium, and has two major functions: as a ultimate source of cellular proliferation and differentiation of corneal epithelium, and as a barrier to separate the corneal epithelium and conjunctive epithelium and to prevent conjunctival growth in the event of corneal epithelial defects. Limbal transplantation restores stem cells, whereas amniotic membrane transplantation restores basement membrane and stroma.

Indira *et al.* (2000) investigated the use of fresh amnion and radiation-sterilized freeze-dried amniotic membrane as transplantation agents for ocular surface reconstruction. The radiation-sterilized freeze-dried amniotic membranes produced by the BATAN Research Tissue Bank were used in this work.

Limbal stem cell transplantation with amniotic membrane was performed on two groups of patients: group A received fresh amnions, while group B received freeze-dried and radiation-sterilized amniotic membranes. Each group consisted of 2 patients with large symblepharon; 2 patients with large conjunctival tumor; 7 and 8 patients with corneal ulcer for groups A and B, respectively; and 1 patient with Stevens–Johnson syndrome. All of the patients had corneal disease with limbal deficiency.

The mean healing time for patients with large conjunctival tumor using fresh amniotic membrane transplantation was 4 weeks (SD, 1.41); and for those using freeze-dried amnion, 5 weeks (SD, 1.95). The mean healing

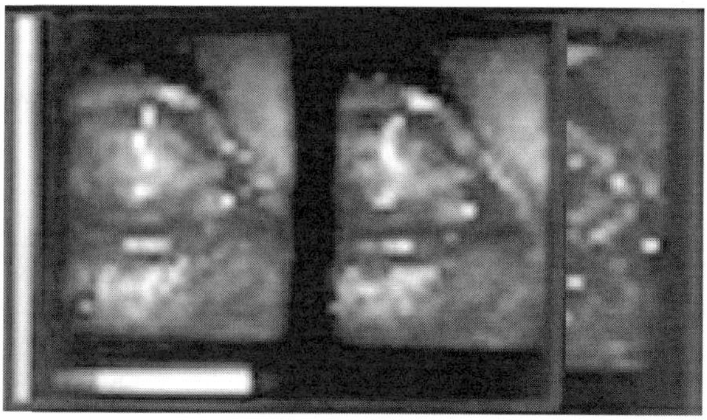

Fig. 2. Patient with large symblepharon (left) before freeze-dried amnion transplantation, and (right) 6 weeks after amnion transplantation (Cicendo Eye Hospital, Bandung, Indonesia).

time for patients with severe corneal defect using fresh amniotic membrane transplantation was 3.43 weeks (SD, 2.44); and for those using freeze-dried amniotic membrane, 3.38 weeks (SD, 2.11). No significant difference in the healing time of defects by transplanted fresh and freeze-dried amnions was detected. Both fresh and freeze-dried amniotic membranes can be used as transplantation agents for ocular surface reconstruction (Fig. 2).

Conclusion

Radiation-sterilized freeze-dried amnion membrane transplantation can be considered as an alternative procedure for ocular surface reconstruction, for example in treating corneal defects to promote corneal healing. Multilayered amnion membrane transplantation (MAMT) using freeze-dried amnion membrane appears to be a safe and effective method to restore a stable corneal epithelium to corneal epithelial defects, as well as an adequate base for initiating the filling of large corneal ulcers. No significant difference was detected in the healing time of corneal defects between using fresh and radiation-sterilized freeze-dried amnion grafts for ocular surgery transplantation.

References

De Roth A (1940). Plastic repair of conjunctival defects with fetal membrane. *Arch Ophthalmol* **23**:522–525.

Getry Sukmawati Ibrahim S (2006). Multilayered amniotic membrane transplantation for the treatment of corneal epithelial defects and ulcers. Department of Ophthalmology, Faculty of Medicine, Andalas University/M. Djamil Hospital, Padang Indonesia (to be published).

Hilmy N, Febrida A, and Basril A (2000). Validation of radiation sterilization dose for lyophilized amnion and bone grafts. *Cell Tissue Bank* **1**(2):143–148.

Hilmy N, Febrida A, and Basril A (2003). Indonesia: statistical sampling technique in validation of radiation sterilization dose of biological tissue. *Cell Tissue Bank* **2**(2):185–191.

Indira S, Laksmi T, and Bambang S (2000). Freeze dried and fresh amniotic membranes with limbal stem cell transplantation in severe conjunctival tumor and corneal defect. In: *8th International Conference on Tissue Banking*, Bali, Indonesia, p. 98.

International Atomic Energy Agency (IAEA) (2004). Code of Practice for the Radiation Sterilization of Tissue Allografts, IAEA, Vienna.

International Atomic Energy Agency and National University Singapore (IAEA/NUS) (1997). Module 4: Procurement. Multimedia Distance Learning Package on Tissue Banking, Interregional Training Centre, Singapore.

International Standards Organization (ISO) (1995). Sterilization of Medical Devices — Microbiological Methods, ISO 11737-1, 1995, Geneva.

Komolsuradej W, Tesavibul N, and Prabhasawat P (2001). Single and multilayer amniotic membrane transplantation for persistent corneal epithelial defect. *Br J Ophthalmol* **85**:1455–1463.

Kruse FE, Rohrschneider K, and Volcker HE (1999). Multilayer amniotic membrane transplantation for reconstruction of deep corneal ulcers. *Ophthalmology* **106**:1504–1511.

Lavery FS (1946). Lime burn of conjunctiva and cornea treated with amnioplastin graft. *Trans Ophthalmol Soc UK* **66**:668.

Lee SH and Tseng SGD (1997). Amniotic membrane transplantation for persistent epithelial defects with ulceration. *Am J Ophthalmol* **123**:303–312.

Prabhasawat P, Barton K, Burkett G, and Tseng SCG (1997). Comparison of conjunctival autografts, amniotic membrane grafts, and primary closure for pterygium excision. *Ophthalmology* **104**:974–985.

Prasad JK, Feller I, and Thompson PD (1986). Use of amnion for the treatment of Stevens–Johnson syndrome. *J Trauma* **26**:945–946.

Sorsby A and Symons HM (1946). Amniotic membrane grafts in caustic burns of the eye (burns of second degree). *Br J Ophthalmol* **30**:337–345.

Sunarti R and Heryati S (2006). Freeze dried amniotic transplantation in corneal ulcer management. Cicendo Eye Hospital, Faculty of Medicine, Padjajaran University, Bandung, Indonesia (to be published).

Tseng SCG (2005). Literature summary on uses of amniotic membrane in ocular surface reconstruction, available at http://www.ocularsurface.com/

Chapter 26

Clinical Applications of Irradiated Amnion Grafts: Use of Amnion in Plastic Surgery

Ahmad Sukari Halim, Aik-Ming Leow, Aravazhi Ananda Dorai and Wan Azman Wan Sulaiman

Reconstructive Sciences Department
School of Medical Sciences, Health Campus
Universiti of Science Malaysia
16150 Kubang Kerian, Kelantan
Malaysia

Introduction

A plethora of (mostly beneficial) synthetic dressings are available, and they account for a substantial portion of any healthcare budget. One of the natural-occurring products — the human afterbirth — is constantly available worldwide, but is almost always discarded despite the established efficacy of its membranes as a true biological dressing (Trelford and Trelford-Sauder 1979; Matthews *et al.* 1982).

In 1910, William Thornton — then a final-year medical student at the Johns Hopkins Hospital, Baltimore, MD — suggested to Dr Staige Davis that fetal membranes might be useful for wound healing. Although the membrane used at that time did not provide permanent cover on the only recorded case in which Davis tested this hypothesis, he was enthusiastic about the concept and recommended further investigations (Davis 1910).

The terms "amniotic membrane" and "amnion" are used loosely in medical literature. Failure to recognize the appropriate terminology has bedeviled the interpretation of clinical results and their outcomes, as highlighted by Trelford and Trelford-Sauder (1979). Thus, these terminologies are important for an accurate definition of clinical practice and subsequent assessment of results. The term "extraembryonic tissue" (EET) refers to placenta, amnion, and chorion. "Extraembryonic membrane" (EEM) or amniotic membrane denotes a general name encompassing the amnion (inner membrane) and the chorion (outer membrane), which is in contact with the maternal decidua during gestation. Hence, the term "amnion" is reserved for the inner layer of the EEM obtained when the amnion epithelium and its underlying layers are stripped from the chorion without using any elaborate separation techniques, although this does not result in absolute anatomical separation in histological terms (Matthews *et al.* 1982).

Procurement of amnion for clinical usage

The real possibility of transmitting diseases via human blood, sera, and tissue products in the modern era cannot be ignored. Therefore, all potential placenta donors should be stringently screened for the possibility of blood-borne diseases such as HIV, HBsAg, HCV, syphilis, gonorrhoea, toxoplasmosis, and cytomegalovirus.

To obtain the membranes, EEM is cut from the edge of the placenta and the reflected portion of the membrane is stripped from the placental surface to the base of the umbilical cord. Strict aseptic techniques should be exercised throughout the procedure. Ideally, only membranes obtained from cesarean sections should be used, but vaginally delivered tissue has been widely applied without complications. For vaginally delivered tissue, the amniotic membrane should be ruptured less than 12 h before delivery. Various conditions whereby the membranes are not suitable include meconium-stained or dysmorphic membranes, membranes from mothers with seropositive blood or a history of venereal disease, endometriosis, prolonged labor, and toxemia. The membranes obtained are thoroughly rinsed in normal saline to remove all blood traces, once in 0.025% sodium hypochlorite, and then again several more times in normal saline before refrigeration at 4°C (Robson and Krizek 1973). The addition of antibiotics is optional (Shun and Ramsey-Stewart 1983).

Type of amnion preparations available for clinical application

Fresh amnions are mostly used in clinical applications. However, dried (Rao and Chandrasekharam 1981), frozen (Colocho *et al.* 1974), irradiated

(Rao and Chandrasekharam 1981), and lyophilized (Burgos and Sergeant 1983) preparations have also been used.

Radiation-sterilized air-dried human amnion

Air- and freeze-dried human amnions have almost similar physical properties, and both have comparable effectiveness as a wound dressing. However, air-dried human amnion is cheaper to prepare and easier to handle. Over a period of 15 years, the National Tissue Bank at the University of Science, Malaysia — in collaboration with the Malaysian Nuclear Agency (NM) — has modified a technique for preparing amniotic membranes that is cost-effective, high in quality, and safe.

The procurement and preparation of human amnions for clinical application are guided by stringent screening protocols, strict aseptic preparation, and gamma irradiation at 25 kGy or lower (according to the bioburden) to achieve a sterility assurance level of 10^{-6}. The radiation of amnion does not seem to cause any damage to its physical or chemical properties. The advantages of air- and freeze-dried amnions in radiation-sterilized packs are that they are safe, ready to be used, and long in life span compared to fresh amnions (Hasim and Yusof 1994).

Specific features of amnion relevant to plastic surgical practice

Skin substitutes and biological dressings play a major role in plastic and reconstructive surgery. The histological characteristics of amnion are quite similar to those of skin. Normal amnion is 0.02–0.05 mm thick, which is only one third of the thickness of the stratum corneum epidermis (Rao and Chandrasekharam 1981).

Among the various types of biological dressings, human amnion membrane plays a vital role in facilitating wound healing. Amnion seems to satisfy all of the criteria for an ideal biological dressing. It is thin and elastic, and adheres to the wound surface. It provides an effective vapor barrier, a durable cover for raw surfaces, and substantial pain relief with potential bacteriostatic properties; in addition, it facilitates rapid re-epithelization (Rao and Chandrasekharam 1981; Colocho *et al.* 1974; Talmi *et al.* 1990; Unger and Roberts 1976). One of the most important principles in plastic surgery is to achieve rapid and complete wound healing in the shortest possible time. Any method that promotes and enhances rapid wound healing has an enormous potential for research and clinical use. Human amnion membrane has an inherent angiogenic property to increase the rate of healing and epithelialization.

Human amnion membrane has long been used for various clinical applications in the plastic surgery field, and is widely used to treat superficial and partial-thickness burns in many centers worldwide (Subrahmanyam 1995). It is also used as a biological dressing in the treatment of chronic ulcers and pressure sores (Ward *et al.* 1989). Moreover, skin graft donor sites can be effectively treated using human amnion membrane. Recently, radiation-induced ulcers have been effectively treated using human amnion membrane (Gajiwala and Sharma 2003). Human amnion thus has the potential to become an attractive biomaterial that is inexpensive and easily obtainable.

Factors That Contribute to the Success of Amnion in Plastic Surgical Practice

Antibacterial properties

There are numerous theories on the mechanism of the antibacterial effect observed in EEM and amnion. Many authors have concurred that EEM and amnion are effective biological dressings, since both membranes fall intimately into the contour of the wound to lie in close apposition to its surface (Trelford *et al.* 1973; Gruss and Jirsch 1978; Bose 1979). It has been noted that the degree of bacterial contamination is inversely proportional to the number of leucocytes beneath a graft (Gruss and Jirsch 1978). Saymen *et al.* (1973) found that leucocytes migrate toward the surface of a covered wound and away from an uncovered wound. Therefore, the precise elimination of dead space is considered important, and amnion alone — being thinner and more pliable than EEM — is probably the most potentially effective dressing available. It has been shown that the surface pH falls after covering with amnion and that the temperature in the underlying granulation tissue rises, increasing phagocytosis and reducing the exudation of interstitial fluid.

Robson and Krizek (1973) found that EEM is superior to allograft (homograft) and xenograft (heterograft) skin. It was as effective as autograft skin in lowering the bacterial count when applied to 20% rat scalds topically inoculated with 10^8 *Pseudomonas aeruginosa*. They concluded that no antibacterial substance exists; however, a substance that enhances leukotaxis or angiogenesis, with subsequent leukotaxis and promotion of host defense mechanisms, would be important. Similarly, a substance depressing the normal host rejection to a "foreign" surface dressing and thus permitting continued close surface adherence would achieve an additional antibacterial effect. The presence of a weak antibiotic-like substance in amniotic fluid has also been demonstrated, and the possibility of its elaboration in EEM epithelium remains strong (Galask and Synder 1970; Sachs and Stern 1970).

Effect of amnion on vessel development

The vascular response of amnion on the wound bed has been extensively studied using standard histological and immunohistological staining techniques (Faulk *et al.* 1980). It was found that there was a considerable proliferation of capillary vessels towards the surface of leg ulcers following 5 days of tissue-culture–preserved EEM application. The blood vessel walls became thinner and more regular, and their lumina were observed to be more consistently patent. Increased vascularity in the burns to which EEM was applied was also microscopically noted (Kirschbaum and Hernandez 1963). Proteins elaborated by amniotic epithelial cells have angiogenic effects, but the precise mode of action remains unknown (Burgos 1983).

Alterations in connective tissues

Studies have shown that reticulin stains are able to reveal a marked loosening of the thick, tightly-woven tissue pattern often seen in the bed of chronic refractory skin ulcers (Faulk *et al.* 1980).With this tight, fibrous matrix, blood vessels are formed in groups, their lumina are often occluded, and their walls are thickened with a tissue density similar to that of the bands seen in the interstitium. Five days of EEM application resulted in loosening of the connective tissue matrix, thinning and shortening of the interstitial fibers, and a more widespread dispersal of smaller blood vessels with better defined walls and more consistent patency (Faulk *et al.* 1980).

Immunosuppressive role of amnion

Elucidation of the fetomaternal relationship has led to a comparison of the fetus with the existence of a parasite that successfully avoids host rejection

(Faulk and Galbraith 1979). A glycoprotein occurring in trophoblast and amniochorion is considered to be very important in suppressing the detection of the fetus as "foreign" to the mother by acting on maternal lymphocytes and preventing rejection throughout pregnancy (McIntyre and Faulk 1979). The role of immunodiagnostic techniques continues to be important in the effort to ascertain the precise action of immunobiologically active glycoproteins of EET as well as in the study of changes in the granulation tissue itself.

Biological Functions and Benefits of Amnion as Wound Dressing

The biological functions and benefits of amnion as a wound dressing include the following:

- Decrease of the bacterial count in the wound
- Reduction of fluid loss
- Promotion of wound healing
- Protection of growing epithelium
- Tight adherence to the wound surface, increase in mobility, and diminished pain
- Help in predicting the readiness for grafting
- Preparation of skin defects for closure
- Decrease in physiological stress for the patient
- Stimulation of neovascularization

Uses of Amnion in Plastic Surgery

Amnion can be used in plastic surgery for the following conditions:

- Burns
- Treatment of leg ulcers
- Extensive skin loss in Stevens–Johnson syndrome
- Dressing for split-thickness skin graft donor sites
- Reconstruction of pelvic floor following pelvic exenteration
- Oral cavity reconstruction
- Flap dressing (temporary dressing following flap necrosis)
- Neurolysis and tenolysis

- Vaginal epithelialization
- Intra-abdominal and peritoneal defects
- Intracranial implantation
- Replacement of nasal mucosa in Rendu–Osler–Weber disease
- Tissue engineering (as a carrier for keratinocytes and fibroblasts)

Below are some specific clinical applications of amnion in plastic surgery.

Burns and Stevens–Johnson syndrome

Burn injuries cause a significant loss of the protective layer of the skin's barrier to infection. The loss of this protective layer can lead to several detrimental effects. Superficial and partial-thickness burns usually heal by 5–21 days. The ideal dressing material is one that provides a moist wound environment and does not interfere with the process of epithelialization. The dressing material should also be conformable and well adherent to the wound bed.

Human amnion membrane is a temporary biological dressing that is thin, pliable, and adheres easily to the surface of the burn wound. It can be easily applied after the first 24–72 h of burn injury after the edema has reduced. It remains attached to the burn wound until the wound has completely healed. A secondary dressing is needed to absorb the moisture and exudate from the wound. Dressing changes are also not frequently required if the secondary layer is adequate. The dressing changes are normally done every 3–5 days, depending on the amount of exudates. During dressing changes, if the amnion remains well adhered to the wound surface, it means that the wound has not completely epithelialized; if the amnion membrane peels off on its own, then it clearly means that the wound has healed well. Being semipermeable in nature, the amnion membrane allows exchange of gases and liquids across the membrane.

There are many advantages to using amnion membrane in burn injuries. It forms a protective layer against microorganisms that can enter the wound from the environment. It also minimizes the loss of body fluids and proteins and thereby reduces the incidence of electrolyte imbalance, which can be a major problem in burns. Furthermore, it provides an ideal substrate for rapid wound healing, and hence significantly reduces hypertrophic scar formation and contractures. Studies have shown that the formation of keloids and contractures were significantly reduced when the burn wounds were treated with fresh amniotic membrane (Sinha 1990).

One of the most significant advantages of using amnion membrane in acute burns is its painless application and removal without requiring analgesia. The subsequent dressing changes are also relatively painless, as the amnion membrane usually sticks well to the burn wound and only the outer layer needs to be changed. Ultimately, the process of epithelialization is not disturbed and rapid wound healing occurs. Hence, as the wound surface is not exposed during each dressing change, bleeding from the wound is minimized. As amnion membrane is readily available and processed, significant reduction in hospitalization costs is also possible (Subrahmanyam 1995).

Stevens–Johnson syndrome is a rare immunological condition characterized by an extensive loss of skin and mucosal surfaces [Fig. 1(a)]. These skin defects are capable of completely re-epithelializing if covered with a good dressing [Fig. 1(b)]. The fact that this condition requires protection from external contamination and protection for the native skin to recover makes amnion membrane one of the preferred biological dressings in the treatment of Stevens–Johnson syndrome [Fig. 1(c)].

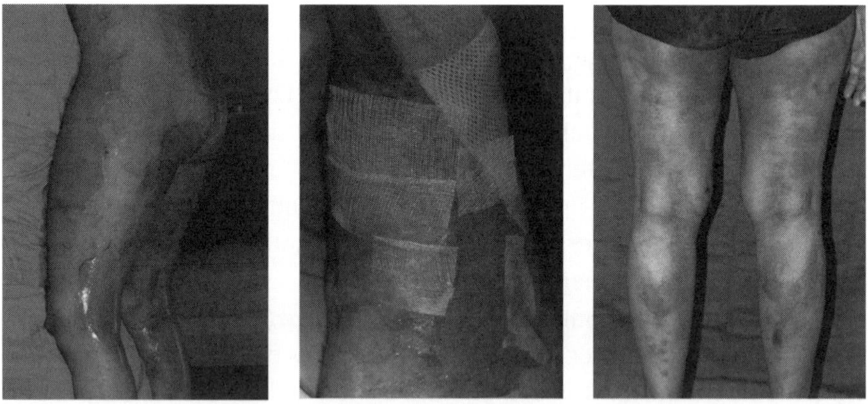

(a) (b) (c)

Fig. 1. Stevens–Johnson syndrome. (a) Prior to amnion application. (b) Immediately after amnion application. (c) Results after wound healing.

Dressing for split-thickness skin graft donor site

Below are some advantages of using radiation-sterilized air-dried human amnion as a biological dressing for split-thickness skin graft donor site.

Wafer-thin, elastic, and lightweight

These criteria are especially useful in children, avoiding bulky dressings that may be uncomfortable and may cause respiratory embarrassment when applied over the torso and abdomen (Rao and Chandrasekharam 1981) [Fig. 2(a)].

Adherence of the membrane to the wound surface

The bond that is established between the amnion and the wound surface is biological, not mechanical. It has been considered to be a fibrin–elastin biological bond (Burleson and Eiseman 1972). This property helps to protect the fragile donor wound surface and allows re-epithelialization to take control until the amnion is readily peeled off when the wound is completely healed [Figs. 2(b) and 2(c)].

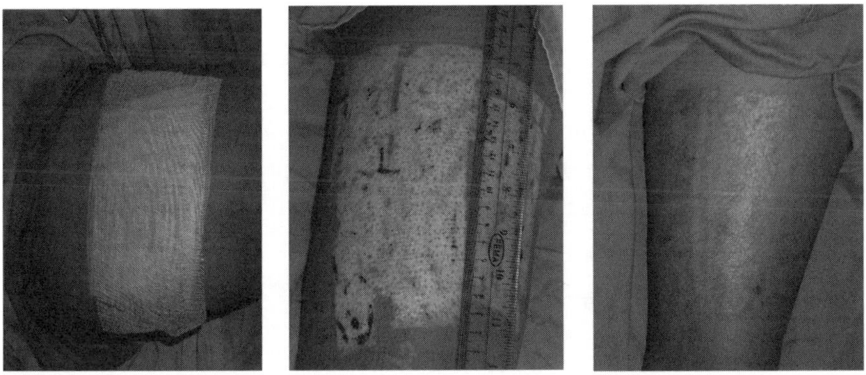

(a) (b) (c)

Fig. 2. Human amnion as biological dressing for split-thickness skin graft (SSG) donor site. (a) Dried human amnion is thin, elastic, and light. (b) SSG donor site treated with amnion at postoperative day 10. (c) SSG donor site treated with amnion at postoperative 3 months.

Effective vapor barrier

The structure of the amnion resembles the stratum corneum epidermis of the skin, which is a natural vapor barrier. It is important to note that amnion does not influence the shift of fluid in the extracellular space from plasma into the interstitial compartment. By preventing evaporation from the wound surface, insensible losses are prevented, thus reducing the quantity of fluid that needs to be replaced in cases of burn injuries (Gump and Kinney 1970). Furthermore, by preventing evaporation from the wound surface, the temperature regulation mechanism is not overstrained and the caloric requirement needed to maintain the temperature is also correspondingly reduced. The maintenance of a moist environment within the donor wound surface by the amnion cannot be overstated, as the moist environment facilitates rapid epithelialization and wound healing (Winter 1962).

Significant reduction of pain at the donor site

Good adherence of the amnion on the donor wound surface and the maintenance of a moist environment shield the exposed nerve endings from external elements. This significantly reduces the pain at the donor site and the requirement of analgesics.

Bacteriostatic activity

Many theories on the bacteriostatic activity of amnion have been reported. It is interesting to note that the drying process of amnion or the removal of chorion does not alter the immunologic properties of the amnion. This indicates that the dried amnion retains all of the antibodies in a dormant state and that the drying, irradiation, and storage processes do not destroy them (Rao and Chandrasekharam 1981).

Adjunct dressing in flap surgery

Flap surgery is the process of transferring a tissue with its own vascular supply from one area (donor site) to a wound defect (recipient site). Flaps are always at risk of failure from reversible congestion to irreversible flap necrosis. Continuous monitoring is vital to avoid necrosis. Flap color is one of the most important clinical parameters to monitor flap wellbeing.

Amnion dressing offers a translucent dressing when in contact with the wound bed, thus facilitating continuous flap monitoring [Fig. 3(a)]. It contours well with the wound bed, resulting in easy application and holistic flap monitoring comparable with other dressings. Amnion adheres well to the wound, and acts as a protective barrier against wound contamination while keeping the wound moist [Fig. 3(b)]. Amnion can also be used as a dressing material for flap donor site wounds (Fig. 4), with the additional advantage of pain reduction.

Traumatic soft tissue injury

Abrasion injury can be described as partial skin loss similar to partial-thickness burn [Fig. 5(a)]. It ranges from epidermal loss to deep dermal loss.

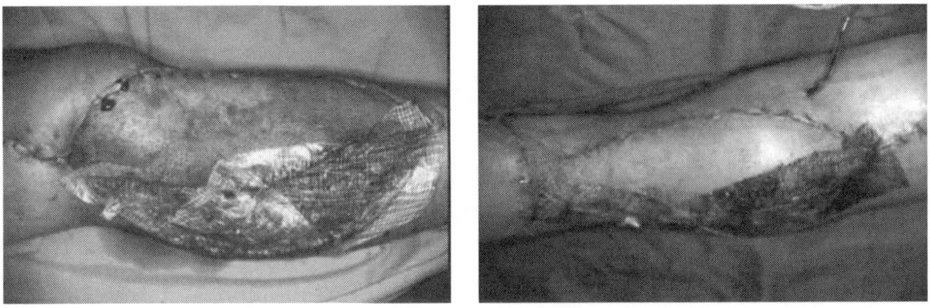

(a) (b)

Fig. 3. Application of amnion on residual wound of flap recipient site. (a) Immediately after application on a revised flap. (b) Three days after amnion application on the residual wound of another free fibula flap.

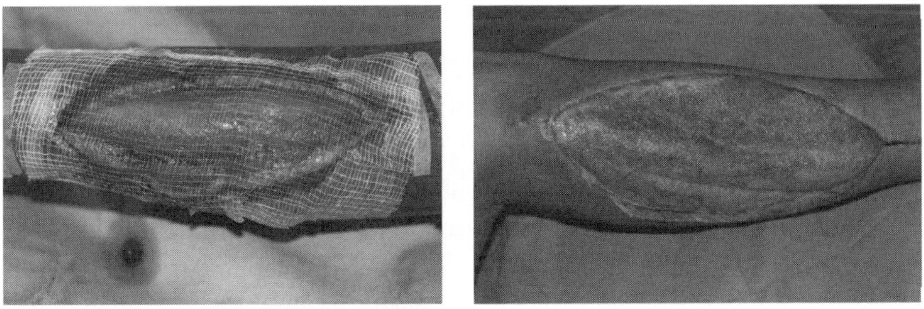

(a) (b)

Fig. 4. Amnion as a flap donor site dressing material. (a) Immediately after application. (b) Five days after application on another patient.

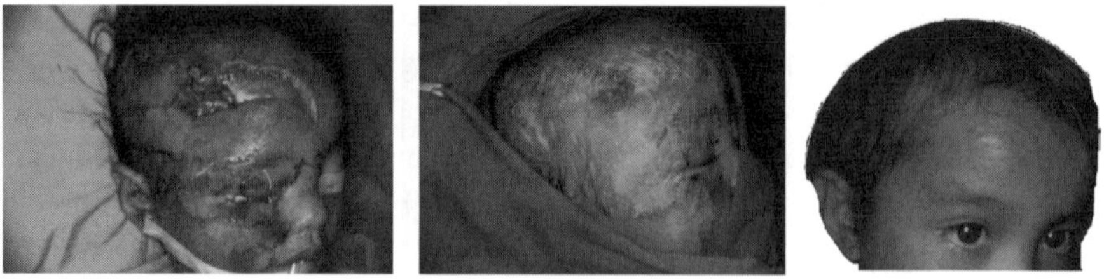

(a) (b) (c)

Fig. 5. Facial trauma with laceration and abrasion wound. (a) Wound prior to repair. (b) Immediately after repair and application of amnion. (c) Results 3 months after injury with minimal scarring.

It heals by re-epithelization with minimal-to-moderate scarring, depending on its thickness.

Amnion is suitable as an abrasion wound dressing material because it contours well with the wound, resulting in maximum wound–amnion contact [Fig. 5(b)]. It keeps the wound moist for better re-epithelization and as a barrier of contamination. Its translucency gives an extra advantage of wound inspection without the need to change the dressing. The end result of abrasion managed with amnion dressing is comparable with other commercial dressings [Fig. 5(c)].

However, amnion is less favorable when used in deep or contaminated abrasion because amnion has minimal absorptive capacity and is biodegradable, thus leaving its outer linen layer impregnated into the granulating wound. Intense tissue reaction can give rise to unfavorable scarring.

Base in tissue engineering

Human amniotic membrane is the innermost layer of the placental membranes. It is a thin semitransparent membrane. It is tough and devoid of blood vessels, lymphatics, and nerves. The amnion comprises a single layer of ectodermally derived columnar epithelial cells, which adhere to a basement membrane largely composed of collagen I, collagen III, collagen IV, laminin, and fibronectin, which in turn is attached to an underlying layer of connective tissue. The connective tissue has three components: an acellular compact layer composed of reticular fibers; a fibroblast layer, which is a loose reticular network containing sporadic fibroblasts; and a spongy layer, which is in contact with the underlying chorion and consists of a complex network of fine fibrils surrounded by mucus.

Amnion cells produce and release a large variety of growth factors. These include epidermal growth factor, transforming growth factor, insulin-like growth factor, hepatocyte growth factor, nerve growth factor, and vascular endothelial growth factor, all of which have been attributed to the proliferative influence of the amnion epithelium. The epithelium of the amnion is capable of storing lipids and glycogen as well as hemosiderin (Rejzek *et al.* 2001).

Tissue engineering methods designed to restore diseased and damaged tissues depend on the presence of a matrix structure that is amenable to cell growth and proliferation. This means that amnion membrane has the potential to become a scaffold for cell culture (Hodde 2002). The matrix component of the amnion membrane has been proven to be biocompatible *in vitro*, and has no adverse effects on cellular proliferation or morphology (Wilshaw *et al.* 2006). The amnion membrane thus has immense potential to be used as a delivery system for epithelial cells, i.e. autologous cells can be grown to confluence and later be returned to the patient as living tissue. The culture of human corneal epithelial cells on amnion membrane has also been well established (Kobayashi *et al.* 2006).

The goal of tissue engineering is to incite the formation of tissue structures that humans are incapable of regenerating on their own as effectively and efficiently as possible while ensuring the safety, minimizing the morbidity, and maximizing the quality of life for the recipient. Naturally occurring biopolymer scaffold materials that interact with the host and fasten tissue regeneration are viable alternatives to synthetic polymers for tissue engineering cell growth substrates.

Conclusion

Amnion comes close to the description of the ideal biological dressing. Being readily available, inexpensive to use, easily processed and stored, low in antigenicity and with antimicrobial potential, and able to enhance epithelialization with marked relief of pain, amnion is suited for temporary or long-term coverage of wounds in various clinical conditions. Therefore, with health service finances increasingly stretched to provide adequate care, it is time for surgeons and patients alike to overcome an almost primitive reluctance to make use of amnion for wound healing when so much evidence indicates its merits. Indeed, this truly biological dressing is needlessly going to waste.

References

Bose B (1979). Burn wound dressing with human amniotic membrane. *Ann R Coll Surg Engl* **61**:444–447.

Burgos H (1983). Angiogenic and growth factors in human amniochorion and placenta. *Eur J Clin Invest* **13**:289–296.

Burgos H and Sergeant RJ (1983). Lyophilized human amniotic membranes used in reconstruction of the ear (letter). *J R Soc Med* **76**:433.

Burleson R and Eiseman B (1972). Nature of bond between partial-thickness skin and wound granulations. *Surgery* **72**:315–322.

Colocho G, Graham 3rd WP, Greene AE, Matheson DW, and Lynch D (1974). Human amniotic membrane as a physiological wound dressing. *Arch Surg* **109**:370–373.

Davis JS (1910). Skin transplantation with a review of 550 cases at the Johns Hopkins Hospital. *Johns Hopkins Med J* **15**:307–395.

Faulk WP and Galbraith GMP (1979). Trophoblast transferrin and transferrin receptors in the host–parasite relationship of human pregnancy. *Proc R Soc Lond B Biol Sci* **204**:83–97.

Faulk WP, Matthews RN, Stevens PJ, Bennett JP, Burgos H, and Hsi BL (1980). Human amnion as an adjunct in wound healing. *Lancet* **1**:1156–1158.

Gajiwala AL and Sharma V (2003). Use of irradiated amnion as a biological dressing in the treatment of radiation induced ulcers. *Cell Tissue Bank* **4**:147–150.

Galask RP and Synder IS (1970). Antimicrobials in amniotic fluid. *Am J Obstet Gynecol* **106**:59–65.

Gruss JS and Jirsch DW (1978). Human amniotic membranes: a versatile wound dressing. *Can Med Assoc J* **118**:237–240.

Gump FE and Kinney JM (1970). Caloric and fluid losses through the burn wound. *Surg Clin North Am* **50**:1235–1248.

Hasim M and Yusof N (1994). Radiation sterilization of amnion and its clinical use. In: *3rd European Conference on Tissue Banking and Clinical Application of Grafts*, Vienna, Austria.

Hodde J (2002). Naturally occurring scaffolds for soft tissue repair and regeneration. *Tissue Eng* **8**:295–308.

Kirschbaum SM and Hernandez H (1963). Use of amnion in extensive burns. In: Broadbent TR (ed.), *Proceedings of the 3rd International Congress in Plastic Surgery*, Excerpta Medica, Amsterdam, pp. 152–162.

Kobayashi A, Yoshita T, and Sugiyama K (2006). In vivo confocal microscopic analysis of human corneal epithelial sheet cultured on amniotic membrane. *Ophthalmic Surg Lasers Imaging* **37**:304–309.

Matthews RN, Faulk WP, and Bennett JP (1982). A review of the role of amniotic membranes in surgical practice. In: Wynn RM (ed.), *Obstetrics and Gynaecology Annual,* Appleton-Century-Crofts, New York, pp. 31–58.

McIntyre JA and Faulk WP (1979). Antigens of human trophoblasts: effects of heterologous and anti-trophoblast sera on lymphocyte responses in vitro. *J Exp Med* **149**:824–836.

Rao TV and Chandrasekharam V (1981). Use of dry human bovine amnion as a biological dressing. *Arch Surg* **116**:891–896.

Rejzek A, Weyer F, Eichberger R, and Gebhart W (2001). Physical changes of amniotic membranes through glycerolization for the uses as an epidermal substitute. Light and electron microscopic studies. *Cell Tissue Bank* **2**:95–102.

Robson MC and Krizek TJ (1973). Amniotic membranes as a temporary wound dressing. *Surg Gynecol Obstet* **136**:904–906.

Sachs BP and Stern CMM (1970). Activity and characterization of a low molecular weight fraction in human amniotic fluid with broad spectrum antibiotic activity. *Br J Obstet Gynaecol* **86**:81–86.

Saymen DG, Nathan P, Holder IA, Hill EO, and Macmillan BG (1973). Control of surface wound infection: skin versus synthetic grafts. *Appl Environ Microbiol* **25**:921–934.

Shun A and Ramsey-Stewart G (1983). Human amnion in the treatment of chronic ulceration of the legs. *Med J Aust* **2**:279–283.

Sinha R (1990). Amniotic membrane in the treatment of burn injury. *Indian J Surg* **52**:11–17.

Subrahmanyam M (1995). Amniotic membrane as a cover for microskin grafts. *Br J Plast Surg* **48**:477–478.

Talmi YP, Finkelstein Y, and Zohar Y (1990). Use of human amniotic membrane as a biological dressing. *Eur J Plast Surg* **13**:160–162.

Trelford JD, Hanson FW, and Anderson DG (1973). Amniotic membrane as a living surgical dressing in human patients. *Oncology* **28**:358–364.

Trelford JD and Trelford-Sauder M (1979). The amnion in surgery, past and present. *Am J Obstet Gynecol* **134**:833–845.

Unger MG and Roberts M (1976). Lyophilized amniotic membranes on graft donor sites. *Br J Plast Surg* **29**:99–101.

Ward DJ, Bennett JP, Burgos H, and Fabre J (1989). The healing of chronic venous leg ulcers with prepared human amnion. *Br J Plast Surg* **42**:463–467.

Wilshaw SP, Kearney JN, Fisher J, and Ingham E (2006). Production of an acellular amniotic membrane matrix for use in tissue engineering. *Tissue Eng* **12**:2117–2129.

Winter GB (1962). Formation of the scab and the rate of epithelialization of superficial wounds in the skin of the young domestic pig. *Nature* **193**:293–294.

APPENDICES

APPENDIX 1

Standards for Tissue Banking

Asia Pacific Association of Surgical Tissue Banks

ASIA PACIFIC ASSOCIATION FOR SURGICAL TISSUE BANKS

STANDARDS FOR TISSUE BANKING

1st Edition

Printing Date: April 2007

These *Standards* are reviewed periodically and revised to incorporate the latest in tissue banking and transplantation techniques that would affect tissue banking. The reader is advised to use the most recent version.

ISBN No: 978-981-05-7404-8
Printed in Singapore

ASIA PACIFIC ASSOCIATION FOR SURGICAL TISSUE BANKS

STANDARDS FOR TISSUE BANKING

Standards Sub-Committee

Chairman:

Aziz Nather (Singapore)

Members:

Norimah Yusof (Malaysia)

Nazly Hilmy (Indonesia)

Yong-Koo Kang (Korea)

Astrid L Gajiwala (India)

Lyn Ireland (Australia)

Shekhar Kumta (Hong Kong)

Chang-Joon Yim (Korea)

Acknowledgements

The Association acknowledges the contributions of the International Atomic Energy Agency under the Interregional Project of Tissue Banking led by Mr. Jorge Morales and Professor Glyn O. Phillips for organising several workshops involving experts from American Association of Tissue Banks, European Association of Tissue Banks and the Therapeutics Goods Administration Act, to develop IAEA International Standards on Tissue Banking designed as a basic template to be used by Asia Pacific Association for Surgical Tissue Banks (APASTB) and the Latin American Association of Tissue Banks (ALABAT) to develop their own *Standards*.

Preface

Recent advances in Medical Science and Biotechnology have led to making transplantation of cells and tissue from one human being into another more safe to restore form and function and improve the quality of life. The act of donating tissues to help the suffering of fellow human beings is a humanitarian act of the highest significance. The procurement, processing and transplantation of such tissues must comply with the highest quality standards to make safe tissue transplantation practice possible.

APASTB has, for a long time, aspired to produce *Standards* that could be implemented and adopted universally by all countries in the region. The Standards Sub-Committee was formed in 2000 in Kuala Lumpur for this purpose. Several meetings with long deliberations have been held. The first draft was produced in Bali in 2000, the second in Seoul, Korea in 2002, the third in Hong Kong in 2004, before finalising a first edition of the *Standards* in Mumbai in November 2006. These *Standards* will be reviewed periodically and new editions will be produced in the future as and when required.

The *Standards* establish performance requirements for all aspects of tissue banking ranging from donor selection criteria, procurement, processing, storage, packaging, labelling and distribution of human musculoskeletal tissues, skin and amnion. APASTB hopes that all tissue banks in the region will comply with the *Standards* established for tissue bank functions relating to donors, tissues and records management. The *Standards* do not encompass the clinical use of cells and tissues.

The production of the first edition of these *Standards* marks an important milestone in the history of APASTB. In the near future, the Association strives to provide accreditation to tissue banks in the region based on the *Standards* it has produced and adopted.

Aziz Nather
Chairman, Standards Sub-Committee, APASTB

Contents

APASTB STANDARDS FOR TISSUE BANKS

SECTION A: GENERAL AND ORGANISATIONAL POLICIES

A 1.000 INTRODUCTION

A 1.100 General

A 1.110 *Scope*

These Standards apply to human tissues used for therapeutic purposes, excluding reproductive and genetically modified tissues. It does not apply to animal tissues.

A 1.120 *Purpose of the Standards*

These standards brings together the current state of the art and practice on selection of donors, tissue retrieval, testing, processing, storage, labelling and distribution of processed tissue, in order to provide safe tissues of reliable quality while respecting the ethical rules.

A 1.200 Definitions

See Annex 1.

A 2.000 ETHICAL AND LEGAL RULES

A 2.100 General

In each country, the applicable Inter-governmental, National, Regional and Local Law or Regulation governing consent and retrieval of tissues from living or cadaver donors shall be followed.

A 2.200 Permission for Tissue Retrieval

If there is no applicable Inter-governmental, National, Regional and Local Law or Regulation, the following principles shall be applied:

A 2.210 *Living Donor Consent*

A 2.211 *Voluntary Donation of Tissue*

- Appropriate medical investigation shall be made to evaluate and reduce the risk to the health of donor and recipient.
- The donor must be given appropriate information before the removal about the possible consequences of this removal, in particular medical, social and psychological, as well as the importance of the donation for the recipient. An Informed Consent in writing shall be obtained from the living donor. Consent before an official body may be necessary according to applicable Inter-governmental, National, Regional and Local Law or Regulation.
- In case of a minor or otherwise legally incapacitated person, Informed Consent shall be obtained from his legal representative, if the donor does not object to it. The appropriate authority shall be consulted in accordance to applicable Inter-governmental, National, Regional and Local Law or Regulation.
- The donation of substances, which cannot regenerate, is usually confined to transplantation between family related persons and restricted to major and capable persons.

A 2.212 *Collection of Surgical Residues*

- Surgical residues are collected during a surgical procedure where the material is collected for therapeutic purpose other than to obtain tissue (e.g. femoral head, skin and amnion).
- Informed Consent shall be obtained from the donor according to applicable Regulation.

A 2.213 *Non-Living Donor Consent*

- No removal of tissue will take place when there was an open or presumed objection on the part of the deceased.
- Permission or confirmation of the absence of objection for tissue donation shall be obtained from the next of kin.

- In case of a minor or legally incapacitated person, the consent of his legal representative is required.
- Removal of tissue can be effected if it does not interfere with a forensic examination or autopsy as required by Law.

A 2.214 *Consent Documentation*

Consent for tissue donation shall be documented. The consent form shall specify whether there is a general permission for organs and / or tissues or permission for specified organs and / or tissues only.

A 2.300 Monetary Inducement for Donation

A 2.310 *Prohibition of Payment to Donor*

Monetary payment or advantages for the donation shall not be made to living donors, cadaver donor's next of kin or any donor-related party.

A 2.320 *Compensation for Donation-Related Expenses*

Donors or their family shall not be financially responsible for expenses related to retrieval of tissues.

A 2.400 Anonymity

Anonymity between donor and unrelated recipient shall be strictly preserved. Anonymity between donor and recipient shall allow tracking of tissues, through anonymous identification numbers.

A 3.000 ORGANISATION OF A TISSUE BANK

A 3.100 Institutional Identity

A 3.110 *General*

The purpose of a Tissue Bank shall be clearly established and documented. The Tissue Bank shall state whether it is a free standing entity or part of an Institution.

A 3.120 *Authorisation, Licensing or Registration*

The Tissue Bank shall comply with all applicable Inter-governmental, National, Regional and Local Law or Regulation for authorisation, licensing or registration.

A 3.130 *Collaboration with other Organisations*

A 3.131 *Written Agreement – Contract*

Each Tissue Bank shall have written agreements or contracts with all other organisations, which perform donor screening services, tissue retrieval, processing or distribution for the Tissue Bank.

Tissue Banks which contract for laboratory services shall verify the laboratory licensing or accreditation, according to applicable Intergovernmental, National, Regional and Local Law or Regulation.

A 3.132 *On-site Audit*

The Tissue Bank shall maintain documentation for the services performed for the Tissue Bank. Such documentation shall itemise all operational systems, which were audited to determine compliance with Standards or applicable Regulation.

A 3.200 Personnel

A 3.210 *Medical Director*

A 3.211 *Qualification*

The Medical Director shall be qualified by training and experiences for the scope of activities being pursued in accordance with applicable Intergovernmental, National, Regional and Local Law or Regulation.

A 3.212 *Responsibilities*

The Medical Director shall be responsible for medical operations, including compliance with these Standards. His/Her responsibilities include determining what tissues are to be collected, define donor screening policies and prescribe technically acceptable means for their processing, Quality Assurance, storage and distribution. The Medical Director shall be responsible for policies and procedures regarding donor suitability and adverse events.

A 3.220 *Administrative Director*

The Administrative Director, when applicable, shall be responsible for administration, management, and other general activities. The Administrative Director shall not be responsible for medical activities.

A 3.230 *Staff*

A 3.231 *General*

The Tissue Bank shall have sufficient personnel for pursuing the various tasks.

A 3.232 *Qualification*

The Tissue Bank staff must possess the educational background, experience and training, sufficient to assure assigned tasks are performed in accordance with the Tissue Banks established procedures.

A 3.233 *Responsibilities*

The technical staff shall be responsible for implementation of policies and procedures as established by the Medical Director. The duties of each staff member shall be described in a written job description. Staff must demonstrate competency in operations to which they are assigned.

A 3.240 *Medical Advisory Board*

It is recommended that a Tissue Bank set up a Medical Advisory Board to provide medico-technical and scientific advice (external from the Tissue Bank).

A 3.250 *Training*

The scope of activities, specific staff responsibilities and reporting structure shall be established by the Medical Director. The Medical Director shall ensure that all staff members have adequate training to perform their duties safely and competently. The Medical Director shall be responsible for ensuring that technical staff maintains their competency by participation in training courses and technical meetings or other educational programmes. All staff shall review applicable institutional policies and procedures annually and when changes are made.

A 3.300 Quality Management System

In order to reduce the risk for patients by the transplantation of tissues to an acceptable level, it is necessary to operate an effective Quality Management System.

The System may include extensive testing of donor blood and tissue samples, but this alone is not sufficient guarantee of safety and efficacy and the System should include other management and control measures.

Those involved in procuring, processing and supplying tissues for transplantation shall, in addition, implement a risk analysis of procedures prone to error to disease transmission. This QA procedure should be used to develop safe procedures and implement a Quality Management System based on clearly identified requirements for tissues.

A 3.310 *Quality Requirements*

The Quality Requirements form the basis of all Quality Assurance and Quality Control Programmes. It is necessary to define the Quality Requirements not only for the final product, but also for the starting material collected, reagents and equipment used, staff competencies, testing techniques, packaging materials, labels and process intermediates.

These Quality Requirements are best prescribed and quantified in written specifications. These specifications determine the Quality Control testing or inspection performed on which release decisions are based.

The Quality Requirements will be based on characteristics that effect both patient safety and maintaining the clinical effectiveness of the product.

A 3.320 *Quality Management*

It is recognised that quality has to be managed in an organisation and that a systematic approach is the only way to ensure that the quality of products produced and services delivered consistently meets the Quality Requirements. The high level of Quality Assurance required for safety, critical therapeutic medical products and clinical services can only be achieved through the implementation of an effective Quality Management.

The International Standard for Quality Management is the ISO 9000 series. Specific principles to be incorporated into the Quality Systems covering the manufacture and Quality Control of medicines are known as Good Manufacturing Practice (GMP). The ISO Standards, GMP or other applicable Standards and other applicable Inter-governmental, National, Regional and Local Law or Regulation, should be consulted when developing a Quality Management for Tissue Banking organisations and other procurement organisations.

A 3.330 *The Basic Elements of an Appropriate Quality Management System*

A 3.331 *Organisational Structure and Accountability*

- This is necessary to achieve the Quality Requirements and for reviewing the effectiveness of the arrangements for Quality Assurance. There should be a suitably qualified and experienced member of staff appointed who verifies that the Quality Requirements are being met, and that there is compliance with the Quality Management System.
- The Quality Manager should be a designated individual who should be independent of production (not directly responsible for or involved in the procurement, processing and testing of tissue) and preferably of other responsibilities within the Tissue Bank.

The Quality Manager should be generally familiar with the specific work being reviewed and be responsible for each Quality Assurance review. This individual should report, for his function, specifically to this Medical Director and/or his/her designee.

Where a Tissue Bank is operated within a large organisation with its own Quality Department and possibly its own Quality Manager then strong working links should exist between the Tissue Bank's Quality Manager and the relevant Quality Department staff, as well as to the Medical Director.

A 3.332 *Documentation*

• *Rationale*

The objectives of thorough documentation are to define the system of information and control, to minimise the risk of misinterpretation and error inherent in oral or casually written communication and to provide unambiguous procedures to be followed.

Documents should clearly state the Quality Requirements, organisational structures and responsibilities, the organisation's policies and standards, the management and technical procedures employed and the records required.

• *General*

All procedures in the processing of tissue should be documented and the documents controlled.

Documentation should be legible, readily identifiable and retrievable.

Documentation should clearly identify the way in which it is to be used and by whom.

Documentation should be available to staff to cover all procedures.

Any correction should be handwritten clearly and legibly in permanent ink and signed and dated by an authorised person.

• *Control of Documentation*

The system for document control should identify the current revision status of any document and the holder of the document.

The system in place should demonstrate that all controlled documents meet the following criteria:

- They are current and authorised.
- They are reviewed at regular intervals.
- Multiple copies are controlled with a distribution list.
- Obsolete documents are removed and controlled to prevent further use.
- Changes to documents should be acted upon promptly. They should be reviewed, dated and signed by the authorised person and formally implemented.

• *Storage and Retention of Documentation*

Documented procedures should be established and maintained for identification, collection, filing, storage, retrieval and maintenance of all documents.

Master copies of obsolete copies should be archived in a secure and safe environment for not less than 10 years or in accordance with applicable Inter-governmental, National, Regional and Local Law or Regulation.

A 3.333 *Control of Processes (SOPs)*

- Written instructions of Standard Operating Procedures (SOPs) shall be produced where it is essential that tasks must be performed in a consistent way. Equipment, processes and procedures shall be validated as effective before being implemented or changed.

Equipment essential to the quality of the product shall be routinely serviced and calibrated, if appropriate. The processing environment and staff performing processes shall meet minimum, prescribed Standards of cleanliness and hygiene.

- The Tissue Bank shall maintain a SOPs Manual which details in writing all aspects of these Standards. The SOPs shall be utilised to ensure that all material released for transplantation meet at least minimum requirements defined by professional Standards and applicable Inter-governmental, National, Regional and Local Law or Regulation.

  The SOPs Manuals should include, where relevant, but should not be limited to the following:

  - Standard procedures for donor screening, consent, retrieval, processing, preservation, testing, storage and distribution
  - Quality Assurance and Quality Control Policies
  - Laboratory procedures for tests performed in-house and in contracted laboratories
  - Specifications for materials used including supply, reagents, storage media and packaging materials
  - Personnel and facility safety procedures
  - Standard procedures for facility maintenance, cleaning and waste disposal procedures
  - Methods for verification of the effectiveness of sterilisation procedures
  - Equipment maintenance, calibration and validation procedures
  - Environmental and microbiological conditions and the methods used for controlling, testing and verification
  - Physiological and physical test specifications for materials
  - Methods for determination of shelf life, storage temperature and assigning expiry dates of tissues
  - Determination of insert and or label text
  - Policies and procedures for exceptional release of material
  - Procedures for adverse events reporting and corrective actions
  - Donor/recipient tracking and product recall policies and procedures

- All SOPs, their modification and associated process-validation studies shall be reviewed and approved by either the Medical or Administrative

Director as dictated by content. All medically related SOPs shall be reviewed and approved by the Medical Director.

Copies of the SOPs Manual shall be available to all staff, and to authorised individuals for inspections upon request. Upon implementation, all SOPs shall be followed as written. SOPs shall be updated at regular intervals to reflect modifications or changes. The authorised person, depending on the content shall approve each modification or change.

Appropriate training shall be provided to pertinent staff. Obsolete SOPs Manuals shall be archived for a minimum of 10 years taking into account the shelf life of the material.

A 3.334 *Record Keeping*

• *General*

Records shall be confidential, accurate, complete, legible and indelible. All donor, processing, storage, and distribution records should be maintained for 10 years or in accordance with applicable Inter-governmental, National, Regional and Local Law or Regulation.

Records shall hold all information that identifies the origins of the product and to demonstrate that the product meets all the Quality Requirements. Records shall show that all the required processing steps and all Quality Control tests have been performed correctly by trained staff and that the product has only been released for use after the correct authorisation.

Records shall also demonstrate correct handling and storage of materials and track the final status of products, whether transplanted, discarded or used for research. The use and storage of records shall be controlled.

• *Contract Records*

When two or more Tissue Banks participate in tissue procurement, processing, storage or distribution functions, the relationships and responsibilities of each shall be documented and ensure compliance with relevant scientific and quality professional Standards by all parties. Tissue Banks should perform on-site audits of contract laboratories to ensure their compliance with relevant scientific and professional Standards, Technical Manuals and the Tissue Bank's own requirements.

• *Donor Tracking*

Each component shall be assigned one unique identifier that shall serve as a lot number to identify the material during all steps from collection to distribution and utilisation. This unique number shall link the final packaged material to the donor. This number shall be used to link the donor to all tests, records, organs and other material, and for tracking purposes to the recipient.

Records shall include identification and evaluation of the donor, blood testing and micro-biological evaluation of the donor, conditions under which the material is procured, processed, tested and stored and its final destination.

Records shall indicate the dates and identity of staff involved in each significant step of the operation.

• *Inventory*

A record of unprocessed, processed, quarantined and distributed tissues shall be maintained.

• *Recipient Adverse Events and Non-compliances*

An adverse events file shall be maintained including any non-compliance.

• *Electronic Records*

If a computer record-keeping system is used, there shall be a system to ensure the authenticity, integrity and confidentiality of all records but retain the ability to generate true paper copies.

A description of the system, its function and specified requirements must be documented. The system shall record the identity of persons entering or confirming critical data.

Alteration to the system or programme shall only be made in accordance with defined procedures. When the release of finished batches is conducted by computerised systems it must identify and record the person (s) releasing the batches.

Alternative management systems should be available to cope with failures in computerised systems.

A 3.340 *Methods for Detecting, Correcting and Preventing Quality Failures from Recurring*

A 3.341 *Quality Failures*

Quality failures include in-use product deficiencies (complaints, adverse events, etc.), failures to meet Quality Control specifications and non-compliance with procedures. Methods for detecting failures include Quality Control tests, inspections, Quality Audits, staff and end-user feedback. The ability to trace, locate, quarantine and recall materials, consumables and products at any stage, is essential to patient safety. Serious failures shall be thoroughly registered, investigated and appropriate changes to specifications, systems and procedures implemented to prevent further failures of a similar nature.

The matter must be reported to Tissue Bank Administration Board. Corrective action must be taken by the tissue bank and a full report of the corrective action must be submitted to the board. The Board must be satisfied with the corrective action.

A 3.342 *Audit*

The Tissue Bank shall participate in an Audit Programme. Quality Assurance staff shall perform internal audits. Focused audits shall be conducted to monitor critical areas and when problems with quality have been identified. Regular audits shall be performed by qualified staff who do not have direct responsibility for the processes being audited.

A 3.350 *Competency*

The educational and training requirements for each member of staff shall be determined and specified. There shall be regular and formal appraisal of staff competency. Training and education shall include the requirements for quality, Standards of Practice and Good Hygiene as well as appropriate continuing professional development. Records of training shall be maintained up to date.

A 3.400 Facilities and Equipment

A 3.410 *General*

The facilities of the Tissue Bank shall be of suitable size and location and shall be designed and equipped for the specialised purposes for which they are to be used.

A 3.420 *Design*

The design of the facilities shall prevent errors and cross-contamination. Critical procedures shall be performed in designated areas of adequate size.

A 3.430 *Security*

Access to the Tissue Bank shall be limited to authorised persons.

A 3.440 *Environmental Monitoring*

Environmental monitoring procedures shall be established, when appropriate, as part of the Quality Assurance Programme. The procedures shall include acceptable test parameters. The monitoring may include particulate air samplings and work surface cultures. Each monitoring activity shall be documented.

A 3.450 *Sanitation*

Facilities used for retrieval, processing or preservation, shall be subjected to routine, scheduled and documented cleaning procedures.

A 3.460 *Equipment and Instruments*

Equipment and instruments shall be of appropriate quality for their intended function. Equipment and non-disposable supplies that come into contact with tissue shall be constructed so surfaces do not alter the safety or quality of the material.

Equipment shall be designed, manufactured and qualified for appropriate cleaning and shall be sterilised or decontaminated after each use. Multiple uses of disposable instruments for several donors shall be excluded.

There shall be SOPs for monitoring, inspection, maintenance, calibration, and cleaning procedures for each piece of equipment. Storage equipment shall be inspected on a regularly scheduled basis. Appropriate certification and maintenance records shall be maintained for equipment and instruments.

A 3.470 *Environmental Safety*

A 3.471 *General*

Each Tissue Bank shall provide and promote a safe work environment by developing, implementing and enforcing safety procedures. Safety precautions and procedures for maintaining a safe work environment shall be included in the SOPs Manual and shall conform to applicable Inter-governmental, National, Regional and Local Law or Regulation.

A 3.472 *Safety Procedures*

Safety procedures shall include, but are not limited to the following:

- Instructions for fire prevention and evacuation routes in case of fire or natural disaster
- Procedures for prevention of worker injury including possible exposure to biohazards material
- Procedures for proper storage, handling and utilisation of hazardous materials, reagents and supplies
- Procedures outlining the steps to be followed in cleaning biohazard spills
- Hazardous material training including chemical, biological and radioactive hazards
- Immunisation: appropriate vaccinations should be offered to all non-immune personnel whose job-related responsibilities involve potential exposure to blood-borne pathogens. Personnel files should include documentation of receipt of vaccination or refusal of vaccination
- Personnel: personnel engaged in the retrieval, processing, preservation and packaging of tissues shall be suitable attired to minimise the spread of transmissible pathogens among and between donors, tissue and staff. Any staff member with a serious infectious condition shall be excluded from the Tissue Banking activities until the condition is resolved.

A 3.473 *Waste Disposal*

Human tissue and other hazardous waste items shall be disposed of in such a manner so as to prevent hazards to Tissue Bank personnel or the environment and shall conform to applicable Inter-governmental, National, Regional and Local Law or Regulation. Dignified and proper disposal procedures shall be applied to human remains.

SECTION B: IMPLEMENTATION

B 1.000 DONOR SELECTION

B 1.100 General

The suitability of a specific donor for tissue allograft donation is based upon medical and behavioural history, medical records review, physical examination, cadaveric donor autopsy findings (if an autopsy is performed) and laboratory tests.

B 1.200 Medical and Behavioural History

B 1.210 *Donor History Review*

Donor evaluation includes an interview of the potential living donor or the cadaveric donor's next of kin, performed by suitably trained personnel, using a questionnaire.

A qualified physician shall approve the donor evaluation process.

B 1.220 *Exclusion Criteria*

B 1.221 *General Contraindications*

The following conditions contraindicate the use of tissues for therapeutic purposes:

- History of chronic viral Hepatitis.
- Presence of active viral Hepatitis or jaundice of unknown etiology.
- History of, or clinical evidence, or suspicion, or laboratory evidence of HIV infection.
- Risk factors for HIV, HBV and HCV have to be assessed by the Medical Director according to existing National Regulations taking into account national epidemiology. Annex 2 includes a generally agreed list of risk factors.
- Presence or suspicion of central degenerative neurological diseases of possible infectious origin, including dementia (e.g. Alzheimer's

Disease, Creutzfeldt-Jakob Disease or familial history of Creutzfeldt-Jakob Disease and Multiple Sclerosis).

- Use of all native human pituitary derived hormones (e.g. growth hormone), possible history of dura-mater allograft, including unspecified intracranial surgery.
- Septicemia and systemic viral disease or mycosis or active tuberculosis at the time of procurement preclude procurement of tissues. In case of other active bacterial infection, tissue may be used only if processed using a validated method for bacterial inactivation and after approval by the Medical Director.
- Presence or history of malignant disease. Exceptions may include primary basal cell carcinoma of the skin, histologically proven and unmetastatic primary brain tumour (see Annex 3).
- Significant history of connective tissue disease (e.g. systemic lupus erythematosus and rheumatoid arthritis) or any immunosuppressive treatment.
- Significant exposure to a toxic substance that may be transferred in toxic doses or damage the tissue (e.g. cyanide, lead, mercury and gold).
- Presence or evidence of infection or prior irradiation at the site of donation.
- Unknown cause of death.

B 1.222 *Specific Tissue Selection Criteria*

Cornea donors with solid extra-ocular malignancies are generally accepted.

B 1.300 Physical Examination

Prior to procurement of tissue, the donor body shall be examined for general exclusion signs and for signs of infection, trauma or medical intervention over donor sites that can affect the quality of the donated tissue.

B 1.400 Cadaveric Donor Autopsy Report

If an autopsy is performed, the results shall be reviewed by the Medical Director or designee before tissue is released for distribution.

B 1.500 Transmissible Diseases Blood Tests

B 1.510 *General*

B 1.511 *Law and Practice*

Tissues shall be tested for transmissible diseases in compliance with Law and practice in the country concerned. In the case of living donors, applicable consent procedure for blood testing shall be followed.

B 1.512 *Tests*

Tests shall be performed and found acceptable on properly identified blood samples from the donor using recognized, and if applicable, licensed tests and according to manufacturer's instructions. Tests shall be performed by a qualified, and if applicable, licensed laboratory and according to Good Laboratory Practice (GLP).

B 1.513 *Timing of Blood Sampling*

Blood for donor screening for deceased donors should be taken at the time of procurement or within 24 hours after death at the latest.

Blood for donor screening for living donors should be taken at the time of procurement or within 7 days of the procurement.

B 1.514 *Recent Blood Transfusion*

For potential tissue donors who have received blood, blood components, or plasma volume expanders within 48 hours prior to death, if there is an expected hemodilution of more than 50%, based on calculation algorithm (see example of algorithm in Annex 4), a pre-transfusion blood sample shall be tested.

B 1.515 *Notification of Confirmed Positive Test Results*

The donor's physician shall be notified in accordance with State Laws of confirmed positive results having clinical significance.

Confirmed positive donor infectious disease tests shall be reported to Local/National Health Authorities, when required.

B 1.516 *Donor Serum Archive*

A sample of donor serum shall be securely sealed and stored frozen in a proper manner until 5 years after the expiration date of the tissue or according to applicable Inter-governmental, National, Regional and Local Law or Regulation.

B 1.520 *Blood Tests*

B 1.521 *Minimum Blood Tests*

Minimum Blood Tests shall include:

- Human Immunodeficiency Virus Antibodies (HIV-1/2-Ab)
- Hepatitis B Virus Surface Antigen (HBs-Ag)
- Hepatitis C Virus Antibodies (HCV-Ab)
- Syphilis: nonspecific (eg. VDRL) or preferably specific (eg. TPHA)

B 1.522 *Optional Blood Tests*

Optional Blood Tests could be necessary for compliance with applicable Inter-governmental, National, Regional and Local Law or Regulation and/or to screen for endemic diseases:

- Hepatitis B core antibodies (HBc-Ab): HBc-Ab should be negative for tissue validation. Though, if the HBc-Ab test is positive and the HBs-Ag is negative, confirmation cascade should be entered.

  If the antibodies against the surface antigen are found (HBs-Ab), the donor can then be considered to have been recovered from an infection and the tissue can be used for transplantation.
- Antigen test for HIV (p24 antigen) or HCV or validated Molecular Biology Test for HIV and HCV (e.g. PCR), if performed by an experienced laboratory.
- Antibody to HTLV 1: depending on the prevalence in some regions.
- Cytomegalovirus (CMV), Ebstein-Barr Virus (EBV) and Toxoplasmosis Antibodies: for immunosuppressed patients.
- Alanine Aminotransferase (ALT) for Living Donors: In addition to the general testing requirements, testing living donors of tissue for Alanine Aminotransferase (ALT) is recommended.

B 1.523 *Living Donors Retesting*

Retesting of living donors for HIV and HCV at 180 days is recommended. If another method of increasing safety, rather than retesting (antigen testing, Molecular Biology or viral inactivation method) is used (and allowed by applicable Regulation), it shall be documented and validated.

B 1.530 *Exclusion Criteria*

B 1.531 *General Exclusion Criteria*

Positive results for HIV_1, HIV_2, Hepatitis B, Hepatitis C and Syphilis are reasons for exclusion.

B 1.532 *Specific Exclusion Criteria*

In life threatening situations for the recipient (e.g. related HPC donation), positive results for Hepatitis are no reason for exclusion, in accordance to applicable Regulations. In these situations, tissues with a higher risk for recipient may be offered as long as full information is given to the recipient or, if it is not possible, to his relatives.

B 1.600 Bacteriological Studies of Donor and Tissues

B 1.610 *Bacteriological Testing Methods*

Representative samples of each retrieved tissue have to be cultured, if the tissues are to be aseptically processed without terminal sterilisation. Samples shall be taken prior to exposure of the tissue to antibiotic containing solution.

The culture technique shall allow for the growth of both aerobic and anaerobic bacteria as well as fungi. Results shall be documented in the donor record.

Blood culture, if procurement is performed on a cadaver donor, may be useful in evaluating the state of the cadaver and interpretating the cultures performed on the grafts themselves. They shall be reviewed by the Medical Director or designee.

B 1.620 *Bacteriological Bioburden Limits*

If bacteriological testing of tissue samples obtained at the time of donation reveals growth of low virulence microorganisms, which are commonly considered nonpathogenic, the tissue may not be distributed without being further processed in a way that effectively decontaminates the tissue.

Tissue from which high virulence microorganisms have been isolated are not acceptable for transplantation, unless the procedure has been validated to effectively inactivate the organisms without harmful potential effects, taking in account possible endotoxins.

B 1.700 Non Microbiological Tests

Non-microbiological tests depend upon the tissues and cells to be transplanted.

Haematopoietic Progenitor Cell donor selection requires as a minimum:

- ABO Blood Group and Rhesus Group
- Human Leucocyte Antigen Typing (HLA)
- Whole Blood Cell Count

B 1.800 Age Criteria

Donor age criteria for each type of tissue shall be established and recorded by the Tissue Bank.

B 1.900 Cadaver Donor Retrieval Time Limits

Tissues shall be retrieved as soon after death as is practically possible. Specific time limits vary with each tissue obtained, which shall be determined by the Medical Director. Usually, procurement of tissues should be completed within 12 hours after death (or circulatory arrest if also an organ donor). If the body has been refrigerated within 4 to 6 hours of death, procurement should preferably start within 24 hours and no later than 48 hours.

B 2.000 TISSUE RETRIEVAL

B 2.100 Rationale

There shall be documented procedures, which detail all requirements for retrieval to ensure that these processes are carried out under controlled conditions.

Retrieval shall be performed using techniques appropriate to the specific tissue recovered, taking into consideration the eventual utilisation of the tissue.

B 2.200 Non-Living Donor Tissue Retrieval

B 2.210 *Determination of Death*

Tissue Bank physicians or physicians involved in removal or transplantation shall not pronounce death nor sign the death certificate of any individual from whom tissue will be collected.

Inter-governmental, National, Regional and Local Law or Regulation concerning determination of death shall be respected.

B 2.220 *Donor Identification*

Precise identification of the cadaver donor shall be performed before procurement begins.

B 2.230 *Retrieval Conditions*

B 2.231 *Facility for Retrieval*

Procurement shall be accomplished in an operating room or adequate mortuary facility.

B 2.232 *Procurement Equipment Sterility*

All instruments and equipment used for procurement shall be sterilised between procurements.

B 2.233 *Aseptic or Clean/Non-Sterile Procurement Techniques*

Tissues may be removed using either aseptic or clean/non-sterile procurement techniques:

• *Aseptic technique:*

Aseptic technique shall be observed throughout the procurement procedure. Procurement sites shall be prepared using a standard surgical technique; all methods shall be consistent with standard operating room practice.

• *Clean/non-sterile technique:*

Allografts procured using clean/non-sterile techniques are suitable for transplantation, if efficient validated sterilising methods are used to eliminate pathogens after retrieval.

B 2.234 *Samples for Microbiological Testing*

Samples for microbiological testing shall be taken, where applicable.

B 2.240 *Body Reconstruction*

Following tissue procurement, the donor's body is to be reconstructed to closely approximate its original anatomical configuration and to make usual funeral proceedings possible.

B 2.300 Surgical Residues Collection

Surgical residues shall be collected under aseptic conditions during a surgical procedure in the operating theatre.

B 2.400 Living Donor Tissue Retrieval

Tissues must be removed under conditions representing the least possible risk to the donor, in properly equipped and staffed institutions.

B 2.500 Packaging and Transportation to the Tissue Bank

B 2.510 *Procurement Container*

- Each tissue segment shall be packaged individually as soon as possible after retrieval, using sterile containers in a manner which will prevent contamination.
- Containers shall conform to Inter-governmental, National, Regional and Local Law or Regulation, as appropriate.
- Specified, validated reagents or preservation solution shall be used, as specified in SOPs.
- Procedures shall be used for ensuring and documenting proper temperature storage during transit.

B 2.520 *Procurement Container Integrity*

After filling and closing the container, it shall not be re-opened nor the tissue removed until further processing by the Tissue Bank.

B 2.530 *Procurement Container Label*

- At all times, the container shall be labelled with the donor and tissue identification, in such manner that traceability of tissues will be achieved.

- The container shall be labelled as containing human tissue, the name and address of the shipping facility and the name and address of the intended receiving facility.
- Containers shall comply with additional labelling requirements established by common carriers or by Inter-governmental, National, Regional and Local Law or Regulation.

B 2.600 Retrieval Documentation

Appropriate records of each donation procedure and all tissues retrieved shall be available and kept by the Tissue Bank.

All retrieved tissue shall be provided with an accompanying retrieval form including, at a minimum:

- the donor identity
- the date, time and place of the procedure
- the identity of the person (s) performing the retrieval
- the tissue(s) retrieved
- donor and tissue selection information

B 3.000 TISSUE BANKING GENERAL PROCEDURES

B 3.100 General

B 3.110 *Written Procedures*

The specific methods employed for processing may vary with each type of tissue and with the manner in which it has been retrieved. Each type of tissue shall be prepared according to a written procedure, which shall conform to these Standards and other applicable Standards, resulting in processed tissues appropriate for safe and efficient clinical use.

B 3.120 *Process Validation*

All steps involved during the processing of tissues shall be validated, when appropriate, to demonstrate the effectiveness of procedures.

When computers are used as part of a processing or Quality Management System, the computer software shall be validated.

When validation cannot be adequately evidenced through testing, validation shall be evidenced through documentation demonstrating adequate design, development, verification and maintenance procedures.

B 3.130 *Quality Controls*

Tests and procedures shall be performed to measure, assay or monitor processing, preservation and storage methods, equipments and reagents to ensure compliance with established tolerance limits. Results of all such tests or procedures shall be recorded.

B 3.140 *Records Management*

Appropriate records of each tissue processed shall be kept by the Tissue Bank.

Records shall allow traceability of tissues, including the different steps in the preparation, the date and time of the procedure, the identity of the person performing the procedure and the record of the materials used.

Laboratory results (e.g. microbiology/processing cultures) and other test results used to determine final release shall be archived by the Tissue Bank distributing the tissue.

B 3.200 Unique Tissue Identification Number

Each individual tissue shall be marked with a unique identification number to relate each specimen to the individual donor.

B 3.300 Reagents, Container and Packaging

B 3.310 *Reagents*

The reagents used in preservation and processing shall be of appropriate grade for the intended use, be sterile, if applicable, and conform to existing Regulation. The origin, characteristics and expiration date of reagents shall be monitored and recorded.

B 3.320 *Tissue Container*

The type of tissue container may vary with the type of tissue and processing. They shall maintain the tissue sterility and integrity, withstand the sterilisation and storage methods utilised and avoid the production of toxic residues. They shall conform to applicable Inter-governmental, National, Regional and Local Law or Regulation.

Each tissue container shall be examined visually for damage or evidence of contamination before and after processing and prior to its dispatch.

B 3.330 *Tissue Outer Package*

Packaging shall ensure integrity and effectively prevent contamination of the contents of the final container. It shall conform to applicable Transportation Regulation.

B 3.400 Pooling

Tissue from each donor shall be processed and packaged in such a way as to prevent contact and cross-contamination with tissues from other donors.

If tissues are subsequently treated in batches (e.g. sterilisation), a unique batch number shall be assigned and added to the records of the tissues.

Pooling of donors is not recommended and should only be accepted for specific tissues. The size of the pool should be limited to the minimum number of donors and traceability to each donor has to be ensured. If pooling is used for specific tissues, a fully documented rationale and risk assessment shall be undertaken to document safety.

B 3.500 Environmental Control

Processing steps shall take place in an appropriately controlled environment.

Tissue processing in an Open System shall have the environmental conditions and monitoring of the area clearly defined (such as for a "clean room" or laminar flow cabinet).

Records shall be maintained to demonstrate that the area is monitored for microbiological contamination and air control.

B 3.600 Storage Conditions

B 3.610 *Temperature*

Acceptable temperature ranges for storage shall be established.

Temperature monitoring of storage:

Low temperature (refrigerated or frozen) storage devices and incubators shall be connected to a central alarm system or each shall be equipped with an audible alarm system, that will sound when the temperature deviates from the acceptable storage range.

The alarm system shall be connected to an emergency power source. Continuous recording and daily review of data are recommended.

B 3.620 *Storage of Quarantined or Unprocessed Tissue*

There shall be a system of Quarantine for all tissues to ensure that they cannot be released for clinical use until they have met the defined acceptable criteria for release.

Storage areas of quarantined or unprocessed tissue shall be separate from storage areas of tissue approved for processing or ready for distribution.

The storage areas shall be clearly labelled as containing quarantined, released for processing or processed finished tissue.

B 3.700 Documentation Reviewing and Tissue Inspection

B 3.710 *Incoming Inspection*

Staff shall inspect the tissue container upon arrival from the procurement facility in order to ensure the integrity of the container(s), the presence of proper identification and documentation.

B 3.720 *Review of Donor Eligibility*

The donor's medical history, the physical examination, the results of tissue procurement microbiologic tests and donor blood testing, and if performed, the results of an autopsy, shall be reviewed by the Medical Director or designee.

Quarantined tissues shall be reviewed prior to distribution after all testing has been satisfactorily completed.

B 3.730 *Sizing of Specimens*

Specimen sizing may be made by actual measurements or by imaging sizing techniques.

B 3.740 *Inspection Prior to Release Into Finished Inventory*

Prior to the release of tissue into the Finished Inventory, a final review shall be made of donor suitability, procurement, production, processing records, Quality Control tests, the finished tissue, containers, closures and labels shall be inspected and approved by the Medical Director or designee.

B 3.750 *Final Inspection*

Prior to distribution, final inspection of the container, label and documentation shall be performed to ensure accuracy and integrity.

B 3.800 Non-Conforming Tissues

Tissues failing any portion of the review process shall be maintained in quarantine pending disposal and shall not be released for clinical use.

There shall be a documented policy for discard of tissue unsuitable for clinical use.

B 3.900 Expiry Dates

Expiry dates shall be established for all tissue released from a Tissue Bank. If the dating period is 72 hours or less, the hour of expiration shall be indicated on the label. Otherwise, the dating period ends at midnight of the expiration date.

B 4.000 SPECIFIC PROCESSING PROCEDURES

B 4.100 General

Section A relating to written procedures, process validation, quality control and record management always apply.

All tissues rejected due to the ineligibility of the donor cannot be used for transplantation, even after processing including sterilisation or disinfection.

Even if terminal sterilisation or disinfection using physical or chemical agents are used, the procurement and processing shall be adequate to minimise the microbial content of tissues to enable the subsequent sterilisation-disinfection process to be effective.

Appropriate indicators for sterilisation must be included in each sterilisation batch.

B 4.200 Disinfectant or Antibiotic Immersion

If disinfectants or antibiotics are used after retrieval, the tissues shall be immersed in a disinfectant or in an antibiotic solution following sterility testing and before final packaging. The type of solution used shall be specified on documentation.

B 4.300 Fresh Tissue

Fresh allografts (e.g. small fragments of articular cartilage and skin) are aseptically procured in an operating room.

Fresh Tissue is usually stored refrigerated at 4°C or in accordance with written procedures.

Fresh Tissue shall not be used in a patient until donor blood testing is completed according to these Standards, available bacteriologic results are acceptable and donor suitability has been approved by the Medical Director or designee.

B 4.400 Frozen Tissue

After aseptic procurement in the operating room, frozen tissue are placed in a -40°C or colder controlled environment within 24 hours of procurement. Subsequent manipulation of tissues (e.g. cleaning and cutting) shall be undertaken aseptically.

B 4.500 Cryopreserved Tissue

A cryopreservative solution (e.g. DMSO or Glycerol) is usually added to treat the tissue prior to freezing. Documentation of the concentration of cryoprotectants and nutrients or isotonic solutions in the cryopreservative solution shall be maintained.

Properly packaged specimens are frozen by placing the specimens below −40°C, or may be subjected to control rate freezing using a computer assisted liquid nitrogen freezing device.

If a programmed control-rate freezing method is employed, a record of the freezing profile shall be evaluated, approved and recorded.

B 4.600 Freeze-Dried Tissue

B 4.610 *Freeze-Drying Methods*

Various Protocols of freeze-drying tissues exist. Freeze-drying is a method for preservation, but is not a sterilisation method; sterility shall be assumed by Aseptic Protocol or additional sterilisation.

After a standardised procedure for freeze-drying has been developed, a Quality Control Programme for monitoring the performance of the freeze-dryer shall be documented.

Freeze-dried tissues shall be stored at room temperature or colder.

B 4.620 *Freeze-Drying Controls*

Each freeze-drying cycle must be clearly documented, including length, temperature and vacuum pressure at each step of the cycle.

Representative samples shall be tested for residual water content.

B 4.700 Simply Dehydrated Tissue

B 4.710 *Dehydration Method*

The use of simple dehydration (evaporation) of tissues as a means of preservation shall be controlled in a manner similar to freeze-drying. Temperatures of simple dehydration shall be below 60°C.

B 4.720 *Dehydration Controls*

Each dehydration cycle shall be monitored during operation for temperature.

Following dehydration, representative samples shall be tested for residual moisture.

B 4.800 Irradiated Tissue

B 4.810 *Irradiation Methods*

Commercial or hospital radiation facilities are available for ionising irradiation.

The minimum recommended dose for bacterial decontamination is 15 kGy (kiloGray).

The minimum recommended dose for bacterial sterilisation is 25 kGy (KiloGray).

Viral inactivation would require higher doses and depends on numerous factors. For this reason no specific dose can be recommended, but shall be validated, when applicable.

The used Protocol shall be validated taking in account the initial bioburden, and shall be performed by facilities following Good Irradiation Practices (see IAEA Code of Practice for the Radiation Sterilization of Biological Tissues).

B 4.820 *Irradiation Sterilisation Controls*

Sterilisation by ionising radiation shall be documented. The processing records include the name of the facility and the resultant dosimetry for each batch.

B 4.900 Ethylene Oxide Sterilised Tissue

B 4.910 *Ethylene Oxide Sterilisation Method*

Care should be taken when using ethylene oxide since the residues may have toxic effects already demonstrated for musculo-skeletal allografts in the literature.

Following appropriate processing procedures, the tissues are placed in ethylene oxide permeable containers and exposed to the ethylene oxide gas mixture following the manufacturer's suggested Guidelines. The conditions of exposure may need to be individualised depending upon the nature of the specimens to be sterilised.

A Quality Control Programme shall demonstrate that equipment meets requirements in temperature, humidity and gas concentration for the selected period.

Following ethylene oxide sterilisation, an appropriate aeration procedure shall be followed, to allow removal of residual ethylene oxide and/or its breakdown products (Ethylene Chlorhydrin and Ethylene Glycol).

B 4.920 *Ethylene Oxide Sterilisation Controls*

Chemical indicator strips shall be included in each batch. A validated procedure shall be used to ensure that sterilisation has been achieved.

Monitoring for residual levels of chemicals or their breakdown products shall be conducted from representative samples of the finished tissues of each batch.

B 4.1000 Other Processing Methods

B 4.1010 *Other Inactivation Methods*

Some chemical agents only have a decontamination role. Other agents may have an inactivation effect on specific pathogens. The efficiency of these agents towards the treated type of tissue shall be validated.

The use of chemical and possible presence of trace residuals shall be included in the information accompanying the tissue.

Under specific conditions, heat may be used to decontaminate or sterilise some type of tissues. The used Protocol shall be validated taking in account the initial bioburden and shall be performed by a recognised facility.

B 4.1020 *Bone Demineralisation*

Several methods and procedures for the formation of demineralised bone are available and acceptable.

Controlled quality reagents shall be used.

Residual calcium obtained by the method shall be determined.

B 5.000 LABELLING

B 5.100 General Requirements

B 5.110 *Rationale*

There shall be written procedures designed and followed to ensure that correct labels and labelling are used for tissue identification.

B 5.120 *Nomenclature*

Standard measurement nomenclature shall be used to describe tissues and the processing they have undergone.

B 5.130 *Label Integrity*

The tissue label applied by the Tissue Bank facility shall not be removed, altered or obscured.

B 5.130 *Visual Inspection*

When visual inspection through the container is possible, a sufficient area of the container shall remain uncovered to permit inspection of the contents.

B 5.200 Tissue Containers Labelling

Tissue containers shall be labelled so as to identify, as a minimum:

- The human nature of the contents
- Product description
- Name and address of Tissue Bank
- Tissue identification number
- Expiration date

The following information shall be included on the label, if possible, otherwise on the accompanying documentation:

- Amount of tissue in the container expressed as volume, weight or dimensions or such combination of the foregoing as needed, for an accurate description of the contents.
- Sterilisation or inactivation procedure used, if applicable.
- Batch number, if applicable.
- Potential residuals of added preserving and processing agents/solution (e.g. antibiotics, ETOH, ETO, DMSO).
- Recommended storage conditions.

B 5.300 Package Insert

B 5.310 *General*

All tissues shall be accompanied by a document describing the nature of tissue and processing methods and instructions for proper storage and reconstitution, when appropriate. Specific instructions shall be enclosed with tissue, which require special handling.

B 5.320 *Accompanying Documentation Requirements*

Accompanying documentation shall contain all the information described for container labelling and the following additional information:

- Origin of tissue (country of procurement).
- The nature and results of biological tests performed on the donor using appropriate and licensed tests.
- Processing methods used and results of sterility tests or inactivation controls.
- Special instructions indicated by the particular tissue for storage or implantation. Tissue that is to be reconstituted at or prior to the time of use shall include information on the conditions, under which such tissue shall be stored and reconstituted prior to implantation.
- Indications and contraindications for use of tissue, when necessary.
- Statement that each tissue shall be used for a single patient only.

B 5.400 Tissue Outer Package Labelling

Labelling of the tissue outer package shall conform to Transportation Regulations, when applicable.

B 6.000 DISTRIBUTION

B 6.100 General

Tissues can be distributed for a specific patient to a physician, dentist and other qualified medical professional or to a storage facility located in another institution for local use or distributed to another Tissue Bank.

Distribution for therapeutic use shall be based on medical criteria on equitable bases, in accordance with Inter-governmental, National, Regional and Local Law or Regulation and practice.

There shall be written procedures and documentation for all tissues distributed.

The clinical team using the tissue shall have instructions for contacting the Tissue Bank for any question they have and shall be made aware of the following:

- Action to be taken in the event of loss of integrity of the package
- Action for reporting of adverse event
- Action for the return or the disposal of unsuitable or unused tissue.

B 6.200 Traceability

There shall be an effective system that enables the traceability of tissues between the donor, the processed tissue and the recipient.

It is the responsibility of the hospital tissue storage and distribution facility or clinician to implement recipient records and to inform the Tissue Bank of the destination of tissues (implantation date, surgeon and recipient identification).

Tissue Banks shall maintain records which document the destination of distributed tissue: implantation (date, surgeon and recipient identification), destruction (date and place) and of any adverse event reports.

B 6.300 Transportation

Maintenance of (upper and/or lower parameters) environmental conditions during transit, as defined in the written procedure of the Tissue Bank, shall be ensured.

Use of hazardous elements such as dry ice or liquid nitrogen shall comply with relevant Regulations.

B 6.400 Accompanying Documentation

The release of tissue from storage shall include all documentation originating from the Tissue Bank. Surgeons shall be aware that copies of this documentation shall be maintained in the recipient's medical records.

B 6.500 Return into Inventory

Issued tissues shall not be returned to the Tissue Bank without prior consultations with the Medical Director or designee. Tissue must be in its original unopened container and the storage conditions must have been maintained as required.

B 6.600 Adverse Events

Reports of adverse events shall be evaluated by the institution where the tissue was used and reported immediately to the Tissue Bank.

All adverse events shall be reviewed by the Medical Director and appropriate action documented, in accordance with Inter-governmental, National, Regional and Local Law or Regulation. Identified transmission of disease shall be reported to the Public Health Authorities, processing Institutions, to the donor's personal physician, if clinically relevant and to physicians involved in implantation of the tissue, in accordance with Inter-governmental, National, Regional and Local Law or Regulation on Confidentiality.

When donor to recipient disease transmission through tissue use is discovered, all facilities involved in the procurement and distribution of organs or tissues from the infected donor shall be notified without delay.

Written reports of the investigation of adverse events, including conclusions, follow up and corrective actions, shall be prepared and maintained by the Tissue Bank in an adverse event file.

B 6.700 Recall

A written procedure shall exist for recall of tissues.

B 6.800 Distribution to Storage Facilities Outside the Tissue Bank (Depot).

B 6.810 *General*

When a storage facility is located outside the Tissue Bank, the institution where this facility is located is responsible for establishing acceptable storage and record keeping procedures to ensure the maintenance of the safety and efficacy of tissue from receipt to use and the traceability of tissue and recipients.

The relevant part of these Standards shall be made available to these institutions. These storage facilities (Depot) shall be subjected to Quality Audit and Control from the Tissue Bank.

B 6.820 *Labelling*

Labels on tissue containers shall not be altered, made invisible or removed.

B 6.830 *Storage*

Tissue storage shall conform with Guidelines established by the distributing Tissue Bank.

B 6.840 *Records*

Records shall document, as a minimum, the receival date of tissue and the destination (transplant date, the recipient's identity and transplant surgeon). These destination records shall be transmitted to the Tissue Bank.

B 6.900 Distribution to Another Tissue Bank

The associated Tissue Bank should adhere to these Standards.

B 6.1000 Acquisition of Tissue from Another Tissue Bank

B 6.1010 *Medical Director Approval*

Prior to acquiring tissue from another Tissue Bank, the Medical Director shall ensure that the standards adopted by that tissue bank are comparable to these standards.

B 6.1020 *Labelling*

Labels on processed tissue acquired from another Tissue Bank shall not be altered, made invisible or removed.

B 6.1030 *Distribution Record*

Accompanying documentation from the original Tissue Bank shall be forwarded with the tissue to the clinical team. After implantation, the destination record (transplant date, the recipient's identity and transplant surgeon) shall be forwarded to the original Tissue Bank.

ANNEXES

ANNEX 1: GLOSSARY

ADVERSE EVENTS [Synonym ADVERSE OUTCOME/REACTION]: An undesirable effect or untoward complication in a recipient consequent to or reasonably related to tissue transplantation.

ALLOGRAFT: A graft transplanted between two different individuals of the same species.

ASEPTIC RETRIEVAL: The retrieval of tissue using methods that restrict or minimise contamination with microorganisms from the donor, environment, retrieval personnel and/or equipment.

BRAIN DEATH/BRAIN STEM DEATH: Complete and irreversible cessation of brain stem and brain encephalic functions and certified according to National Laws. Synonym = death.

CLEAN ROOM: A room in which the concentration of airborne particles is monitored and controlled to defined specification limits.

COMPLIANCE: Conforming to established Standards or Regulations.

CONTAINER: An enclosure for one unit of transplantable tissue.

CONTROLLED ENVIRONMENT: An environment, which is controlled with respect to particulate contamination, both viable and non-viable particles. May also include temperature and humidity controls.

CORONER: (See Medical Examiner)

CORRECTIVE ACTION: Steps taken to ameliorate non-compliance.

COST: The actual costs for retrieval, processing, preservation, storage, distribution, education, research and development.

CROSS-CONTAMINATION: The transfer of infectious agents from tissues to other tissue or from one donor's tissue to another donor's tissue.

DEATH: (See Brain Death)

DISINFECTION: A process that reduces the number of viable cellular microorganisms, but does not necessarily destroy all microbial forms, such as spores and viruses.

DISTRIBUTION: Transportation and delivery of tissues for storage or use in recipients.

DONOR MEDICAL HISTORY INTERVIEW: A documented dialogue with an individual or individuals who would be knowledgeable of the donor's relevant medical history and social behaviour; such as the donor, if living, the next of kin, the nearest available relative, a member of the donor's household, other individual with an affinity relationship and/or the primary treating physician. The relevant social history includes questions to elicit whether or not the donor met certain descriptions or engaged in certain activities or behaviours considered to place such an individual at increased risk for HIV and Hepatitis or other diseases.

DONOR REGISTRY: A formal compilation of individual's intent relating to donation that may be maintained by a Governmental agency or private establishment.

DONOR SELECTION/DONOR SCREENING: The evaluation of information about a potential donor to determine whether the donor meets qualifications specified in the SOPs and Standards. This includes but is not limited to, medical social and sexual histories, physical examination and laboratory test results (and autopsy findings, if performed).

DONOR: A living or deceased individual who is the source of tissue for transplantation in accordance with established medical criteria and procedures.

END-USER: A healthcare practitioner who performs transplantation procedures.

FACILITY: Any area used in the procurement, processing, sterilisation, testing, storage or distribution of tissue and tissue components.

FINISHED INVENTORY: Storage of finished tissue.

FINISHED TISSUE: Tissue that has undergone all of the stages of processing, packaging and is approved for distribution.

GIFT DOCUMENT: A legally recognised document in which an individual indicates his/her wishes as they relate to donation of organs and tissues.

GOOD TISSUE BANKING PRACTICES: Practices that meet accepted Standards as defined by relevant Government or professional organisations.

HPC: Haematopoietic Progenitor Cells.

INSPECTION: An examination of a Tissue Bank to ascertain Good Tissue banking Practices.

LABELING MATERIAL: Any printed or written material including labels, advertising, and/or containing information (for example package insert, brochures, pamphlets) related to the tissues.

LABELING: Includes steps taken to identify the material and to attach the appropriate labels on the container or package so that it is clearly visible. Includes the package insert which is the written material accompanying a tissue graft bearing information about the tissue, directions for use and any applicable warnings.

MEDICAL EXAMINER [Synonym Coroner]: Governmental official (usually a pathologist) charged with investigating deaths and determining cause of death.

NATIONAL REGULATORY AUTHORITY [NRA]: A body appointed by the Government with the goal of controlling Tissue Banking practices.

NEXT OF KIN: The person(s) most closely related to a deceased individual as designated by applicable law.

NON-COMPLIANCE: Non-conformance to established standards or regulations.

OPEN SYSTEM: A system which has been breached but where every effort is made to maintain sterility by the use of sterile material and aseptic handling techniques in a clean environment.

ORGAN (See Vascular Organ)

PACKAGING (See Container)

PROCESSING: Any activity performed on tissue, other than tissue recovery, including preparation, preservation for storage and/or removal from storage, to assure the quality and/or sterility of human tissues.

QUALITY: Totality of characteristics of a product, process or system that bear on its ability to satisfy customers or other interested parties.

QUALITY ASSURANCE (part of Quality Management): Planned and systematic actions necessary to provide confidence in fulfilling Quality Requirements (See Quality Requirements).

QUALITY AUDIT: A documented review of procedures, records, personnel functions, equipment, materials, facilities, and/or vendors in order to evaluate adherence to the written SOPs, Standards, or government laws and regulations.

QUALITY CONTROL (part of Quality Management): Operational techniques and activities that are used to fulfil Requirements for Quality.

QUALITY MANAGEMENT: All activities of the overall management function that determine the Quality Policy, Objectives and Responsibilities, and their implementation by means of Quality Planning, Quality Control, Quality Assurance and Quality Improvement, within the Quality System.

QUALITY REQUIREMENTS: Requirements for the characteristics of a product, a process or a system.

QUALITY MANAGEMENT SYSTEM (See Quality Management)

QUARANTINE: The status of retrieved tissue or packaging material, or tissue isolated physically or by other effective means, whilst awaiting a decision on their release or rejection.

RECALL: The requested return of finished tissue known or suspected to be non-compliant to the Tissue Bank, in accordance with the instructions contained in an advisory notice.

RECIPIENT: An individual into whom organs, tissue is transplanted.

RETRIEVAL [synonyms Recovery, Procurement, Removal, Harvest]: The removal of tissues from a donor for the purpose of transplantation.

STANDARD OPERATING PROCEDURES [SOPs]: A group of Standard Operating Procedures detailing the specific policies of a Tissue Bank and the procedures used by the staff/personnel. This includes, but is not limited to procedures to: assess donor suitability and retrieve, process, sterilise, quarantine, release to inventory, label, store, distribute and recall tissue.

STERILISATION: A validated process to destroy, inactivates, or reduces micro-organisms to a sterility assurance level of 10^{-6}.

STERILITY ASSURANCE LEVEL: The probability of detecting an unsterile product, tissue.

STORAGE: Maintenance of tissues in a state ready for distribution.

TERMINAL STERILISATION: Sterilisation that takes place at the end of processing the tissue, in the final packaging.

TISSUE: Human tissue includes all constituted parts of a human body, including surgical residues and amnion, but excluding organs, blood and blood products, as well as reproductive tissues such as sperm, eggs and embryos. New products engineered from human tissue are included. The word "Tissue" in this text applies to all types of tissues, including corneas and to cells.

TISSUE BANK: An entity that provides or engages in one or more services involving tissue from living or cadaveric individuals for transplantation purposes. These services include assessing donor suitability, tissue recovery, tissue processing, sterilisation, storage, labelling and distribution.

TRACEABILITY: The ability to locate tissue during any step of its donation, collection, processing, testing, storage and distribution. It implies the capacity to identify the donor and the medical facility receiving the cells and/or tissue or the recipient.

TRANSPLANTATION: The removal of tissues and/or cells and grafting of these tissues whether immediately or after a period of preservation and/or storage. Transplantation may be from one person to another (allogeneic) or from a person to themselves (autologous).

VALIDATION: Refers to establishing documented evidence that provides a high degree of assurance that a specific process will consistently produce a product meeting its predetermined specifications and quality attributes. A process is validated to evaluate the performance of a system with regard to its effectiveness based on intended use.

VASCULAR ORGANS: Any part of a human body consisting of vascularised, structured arrangement of cells, which removed, cannot be replicated by the body. Example: Heart, liver, lung, kidney, pancreas, intestine.

ANNEX 2: GUIDELINES OF FACTORS TO BE CONSIDERED FOR DETERMINING RISK FOR HUMAN IMMUNODEFICIENCY VIRUS OR B OR C HEPATITIS

- Men who have had sex with another man in the preceding 12 months.
- Persons who report non-medical intravenous, intramuscular or subcutaneous injection of drugs in the preceding 12 months.
- Men and women who have engaged in sex in exchange for money or drugs in the preceding 12 months.
- Persons with a history of chronic Hemodialysis.
- Persons with a history of Haemophilia or related clotting disorders who have received human-derived clotting factor concentrates.
- Persons who were sexual partners of persons having a HIV or B or C Hepatitis history, manifestations, or risk factors previously described, in the past 12 months.
- Percutaneous exposure or contact with an open wound, non-intact skin or mucous membrane to blood thought to be at high risk for carrying HIV or Hepatitis in the preceding 12 months.
- Inmates of correctional systems in past 12 months.
- Diagnosed or treated for Syphilis or Gonorrhea in past 12 months.
- A potential tissue donor who has received a blood transfusion within 12 months prior to death may only be accepted as a tissue donor after individual approval from the Medical Director.
- The donor is not eligible if in a deferral status of any Blood Services Donor Deferral Register. The local blood centre(s) shall be checked each time possible (blood donor card available).
- Tattoo, ear piercing, body piercing, and/or acupuncture, unless by sterile, non-reused needle or equipment, in the preceding 12 months.

ANNEX 3: PRIMARY TUMOURS OF THE CENTRAL NERVOUS SYSTEM: EVALUATION OF A SUITABLE DONOR. A REFERENCE LIST

No Contraindication
- Pituitary Adenoma
- Pinelcytoma
- Hemangioblastoma
- Schwannoma
- Choroid Plexus Papilloma
- Ependimoma
- Oligodendroglioma differentiated
- Craniopharyngioma
- Benign Meningioma
- Pilocytic astrocytoma
- Epidermoid tumours

Contraindication
- Medulloblastoma
- Chordoma
- Glioblastoma multiforme
- Highly anaplastic Oligodendroglioma
- Anaplastic Epidimoma
- Anaplastic Meningioma
- Primary CNS Lymphoma
- Pineoblastoma
- CNS Sarcomas
- Astrocytoma grade II
- Astrocytoma grade III

ANNEX 4: EXAMPLE OF ALGORITHM FOR CALCULATING THE HEMODILUTION OF A DONOR HAVING RECEIVED BLOOD, BLOOD COMPONENTS, OR PLASMA VOLUME EXPANDERS WITHIN 48 HOURS PRIOR TO DEATH

The following equation allows calculation of a potential donor 50% plasma volume:

$$50\% \text{ plasma volume (ml)} = 21 \times \text{donor's body weight (kg)}$$

The equation as been calculated as follows:

$$\text{Total blood volume per kg} = 1\,\text{kg} \times 70\,\text{ml} = 70\,\text{ml}$$

$$\begin{aligned}&\text{Total plasma volume per kg}\\ &\quad = 70\,\text{ml (total blood volume per kg)} \times 1.0\\ &\qquad - 0.40\text{ (normal adult hematocrit)}\\ &\quad = 70\,\text{ml} \times 0.60\\ &\quad = 42\,\text{ml}\end{aligned}$$

$$\begin{aligned}&\quad\ \ 50\%\text{ plasma volume per kg}\\ &\quad = 42\,\text{ml (total plasma volume per kg)} \times 0.50\\ &\quad = 21\,\text{ml per kg}\end{aligned}$$

ANNEX 5: REFERENCES AND CONTACT ADDRESSES

- American Association of Tissue Banks (AATB)
  - Standards for Tissue Banking (1984, 1985, 1987, 1989, 1993, 1996, 1998, 2001)
- Australian Code of Good Manufacturing Practice- Human Blood and Tissues. Therapeutic Goods Administration, 2000.
- Council of Europe
  - Guide on Safety and Quality Assurance for Organs, Tissues and Cells (Version 11. CDSP, Released for Consultation 1/2001)
- European Association of Tissue Banks (EATB)
  - EATB General Standards for Tissue Banking (1995)
  - EATB and EAMST Standards for Musculo-skeletal Tissue Banking (1997, revised1999)
  - EATB Standards for Skin Banking and Banking of Skin Substitutes (1997)
- International Atomic Energy Agency/National University of Singapore Multi-Media Curriculum for Tissue Banking. IAEA/NUS Regional and International Training Centre, National University Hospital, Singapore 1998.
- International Atomic Energy Agency Code of Practice for Radiation Sterilization of Tissue Allografts 2004, IAEA, Vienna.

- Radiation and Tissue Banking. Ed by G.O. Phillips. World Scientific. Singapore, New Jersey, London, Hong Kong. 2000.
- Scientific Basis of Tissue Transplantation. Ed by A Nather. World Scientific. Singapore, New Jersey, London, Hong Kong. 2002.
- UK Code Of Practice for Tissue Banks. Department of Health. United Kingdom. 2001.

CONTACT ADDRESSES:

- Asia-Pacific Surgical Tissue Banking Association
  Professor Yong Koo Kang
  St. Vincent's Hospital,
  Suwon, 440-060, Korea
  Email: ykang@vincent.cuk.ac.kr
- American Association of Tissue Banks (AATB)
  1350 Beverly Road, Suite 220A, McLean, VA 22101, USA
  www.aatb.org
- Council of Europe
  Karl Friedrich Bopp, Health Department, Council of Europe,
  67075 Strasbourg Cedex, France
  www.coe.int
- European Association of Tissue Banks (EATB)
  C/- Dr Heinz Winkler, Vienna AUSTRIA
  www.eatb.de

APPENDIX 2

International Atomic Energy Agency

THE IAEA INT/6/052 PROGRAMME IN RADIATION AND TISSUE BANKING

Code of Practice

Code of Practice for the Radiation Sterilization of Tissue Allografts: Requirements for Validation and Routine Control

2004

International Atomic Energy Agency

Project No: INT/6/052

Code of Practice for the Radiation Sterilization of Tissue Allografts: Requirements for Validation and Routine Control

Contents

Annexes

CODE OF PRACTICE FOR THE RADIATION STERILIZATION OF TISSUE ALLOGRAFTS: REQUIREMENTS FOR VALIDATION AND ROUTINE CONTROL

Preamble

This Code of Practice for the Radiation Sterilization of Tissues Allografts adopts the principles which the International Standards Organization (ISO) applied to the radiation sterilization of health care products. The approach has been adapted to take into account the special features associated with human tissues, and the features which distinguish them from industrially produced sterile health care products.

The Code, as described here, is not applicable if viral contamination is identified. Thus, it is emphasised that the human donors of the tissues must be medically and serologically screened. To further support this screening, it is recommended that autopsy reports are also reviewed if available. This adaptation of established ISO methods can thus only be applied for sterilization of tissue allografts if the radiation sterilization described here is the terminal stage of a careful detailed, documented sequence of procedures, involving:

- donor selection,
- tissue retrieval,
- tissue banking general procedures,
- specific processing procedures,
- labelling and
- distribution,

all of which are conducted according to the IAEA International Standards for Tissue Banks. It shall not be used outside this context.

The methods proposed here for the establishment of a sterilization dose are based on statistical approaches used for the sterilization of health care products (ISO 11137:1995, ISO 13409:1996, ISO 15844:1998, AAMI TIR 27:2001) and modified appropriately for the low numbers of tissue allograft samples typically available.

For a Standard Distribution of Resistance (SDR), the Tissue Bank may elect to substantiate a sterilization dose of 25 kGy for microbial levels up to 1000 colony forming units (cfu) per allograft product.

Alternatively, for the SDR and other microbial distribution, specific sterilization doses may be validated depending on the bioburden levels and radiation resistances (D_{10} values) of the constituent microorganisms.

1. Introduction

International standards have been established for the radiation sterilization of health care products which include medical devices, medicinal products (pharmaceuticals and biologics) and *in vitro* diagnostic products (*ISO 11137:1995 (E)*; *ISO 11737-1:1995*; *ISO 11737-2:1998*; *ISO/TR 13409:1996*, *ISO/TR 15844:1998 and AAMI TIR 27:2001*).

Following intensive studies of the effects of ionising radiation on chemical, physical and biological properties of tissue allografts and their components, these are now radiation sterilized using a variety of methods and practices.

Through its Radiation and Tissue Banking Programme, the International Atomic Energy Agency has sought during the period 2001–2002 to establish a Code of Practice for the Radiation Sterilization of Tissue Allografts and its requirement for validation and routine control of the sterilization of tissues.

Annex A describes the methods for selecting a sterilization dose. Annex B provides three worked examples applying these methods. Annex C gives Tables which contain microbial survival data relating to Standard Distribution of Resistances. Annex D gives a bibliography of key references for the sterilization of tissues by ionising radiation.

This Code sets out the requirements of a process, in order to ensure that the radiation sterilization of tissues produces standardized sterile tissue allografts suitable for safe clinical use. Although the principles adopted here are similar to those used for the sterilization of health care products, there are substantial differences in practice arising from the physical and biological characteristics of tissues.

For health care products, the items for sterilization come usually from large production batches. For example, syringes are uniform in size and have bacterial contamination arising from the production process, usually at low levels. It is the reduction of the microbial bioburden to acceptable low levels which is the purpose of the sterilization process, where such levels are defined by the Sterility Assurance Level (SAL). The inactivation of microorganisms by physical and chemical means follows an exponential law and so the probability of a surviving microorganism can be calculated if the number and type of microorganisms are known and if the lethality of the sterilization process is also known. Two methods are used in ISO 11137:1995 to establish the radiation doses required to achieve low SAL values.

Method 1 of ISO 11137:1995 relies on knowing the bioburden (assuming a Standard Distribution of Resistances) before irradiation and uses this data to establish a verification dose, which will indicate the dose needed for a SAL of 10^{-2}. The method involves a statistical approach to setting the dose based on three batches and hence relatively large numbers of samples are required for both establishing the initial bioburden and the verification dose, both per product batch. A further adaptation of method 1 for a single production batch has also been developed (*ISO/TR 15844–1998*).

In Method 2 of ISO 11137:1995, the bioburden levels are measured after giving a series of incremental doses to the samples, these doses being well below the dose required for a SAL of 10^{-6}. In this method, 280 samples are required to determine the dose to produce a SAL value of 10^{-2}, from which the dose needed to yield a SAL value of 10^{-6} may be extrapolated. No assumptions are made in Method 2 about the distribution of microorganisms and their resistances.

In a later ISO/TR 13409:1996, Method 1 was adapted to allow the use of as few as 10 samples to determine the verification dose. In this modification, the dose needed for a SAL value of 10^{-1} is used to establish the dose required for a SAL value of 10^{-6}. The sole purpose, however, of this modification is to substantiate whether 25 kGy is an appropriate dose to achieve a SAL value of 10^{-6}. In AAMI TIR 27:2001, another method to substantiate the sterilization dose of 25 kGy was developed.

Sterilization of tissue allografts

Tissues used as allografts comprise a wide range of materials and bioburden levels such that the above quality assurance methods developed for health care products cannot be applied without careful and due consideration given to the differences between health care products and tissue allografts.

Tissues which are sterilized currently include: bone, cartilage, ligaments, tendons, fascias, dura mater, heart valves, vessels, skin and amnion. Unlike health care products, the variability in types and levels of bioburden in tissues is much greater than that found for health care products where the levels of microbial contamination are usually low and relatively uniform in type and level.

In addition, tissue allografts are not products of commercial production processes involving large numbers of samples. These differences mean that extra attention must be given to the following:

a) uniformity of sample physical characteristics (shape and density),
b) uniformity of bioburden in sample,
c) donor screening for viral contamination,
d) whether low numbers of samples can be used for sterilization dose setting purposes.

2. Objective

The objective of this Code is to provide the necessary guidance in the use of ionising radiation to sterilize tissue allografts in order to ensure their safe clinical use.

3. Scope

This Code specifies requirements for validation, process control and routine monitoring of the selection of donors, tissue processing, preservation, storage and the radiation sterilization of tissue allografts. They apply to continuous and batch type gamma irradiators using the radioisotopes ^{60}Co and ^{137}Cs, electron beam accelerators and X-rays.

The principles adopted here are similar to those elucidated in ISO 11137:1995 in that statistical approaches to establishing doses to assure sterility of the tissue products are proposed.

4. Normative references

The following Standards contain provisions which are relevant to this Code:

ISO 9001: 2000 *Quality management systems — Requirements.*

ISO 11137: 1995 *Sterilization of health care products — Requirements for validation and routine control — Radiation sterilization.*

ISO 11737-1: 1995 *Sterilization of medical devices — Microbiological methods — Part 1.*

ISO 11737-2: 1998 *Sterilization of medical devices — Microbiological methods — Part 2.*

ISO/TR 13409: 1996 *Sterilization of health care products — Radiation sterilization — Substantiation of 25 kGy as a sterilization dose for small or infrequent production batches.*

ISO/TR 15844: 1998 *Sterilization of health care products — Radiation sterilization — Selection of sterilization dose for a single production batch.*

AAMI *Technical Information Report (TIR 27) : 2001 — Sterilization of health care products — Radiation sterilization — Substantiation of 25 kGy as sterilization dose – Method* VD_{max}.

ISO/ASTM 51261 (*2002*) *Guide for Selection and Calibration of Dosimetry Systems for Radiation Processing.*

IAEA (*May, 2002*) *International Standards for Tissue Banks.*

5. Definitions

The majority of the definitions relating to the sterilization process are given in ISO 11137:1995. The following definitions are particularly useful for this Code and are given below.

***Allograft*:** A graft transplanted between two different individuals of the same species.

***Allograft product*:** An allograft or a collection of allografts within a primary package.

***Absorbed dose*:** The quantity of radiation energy imparted per unit mass of matter. The unit of absorbed dose is the gray (Gy), where 1 gray is equivalent to the absorption of 1 joule per kilogram (1 Gy = 100 rads).

***Batch* (*irradiation*):** Quantity of final product irradiated at the same cycle in a qualified facility.

***Batch* (*production*):** Defined quantity of finished tissue product from a single donor that is intended to be uniform in character and quality, and which has been produced during a same single cycle of processing.

***Bioburden*:** Population of viable microorganisms on tissue allograft and package prior to the sterilization process.

***Distribution*:** Transportation and delivery of tissues for storage or use in recipient.

***Dose mapping*:** An exercise conducted within an irradiation facility to determine the distribution of the radiation dose throughout a load of tissue allograft or simulated items of specified bulk density, arranged in irradiation containers in a defined configuration.

***Dosimeter*:** A device having a reproducible measurable response to radiation, which can be used to measure the absorbed dose in a given material.

***Dosimetry system*:** System used for determining absorbed dose, consisting of dosimeters, measuring instrumentation and procedures for the system's use.

D_{10}: Radiation dose required to inactivate 90 per cent of the homogeneous microbial population where it is assumed that the death of microbes follows first-order kinetics.

***Good Tissue Banking Practice* (*GTBP*):** Practice that meets accepted Standards as defined by relevant Government or professional organizations.

***Irradiator*:** Assembly that permits safe and reliable sterilization processing, including the source of radiation, conveyor and source mechanisms, safety devices and shield.

***Positive test of sterility*:** A test of sterility which exhibits detectable microbial growth after incubation in a suitable culture medium.

***Qualification*:** Obtaining and documenting evidence concerning the processes and products involved in tissue donor selection, tissue retrieval, processing, preservation and radiation sterilization that will produce acceptable tissue allografts.

***Recovery efficiency*:** Measure of the ability of a specified technique to remove microorganisms from a tissue allograft.

***Reference standard dosimeter*:** Dosimeter, of high metrological quality, used as a standard to provide measurements traceable to and consistent with measurements made using primary standard dosimeters.

***Routine dosimeter*:** A dosimeter calibrated against a primary or reference dosimeter and used routinely to make dosimetric measurements.

***Sample Item Portion (SIP)*:** Defined standardized portion of a tissue allograft that is tested.

***Sterile*:** Free of viable micro-organisms

***Sterility Assurance Level (SAL)*:** Probability of a viable microorganism being present on a tissue allograft after sterilization.

***Sterilization*:** A validated process to destroy, inactivate, or reduce microorganisms to a Sterility Assurance Level (SAL) of 10^{-6}. (Sterility is expressed by several national legislations and international standards as a SAL of 10^{-6}).

***Sterilization dose*:** Minimum absorbed dose required to achieve the specified Sterility Assurance Level (SAL).

***Test of sterility*:** Test performed to establish the presence or absence of viable microorganisms on tissue allograft, or portions thereof, when subjected to defined culture conditions.

***Tissue Bank*:** An entity that provides or engages in one or more services involving tissue from living or cadaveric individuals for transplantation purposes. These services include assessing donor suitability, tissue recovery, tissue processing, sterilization, storage, labeling and distribution.

***Validation*:** Refers to establishing documented evidence that provides a high degree of assurance that a specific process will consistently produce a product meeting its predetermined specifications and quality attributes.

A process is validated to evaluate the performance of a system with regard to its effectiveness based on intended use.

***Verification dose*:** Dose of radiation to which tissue allograft, or portions thereof are nominally exposed in the verification dose experiment with the intention of achieving a predetermined Sterility Assurance Level (SAL).

6. Personnel

Responsibility for the validation and routine control for sterilization by irradiation including tissue donor selection, tissue retrieval, processing, preservation, sterilization and storage shall be assigned to qualified personnel in accordance with sub-clauses 6.2.1 and 6.2.2 of ISO 9001:2000, whichever is applicable.

7. Validation of Pre-sterilization Processes

7.1. General

An essential step in the overall radiation sterilization of tissues is rigorous donor selection to eliminate specific contaminants. Full details about donor selection, tissue retrieval, tissue banking general procedures, specific processing procedures, labelling and distribution are given in IAEA International Standards for Tissue Banks. Such tissue donor selection, retrieval, processing and preservation are processes which determine the characteristics of the tissue allograft prior to the radiation sterilization process. The most important characteristics are those relating to use of the tissues as allografts, namely, their physical, chemical and biological properties, the latter including the levels and types of microbial contamination. Validation of these processes shall include the following:

a) qualification of the Tissue Bank facilities,
b) qualification of the tissue donors,
c) qualification of the tissue processing and preservation,
d) certification procedure to review and approve documentation of a), b) and c),
e) maintenance of validation,
f) process specification.

7.2. Qualification of the tissue bank facilities

Tissue Banks shall have facilities to receive procured tissues and to prepare tissue allograft material for sterilization. Such facilities are expected to include laboratories for the processing, preservation and storage of tissues prior to sterilization. These laboratories and the equipment contained therein shall meet international standards enunciated by the various Tissue Bank Professional Associations and now combined in the IAEA International Standards for Tissue Banks.

A regular documented system should be established which demonstrates that these standards are maintained, with special emphasis on the minimisation of contamination by microorganisms throughout the tissue retrieval, transportation, processing, preservation and storage stages to bioburden levels which comply with the IAEA International Standards for Tissue Banks.

Tissue Banks shall also have access to qualified microbiological laboratories to measure the levels of microorganisms on the tissue allografts at various stages in their preparation for the purposes of assessing both the levels of contamination at each stage and also typical bioburden levels of the pre-irradiated tissue allografts. The standards expected of such laboratories are specified in: *ISO 11737-1:1995 and ISO 11737-2:1998.*

The overall purpose of the above facilities contained within Tissue Banks is to demonstrate that they are capable of producing preserved tissue allografts which have acceptably low levels of microorganisms in the preserved product prior to their sterilization by radiation.

7.3. Qualification of tissue donors

The main aim of the tissue donor selection process carried out prior to processing, preservation, storage and sterilization is to produce tissue allografts which are free from transmissible infectious diseases. Such a selection process in order to produce acceptable tissues shall include the following minimal information:

a) time of retrieval of tissue after death of donor, conditions of body storage,
b) age of donor,
c) medical, social and sexual history of donor,
d) physical examination of the body,

e) serological (including molecular biology) tests,
f) analysis of autopsy as required by law.

Such information shall be used to screen donors to minimise the risk of infectious disease transmission from tissue donors to the recipients of the allografts. The information collected shall be comprehensive, verifiable and auditable following Good Practice on Tissue Banking, as specified in the IAEA International Standards for Tissue Banks.

The following serological tests shall be carried out as a minimum on each donor:

a) antibodies to Human Immunodeficiency Virus 1 and 2 (HIV 1, 2),
b) antibodies to Hepatitis C virus (HCV),
c) hepatitis B surface antigen (HBs-Ag),
d) syphilis: non-specific (e.g., VDRL) or preferably specific (e.g., TPHA)

Other tests may be required by statutory regulations or when specific infections are indicated as specified in the IAEA International Standard for Tissue Banks. In using such laboratory-based tests to provide additional assurance that allografts are free of transmissible disease, due consideration should be given to the detection limits of such tests. It should therefore be verified that the combination of processing, preservation and irradiation is capable of reducing the low levels of viral contamination, which might be implied by an otherwise negative test, to an SAL of 10^{-6}.

When addressing the problem of viral contamination, the same basic principles already advanced for the elimination of bacterial contamination need to be applied with regard to donor screening, serology, processing, preservation and sterilization by ionizing radiation. It should be noted that, in general, the D_{10} values for viruses are higher than those for bacteria and other microflora.

7.4. Qualification of tissue processing and preservation

The processing of tissue allograft materials such as bone, cartilage, ligaments, fascias, tendons, dura mater, heart valves and vessels, skin and amnion comprises various stages such as removal of bone marrow, defatting, pasteurisation, antibiotic treatment, percolation and treatment with disinfectants such as hypochlorite, ethyl alcohol and glycerol.

The inclusion of any or all of these stages will depend on a number of factors including:

a) the preferred practice of the Tissue Bank,
b) the nature of the tissue (and its anticipated use in the clinic), and
c) the degree of contamination of the procured tissue.

The preservation of the processed tissue allografts may include:

a) freeze drying,
b) deep freezing,
c) air drying,
d) heat drying and
e) chemical treatment.

An important function of these processes in 7.2 to 7.4 is to produce tissue allografts which have low levels of microbial contamination and in particular less than 1000 cfu per allograft product when it is desired to substantiate a sterilization dose of 25 kGy. In the latter case, for a bioburden of 1000 cfu per allograft product, a 25 kGy dose is sufficient to achieve a SAL of 10^{-6} for a Standard Distribution of Resistances. It should be recognised that microflora can originate from both the environment and the donor, and in the case of the latter, may show substantial variations from donor to donor. The capacity of all of the tissue processing and preservation procedures to remove microorganisms should be checked periodically and documented.

7.5. Maintenance of validation

For each of the qualifications detailed above in 7.2–7.4, a validation process should be specified, which will demonstrate that the standards expected will be maintained. As a minimum, these validation processes shall include:

a) an audit of the origin and history of the procured tissues with reference to 7.3 a) to d),
b) a random, statistically-significant sampling of procured tissues (that is, prior to processing and preservation) followed by a laboratory-based screening for viruses and infectious agents (see 7.3),

c) measures of particle count and microbial contamination in the environment of each of the separate facilities of the Tissue Bank,
d) random, statistically-significant sampling of tissue allografts prior to and after tissue processing and preservation for measurements of bioburden levels,
e) determination of the ability of the tissue processing and preservation procedures to both reduce the levels of microorganisms and to produce the levels of bioburden required for the radiation sterilization process. This should ensure a microbial contamination level of 1000 cfu per allograft product or less when it is required to substantiate a sterilization dose of 25 kGy.

7.6. Process specification

A process specification shall be established for each tissue allograft type. The specification shall include:

a) the tissue allograft type covered by the specification,
b) the parameters covering the selection of tissue for processing,
c) details of the tissue processing and preservation carried out prior to irradiation as appropriate to each tissue type,
d) details of the equipment, laboratory and storage facilities required for each of the processing and preservation stages, particularly with regard to acceptable contamination levels,
e) details of the routine preventative maintenance programme,
f) process documentation identifying every processed tissue, including details of its origin (see 7.3), its processing and preservation, dates of performing all processes, details of process interruptions, details of any deviations from the adopted processing and preservation procedures.

8. Validation of the sterilization process

8.1. General

The guidance given here is based on the procedures specified in previous documents (ISO 11137:1995, ISO/TR 13409:1996, ISO/TR 15844:1998 and AAMI TIR 27:2001) for the sterilization of health care products. More emphasis is given here, however, on the factors which affect the ability of the sterilization process to demonstrate that an appropriate Sterility Assurance Level (SAL) can be achieved with low numbers of tissue allografts, which may have more variability in the types and levels of microbial contamination than is found in health care products and which may also be more variable in size and shape.

More specifically, several approaches to establishing a sterilization dose are proposed for the small numbers of tissue allografts typically processed.

Emphasis is placed on the need to take into account both the variability of bioburden from one tissue donor to another, as well as the variability of size and shape of tissue allografts, which can affect both the accuracy of product dose mapping (and hence the sterilization dose itself) and also the applicability of using Sample Item Portions (SIP) of a tissue allograft product.

Validation of the sterilization process shall include the following elements:

a) qualification of the tissue allografts and their packaging for sterilization,
b) qualification of the irradiation facility,
c) process qualification using a specified tissue allografts or simulated products in qualified equipment,
d) a certification procedure to review and approve documentation of a), b) and c),
e) activities performed to support maintenance of validation.

8.2. Qualification of the tissue allografts for sterilization

Evaluation of the tissue allograft and packaging

Prior to using radiation sterilization for a tissue allograft, the effect that radiation will have on the tissue allograft and its components shall be considered. The key references given in Annex D contain information on this aspect. Similarly, the effect of radiation on the packaging shall also be considered. Guidance on the latter is given in Annex A of ISO 11137:1995. Using such information, a maximum acceptable dose shall be established for each tissue allograft and its packaging.

Sterilization dose selection

A knowledge of the number and resistance to radiation of the microorganism population as it occurs on the tissue allografts shall be obtained and used for determination of the sterilization dose.

For the sterilization of health care products, a reference microbial resistance distribution was adopted in ISO 11137-1:1995 for microorganisms found typically on medical devices.

Studies should be carried out to establish the types of microorganisms that are normally found on the tissue types to be sterilized as well as their numbers and resistance to radiation. Such studies should take account of the distribution of the microorganisms within the tissue allograft itself since this may not be uniform. This should be determined by taking Sample Item Portions (SIP) of the tissue and demonstrating that there are no significant statistical variations in distribution from SIP to SIP.

If such studies show a consistent distribution of microorganisms from one tissue allograft to another, and one which is less resistant than the Standard Distribution of Resistances (SDR) (See Table 1), then a Table similar to B24 in ISO 11137:1995 giving a distribution of resistances appropriate to the allografts may be constructed for the purpose of sterilization dose setting. This would allow the use of appropriate and perhaps lower sterilization doses than would be the case if Method-1 in ISO 11137:1995, based on the SDR in Table 1, were used. In the absence of such studies, the SDR may be used to establish sterilization doses.

To establish a sterilization dose which will give a Sterility Assurance Level (SAL) of 10^{-6}, the methods based on those in ISO 11137:1995, ISO/TR 15844:1998, ISO/TR 13409:1996 and AAMI TIR 27:2001 should be used. A summary of these approaches as they apply to tissue allografts is given in Annex A.

Technical requirements

The technical requirements to generate the information required for selection of the sterilization dose shall be:

a) access to qualified microbiological and dosimetric laboratory services,
b) Microbiological testing performed in accordance with ISO 11737-1:1995 and ISO 11737-2:1998,

c) access to a ^{60}Co or ^{137}Cs radiation source, or electron beam or X-ray irradiators.

Transfer of sterilization dose

The conditions for transferring the sterilization dose between two irradiation facilities are the same as those given in ISO 11137:1995 (Section 6.2.3) and apply equally to tissue allografts.

8.3. Qualification of the irradiation facility

The principles covering the documentation of the irradiation system, its testing, calibration and dose mapping are covered in ISO 11137:1995 (Section 6.3) and apply equally to tissue allografts.

8.4. Qualification of the irradiation process

Determination of the product-loading pattern

The principles given in ISO 11137:1995 (Section 6.4.1) covering this shall also apply for the sterilization of tissue allografts.

Product dose mapping

In general, the guidelines given in ISO 11137:1995 (Section 6.4.2) apply also to tissue allografts. However, it should be recognized that the product dose mapping of relatively uniform (i.e. in shape, size, composition and density) health care products is a more straightforward task than the product dose mapping of tissue allografts, which by their nature are more variable in their physical characteristics. In particular, the density of tissue allografts may vary depending on their water content.

In addition, some tissue allografts may be heterogeneous in their distribution of density within the product, requiring an appropriate number of dosimeters for the dose mapping exercise. A consideration of these factors affecting the actual absorbed dose in tissue allografts must be undertaken so that the level of accuracy in delivering a dose to a particular tissue can be determined.

The acceptability of the accuracy of delivering a dose to tissue allografts will depend on the dose delivered in the verification dose experiments. If, for example, the actual dose delivered at its lowest possible accuracy limit is less than 90% of the verification dose, then the verification test must be repeated at a higher dose.

Similarly, the minimum absorbed dose administered for sterilization should take into account the likely variation in dose delivered so that sterilization can be assured. As a guideline, uncertainties in the delivered dose should be within +/− 10%.

8.5. Maintenance of validation

The guidelines covering calibration of equipment and dosimetric systems, irradiator requalification and sterilization dose auditing are the same as given in ISO 11137:1995 (Section 6.6) and apply equally to tissue allografts.

8.6. Routine sterilization process control

The guidelines covering process specification, tissue allograft handling and packing in the irradiation container, sterilization process documentation are similar to those given in ISO 11137:1995 (Section 7) and apply equally to tissue allografts.

9. Quality, safety and clinical application of the tissue allograft

A programme to demonstrate the quality, safety and clinical application of the tissue allograft throughout its shelf life shall be performed. Sampling procedures appropriate to the tissue type should be devised for this purpose.

10. Documentation and certification procedures

Information gathered or produced while conducting the qualification and validation of the tissue allografts, Tissue Bank facilities and tissue processing, preservation and radiation sterilization procedures shall be documented and reviewed for acceptability by a designated individual or group and retained in accordance with ISO 9001:2000 and the IAEA International Standard for Tissue Banks or revision thereof, whichever is applicable.

11. Management and control

Control of the procedures involved in the selection of tissue donors, tissue processing and preservation prior to sterilization by radiation and the radiation sterilization process itself, shall be fully documented and managed in accordance with ISO 9001:2000 and IAEA International Standard for Tissue Banks, whichever is applicable.

Annex A

Establishing a Sterilization Dose

Scope

This Annex describes the practices and procedures for determining the bioburden levels of the tissue allografts and the application of this information to establish the radiation sterilization dose. It must to be emphasised hat such samples must be the end results of the series of validated donor screening and subsequent procedures as are described in the IAEA International Standards for Tissue Banks.

Selection of tissue allograft products

Tissue allografts can be prepared from a wide range of tissues such as skin, amnion, bone, cartilage tendons and ligaments. If samples can be prepared from these tissues, which are reasonably reproducible in shape, size and composition and also in sufficient numbers for statistical purposes, then the usual sampling procedures apply, as given, for example, in ISO 11137 and ISO/TR 13409. However, if allograft products are both few in number (less than 10) and cannot be considered as identical products then it may be necessary to take multiple Sample Item Portions of a single tissue allograft product for both bioburden analysis prior to sterilization and also for the purpose of establishing a sterilization dose. In such instances, it is important to have confidence in the distribution of microorganisms throughout the sample, obtained, for example, by periodic monitoring of such products.

Sample item portion (SIP)

The SIP shall validly represent the microbial challenge presented to the sterilization process. SIPs may be used both to verify that microorganisms are distributed evenly, bioburden estimation and for establishing a sterilization dose. It is important to ascertain that the SIPs are representative, not only in shape, size and composition but also in bioburden, recognising that the bioburden can originate from both the environment and the donor, the latter of which may vary according to the type of tissue used. Statistical tests should be applied to establish this. At least 20 SIPs should be used (10 for bioburden testing and 10 for the verification dose experiments).

Bioburden determination

Bioburden determination could include the count of aerobic bacteria, spores, yeasts, molds and anaerobic bacteria. Many factors determine the choice of the tests most appropriate for the tissue allograft. At a minimum, the aerobic bacteria and fungi should be counted.

The objective of the bioburden determination is to:

a) determine the total number of viable microorganisms within or on a tissue allograft and the packaging after completion of all processing steps before sterilization,
b) act as an early warning system for possible production problems,
c) calculate the dose necessary for effective radiation sterilization.

The validation of the bioburden estimation requires the determination of the effectiveness and reproducibility of the test method.

The steps to estimate bioburden are the shown in the following flow chart and full details can be found in ISO 11737-1:1995.

Bioburden determination

The objective of the bioburden determination is to: i)Determine the total number of viable microorganisms within or on a tissue allograft and the packaging after completion of all processing steps before sterilizlation, ii) Act as an early warning system for possible processing problems, iii) Calculate the dose necessary for effective radiation sterilization.

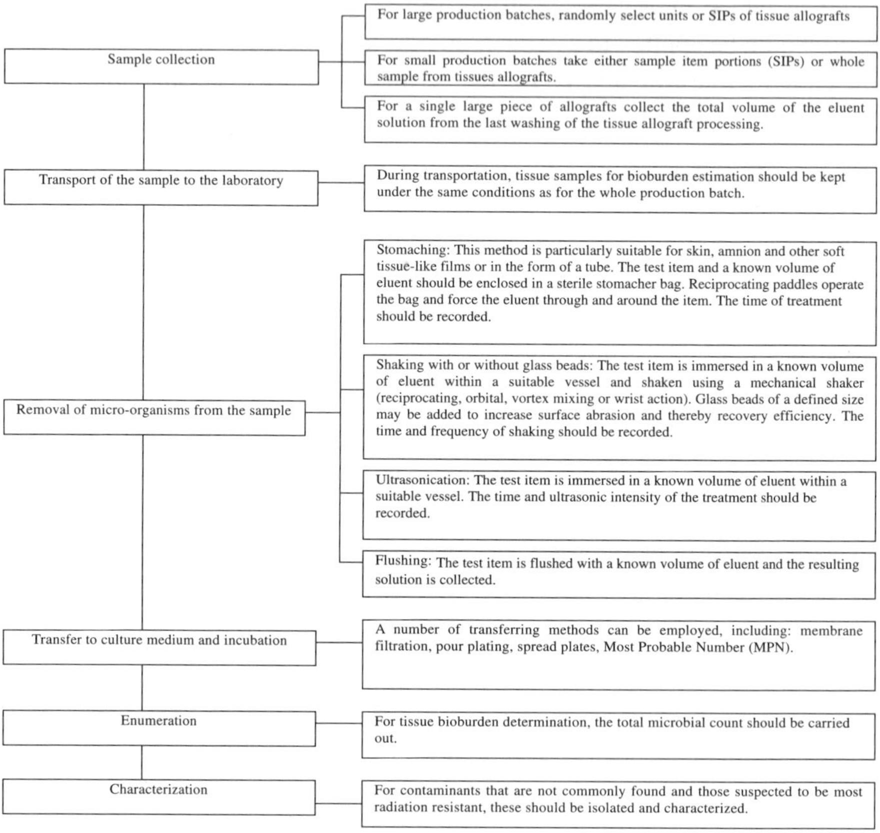

Verification dose experiments

In ISO 11137-1, the concept of establishing a verification dose for a SAL value which is much higher than 10^{-6}, for example, for a SAL value of 10^{-2} was proposed as an experimental method of establishing the sterilization dose corresponding to a SAL of 10^{-6}.

For such verification dose experiments, samples of tissue allografts should be taken from production batches and irradiated at the calculated verification dose. In these experiments it is assumed (and should be demonstrated statistically) that the tissue allograft products are reasonably uniform in shape, size, composition and bioburden distribution. For single batch sizes up to 999, the number of samples required may be obtained from Table 1 of ISO/TR 13409. For minimum batch sizes of 20–79, for example, 10 samples are required for the bioburden determination and 10 for the verification dose experiment. In general, the number of samples required for the bioburden determination and verification dose experiments will depend on the number of batches and the number of samples in each batch. For each circumstance, the number of positive sterility tests allowed in the verification dose experiment should be calculated statistically using an acceptable range of values of probability for 0, 1, 2, 3 etc. positive tests of sterility. For the 100 samples used in Method 1 of ISO 11137, for example, there is a 92% chance of there being 1% positives when up to 2 positives are detected and a 10% chance of accepting a batch with 5.23% positives (*W.A. Taylor and J.M. Hansen, Alternative Sample Sizes for Verification Dose Experiments and Dose Audits, Radiation Physics and Chemistry*, (1999), 54, 65–75).

For the 10 samples taken in ISO/TR 13409:1996 from a batch of 20, up to 1 positive test of sterility is proposed. For 30 or more, up to 2 positive tests of sterility are proposed (ISO/TR 13409:1996) It should be noted here that these latter statistical tests do not offer the same degree of protection as obtained when accepting up to two positive tests of sterility for a sample size of 100. For example, when accepting up to one positive test of sterility in a sample size of ten, there is a 95% chance of accepting a batch with 3.68% positives and a 10% chance of accepting a batch with 33.6% positives. Alternative sampling strategies are now available (see *Taylor and Hansen 1999* above) which include for example, double sampling plans which can minimise sample sizes and yet offer similar protection. For single batches of low sample sizes, protection levels similar to those of the 100 sample approach in ISO 11137 can only be obtained by accepting a small number (possibly even zero) of positive sterility tests. For example, accepting up to one positive for a sample size of 50 offers similar protection.

Hence, in ISO/TR 13409:1996 the verification dose for 10 samples taken from a batch of 20 is that which is required to produce a SAL of 10^{-1} (the reciprocal of the number of SIPs used) and is that dose which will yield not more than one positive test of sterility from the ten irradiated SIPs.

Selection of dose-setting method

In order to calculate the verification doses as well as the doses required to produce a SAL value of 10^{-6} in tissue allografts, one of several approaches may be taken to establish an appropriate verification dose for low sample numbers (up to 100 but typically much less). The methods proposed here for the establishment of a sterilization dose are based on statistical approaches used previously for the sterilization of health care products (ISO 11137:1995, ISO 13409:1996, ISO 15844:1998, AAMI TIR 27:2001) and modified appropriately for the typical low numbers of tissue allografts samples available. For a Standard Distribution of Resistance (SDR), the Tissue Bank may elect to substantiate a sterilization dose of 25 kGy for microbial levels up to 1000 cfu per unit. Alternatively, for the SDR and other microbial distribution, specific sterilization doses may be validated depending on the bioburden levels and radiation resistances (D_{10} values) of the constituent microorganisms. The following diagram shows the available methods:

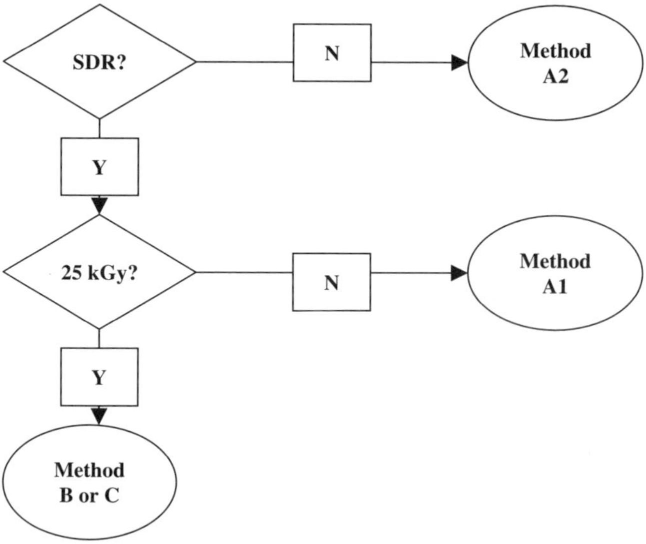

Method A1 *For establishing specific sterilization doses for Standard Distribution of Resistance and other microbial distribution for samples sizes between 10 and 100*, an adaptation of Method 1 of ISO 11137:1995 may be used. Method 1 of ISO 11137 is normally used for multiple batches containing a large number of samples per batch. For batches of 100 samples for example, verification dose experiments are carried out for a SAL of 10^{-2}. A successful experiment (up to 2 positive tests of sterility) will then enable the dose required to achieve a SAL value of 10^{-6} to be calculated from the survival curve of a Standard Distribution of Resistances (SDR). In this Code, an extension of Table 1 of ISO 11137 is given so that verification doses for SAL values between 10^{-2} and 10^{-1} may be found for bioburden levels up to 1000 cfu per allograft product. These SAL values correspond to relative low sample sizes of 10–100. This allows Method 1 of ISO 11137-1 to be used for typical tissue allografts where relatively low numbers of samples are available.

Method A2 A similar approach can also be undertaken when the distribution of microbial radiation resistances is known and different to the SDR. The worked example given later in Annex B uses this approach and, in addition, applies it (with appropriate statistical sampling, see above) to a microbial population which has a different distribution of radiation resistances than the SDR.

However, it should be noted that, for both Methods A1 and A2 above, low bioburden levels combined with low sample numbers, will give rise to an increased probability of failure of the verification dose experiment. In the case of failure, the methods B and C outlined below for substantiation of a 25 kGy sterilization dose may decrease this risk.

Method B *For substantiation of a 25 kGy sterilization dose, the Method in ISO/TR 13409:1996* may be used to calculate the verification dose. This is an accredited method and is essentially a modification of Method 1 of ISO 11137-1 and applies only to a Standard Distribution of Resistances. In this method, the verification dose for a given SAL is approximated to the initial bioburden by a series of linear relationships. Each linear equation is valid for a particular ten-fold domain of bioburden level e.g., 1–10 cfu. The method in ISO/TR 13409:1996 can only be used to substantiate a dose of 25 kGy. It should be noted that the statistical approach allowing up to 1 positive test for sample sizes up to 30 and up to 2 positive tests for sample sizes above 30 does not offer the same level of protection as for the 100 samples in ISO 11137 until the sample size reaches 100. Alternative sampling strategies may be employed (*Taylor and Hansen 1999*) for all the verification dose methods proposed here.

Method C *For substantiation of a 25 kGy sterilization dose*, an alternative and more recent method in AAMI TIR 27 may be used. This method may be adopted as a formal replacement of Method B (ISO/TR 13409) for the use of 25 kGy as a sterilization dose. The modification takes into account how the verification dose varies with bioburden level for a given SAL (and sample size) on the assumption that an SAL of 10^{-6} is to be achieved at 25 kGy. Depending on the actual bioburden levels to be used (1–50 or 51–1000 cfu per allograft product), a linear extrapolation of the appropriate SDR survival curve is made from either (log N_0, 0 kGy) or (log 10^{-2}) to (log 10^{-6}, 25 kGy) for 1–50 cfu and 51–1000 cfu respectively. For bioburden levels less than 1000 cfu per allograft unit, these constructed survival curves represent a more radiation resistant bioburden than would otherwise be the case. The validity of this approach arises from the purpose of the method which is to validate a sterilization dose of 25 kGy. For all bioburden levels below 1000 cfu per allograft product, this means that for the reference microbial resistance distribution given in Table B24 of ISO 11137:1995 for medical devices, a more conservative approach to the calculation of a verification dose is taken. Hence, this modification allows the use of greater verification doses than would be allowed using the formula given in either Method 1 of ISO 11137-1 or in ISO/TR 13409:1996. The result is that there are fewer unexpected and unwarranted failures relative to verification doses experiments carried out using the method in ISO/TR 13409:1996. At a bioburden level of exactly 1000 cfu per allograft product (the maximum in both methods), there is no difference in the outcomes of the methods i.e. the calculated verification doses are identical.

Procedures

a. *Establish test sample sizes*

Select at least 10 allograft products or SIPs, as appropriate, for the determination of the initial bioburden. The number of allograft products or SIPs should be sufficient to represent validly the bioburden on the allograft product(s) to be sterilized.

Select between 10 and 100 allograft products (or SIPs) for the verification dose experiments and record the corresponding verification dose SAL($= 1/n$, where n is the number of allograft products or SIPs used).

b. *Determine the average bioburden*

Using methods such as those in ISO 11737-1:1995 and as described above (Bioburden estimation), determine the average bioburden of at least 10 allograft products or SIPs (the number will depend on the number of batches and the number of samples in the batches). For SIP values less than unity, the bioburden level for the whole product should be calculated and should be less than 1000 cfu per allograft product for verification dose experiments carried out to substantiate a 25 kGy sterilization dose.

c. *Establish the verification dose*

The appropriate verification dose depends on the number of samples (allograft products or SIPs) to be used in the experiment(= 1/ number of samples) The verification dose calculation depends on which of the three methods above is being used, as follows:

Methods A1 and A2 For establishing specific sterilization doses for Standard Distribution of Resistance and other microbial distribution for samples sizes between 10 and 100: (an adaptation of Method 1 of ISO 11137-1:1995)
Calculate the dose required to achieve the required SAL from a knowledge of the initial bioburden level and from the microbial distribution and associated radiation resistances. This may be calculated from the equation,

$$N_{tot} = N_{0(1)} \cdot 10^{-(D/D1)} + N_{0(2)} \cdot 10^{-(D/D2)} + \cdots + N_{0(n)} \cdot 10^{-(D/Dn)}$$

where N_{tot}, represents the numbers of survivors; where $N_{0(i)}$ represents the initial numbers of the various microbial strains i (where $i = 1 - n$), $D1, D2 \cdots D(n)$ represent the D_{10} values of the various microbial strains. D represents the radiation dose and n the number of terms in the equation representing the standard distribution of resistances (For the SDR, $n = 10$).

Method A1 For the reference Standard Distribution of Resistances (K.W. Davis, W.E. Strawderman and J.L. Whitby, 1984, J. Applied Bacteriology 57, 31–50) used in ISO 11137:1995 for medical devices (see Table 1 of Annex C), this equation will produce data similar to Table B1 of ISO 11137:1995 but for SAL values between 10^{-2} and 10^{-1} instead. By equating N_{tot} to the selected SAL value and by using the appropriate D_{10} values for each microbial type (from Table 1 of Annex C) together with their numbers prior to irradiation, the verification dose, D, for SAL values between

10^{-2} and 10^{-1} can be calculated. These values are set out in Table 2a of Annex C. The same calculation can be used to find the sterilization dose for the desired SAL of 10^{-6} and these values are set out in Table 2b of Annex C. In this method, the sterilization dose is then calculated using the bioburden level of the whole product (i.e. SIP = 1) or equivalent for SIP values less than unity. Alternatively, approximate values of the verification doses to achieve the same SAL values may be calculated using the equation given in ISO/TR 13409:1996 (see next paragraph).

Method A2 The same equation above can be adopted to calculate both the verification and sterilization doses where a distribution of microflora which is different to the SDR is to be sterilized. It requires a knowledge of the different proportions of microflora with their respective D_{10} values. A worked example is given in Annex B.

Method B For substantiation of a 25 kGy sterilization dose, Method ISO/TR 13409:1996:

From a knowledge of the average bioburden and the number of samples or SIPs to be used in the verification experiment, the verification dose for a Standard Distribution of Resistances is approximated by the equation;

$$\text{Verification dose at a the selected SAL} = \text{I} + [\text{S} \times \log(\text{bioburden})]$$

where I and S are given in Annex C, Table 3 of this Code. Verification doses are calculated from the bioburden on the SIP. It should be confirmed that the bioburden for the whole sample (SIP = 1) is less than 1000 cfu for the method to be valid.

***Method C For substantiation of a 25 kGy sterilization dose, AAMI TIR 27:2001*:**

The calculation of the verification dose follows the procedures by Kowalski and Tallentire, 1999 (*Radiat. Phys. Chem.*, 54, 55–64) where the bioburden levels refer to either the SIP or whole product whichever is being used in the verification dose experiment:

For bioburden levels of 1 to 50 cfu per allograft product or SIPs

Step 1: $D_{\text{lin}} = 25\,\text{kGy}/(6 + \log N_0)$
Step 2: Verification dose $= D_{\text{lin}}(\log N_0 - \log SAL_{\text{VD}})$

where D_{lin} represents the D_{10} dose for a hypothetical survival curve which is linear between the coordinates (log N_0, 0 kGy) and (log 10^{-6}, 25 kGy) for initial bioburden levels, N_0, up to 1000 cfu per allograft product. This linear plot therefore represents a constructed survival curve in which there is 1 out of 10^6 probability of a survivor at 25 kGy. The method is valid therefore only for the substantiation of a 25 kGy sterilization dose regardless of whether a lower dose could in fact be validated.

For bioburden levels of 51 to 1000 cfu per allograft product or SIPs

Step 1: For a particular value of bioburden, use Table B1 of ISO 11137:1995 to identify the doses (kGy) corresponding to SAL values of 10^{-2} [D(10^{-2})] and 10^{-6} [D(10^{-6})]. From these values, calculate TD_{10} from the following equation:

$$TD_{10} = (Dose_{-6}\,kGy - Dose_{-2}\,kGy)/4$$

where TD_{10} represents the hypothetical D_{10} value for a survival curve for a Standard Distribution of Resistances which has been modified such that it is linear between log 10^{-2} and log 10^{-6} (log SAL values) when plotted against dose, with the log 10^{-6} value being set at 25 kGy. Essentially, this produces a survival curve which is more resistant to radiation than the SDR (for bioburden levels less than 1000 cfu per allograft product) and one which is appropriate to substantiation of a 25 kGy sterilization dose only.

Step 2: Verification dose $= 25\text{kGy} - [TD_{10}(\log SAL_{VD} + 6)]$
where SAL_{VD} is the sterility assurance level at which the verification dose experiment is to be performed.

In AAMI TIR 27, a refinement of the above calculations has been undertaken and as a result values of verification doses for a SAL of 10^{-1} for bioburden values between 0 and 1000 cfu can be found in tabular form in that publication — they are reproduced here in Table 4. For other SAL values the methods of calculation detailed above should be used. In AAMI TIR, the verification dose for SIP values less than unity are calculated from the equation:

$$\text{SIP Verification dose} + (\text{SIP} = 1\text{verification dose})$$
$$+ (\log \text{SIP} * \text{SIP dose reduction factor})$$

Values of the SIP dose reduction factor can be found in Table 4 (for verification doses experiments conducted at a SAL of 10^{-1}).

d. *Perform verification dose experiment*

Irradiate the tissue allografts or SIPs thereof at the verification dose. Irradiation conditions of the samples for verification of the sub-sterilization dose should be the same as the whole batch which is to be sterilized. For example, if the produced tissue batch is irradiated in frozen condition, the samples for the sub-sterilization dose verification studies should be irradiated in the same condition and the frozen condition should be kept during the whole irradiation process.

The defined test sample size (SIP ≤ 1), according to the SAL and batch size, is exposed to radiation at the verification dose. The delivered dose may vary from the calculated verification dose by $+10\%$ but it should not be less than 90% of the calculated verification dose.

Test the tissue allografts for sterility using the methods in ISO 11737-2:1998 and record the number of positive tests of sterility. The irradiated SIPs, of all types of tissue allografts, are transferred to a suitable growth medium to detect total mesophilic aerobic bacteria and incubated at 30+/− 2 C for 14 day. Positive and negative sterility tests results should be registered.

For bone and skin allografts, an additional test is recommended to detect anaerobic bacteria.

e. *Interpretation of results*

For a verification dose experiment performed with up to 30 allograft products or SIPs, statistical verification is accepted if there is no more than one positive test of sterility observed. For 30 to 100 products or SIPs, statistical verification is accepted if there are no more than two positive tests of sterility observed (see ISO/TR 13409:1996). However, it should be noted that the degree of protection in accepting these limits varies according to the sample size taken (see also above).

Where the verification dose experiment is successful, the dose required to produce a SAL of 10^{-6} for the whole allograft product should be calculated for Methods A1 and A2 as indicated above and calculated in Annex C, Table 2b.

For procedures in Methods B and C, a successful verification dose experiment substantiates the use of 25 kGy as a sterilization dose.

Routine use of sterilization doses

The routine use of a sterilization dose calculated in procedure c(i) or of 25 kGy as substantiated by either procedure c(ii) or c(iii) shall only be valid if the tissue selection and tissue processing procedures have been demonstrated to produce tissues allografts with consistent bioburden levels. It should be demonstrated that the level of variation in bioburden, is consistent with the sterilization dose to be used routinely. In such cases, sterilization dose audits should be carried out at regular intervals, at least every three months.

Annex B

Sterilization of Tissue Allografts

Examples of Sterilization Procedures

1. Limited number of amnion samples with low bioburden and low bacterial resistance using Method 1 of ISO 11137:1995 to calculate the verification dose

Introduction

This method uses Method A2 (an adaptation of Method 1 of ISO 11137-1:1995) but applies it to sample sizes of less than 100 in a single production batch. The example chosen consists of a single batch of 20 amnion membranes (5 × 5 cm) from which 10 are used for the bioburden determination and 10 are used for the verification dose experiment. The data used in the example are consistent with data on bioburden levels, bacterial types and distribution found in *Hilmy et al., J.Cell and Tissue Banking (2000) 1, 143–147*. In that study, the most radiation resistant microbes were assumed to have a D_{10} value of 1,8 kGy. i.e. a distribution which differs from the reference microbial resistance distribution in that there are no microbes with a D_{10}value higher than 1,8 kGy. Furthermore, the tissue processing and preservation procedures have produced tissue allografts which are much lower than 1000 cfu per allograft product. For such samples, a sterilization dose which is significantly less than 25 kGy is confirmed from the verification dose experiment.

Procured tissue qualification

(i) Tissue type ...*Amnion samples of 5 × 5 cm*

(ii) Screening of tissue for transmission of disease

Age of donor ...25

Medical, social and sexual history . . .*None to suggest risk of transmissible disease*
Serological tests

HIV (HIV-1,2 Ab)	...*Negative,*
Hepatitis C (HCV-Ab)	...*Negative,*
Hepatitis B (HBs-Ag)	...*Negative,*
Syphillis (VDRL)	...*Negative.*

Tissue processing and preservation qualification

(i) Description of processing technique ...*Hypochlorite*
(ii) Description of preservation technique ...*Lyophilization*
(iii) Typical microbial levels of procured tissue before processing ...*In the range of 5000–10000 cfu per tissue*
(iv) Typical bioburden levels of processed and preserved tissues ...*57 cfu per allograft product (Note 1)*

Note 1: It is noted from the study of Hilmy et al. (see above) that the bioburden levels of the processed tissue (i.e. before sterilization by irradiation) decreased from about 1400 cfu to 120 cfu during the study period 1994 to 1997, with 1998 data showing an average of 57 cfu per allograft product (range 12–160 cfu). Clearly, good processing techniques can have a dramatic effect on the bioburden levels of the tissue being prepared for sterilization by irradiation. The level of reduction used in this example is probably therefore a conservative estimate of the degree of elimination of bacteria.

Qualification of tissue allografts for sterilization

Typical bioburden distribution

The distribution of bacterial resistances given below is assumed to consist entirely of bacteria with a D_{10} value of 1.8 kGy and represents a distribution which is similar but not identical to the Standard Distribution of Resistances. i.e.:

D_{10}(kGy)	1.8
Frequency	1.0

Calculation of the sterilization dose

Stage	Value	Comments
Stage 1		
Production batch size	40	5 × 5 cm amnion samples
Test sample size for bioburden determination	10	
Test sample size for the verification dose experiment	10	Verification dose required for SAL 10^{-1} (= 1/10)
Stage 2		
Obtain samples	20	10 for bioburden; 10 for verification dose experiment
Stage 3		
SIP	1	The whole allograft product is used.
Average bioburden	57	Bioburden results of 15, 91, 99, 30, 30, 99, 8, 84, 91, 23.
Stage 4		
Verification dose calculation	4.96 kGy	Using the bacterial resistance distribution given above (and not the SDR), the survival equation is constructed (see Annex A) and used to calculate the verification dose (D) for a N(tot) value of 0,1 (equivalent to a SAL value of 0,1, the reciprocal of the number of samples used) and where the total initial number of microorganisms per product (SIP = 1) is equal to 57. The survival equation is : $N_{tot} = 5710^{-(D/1.8)}$ From this data, the verification dose is calculated as 4.96 kGy.
Stage 5		
Verification dose experiments	5.0 kGy (delivered dose) 1 positive/10 samples	The sterility test yielded one positive test out of ten and therefore the verification dose experiment was successful *(but note that the level of protection is significantly less than allowing up to 2 positives for a sample size of 100, see Annex A)* and the sterilization dose for SAL = 10^{-6} can be calculated from the survival equation given above(= 13.96 kGy). *Note : In the case that a SIP < 1 was taken instead, the bioburden for the whole product should be used to calculate the sterilization dose.*

Conclusion

This example shows how the combination of good tissue processing and preservation and sterilization by ionising radiation, for samples which are known to have bacterial contamination relatively susceptible to radiation, can allow the use of a sterilization dose which is much less than 25 kGy.

2. Limited number of amnion samples requiring only substantiation of 25 kGy as a sterilization dose

Introduction

In this example, it is assumed that there is a Standard Distribution of Resistances which defines the bacterial contamination of the tissue allografts. The example chosen consists of a single batch of 40 amnion membranes (5 × 5 cm) from which 10 are used for the bioburden determination and 10 are used for the verification dose experiment. The data used in the example are consistent with data on bioburden levels, bacterial types and distribution found in *Hilmy et al., J.Cell and Tissue Banking (2000) 1, 143–147.* Furthermore, for the limited number of samples to be tested, it is required only to establish that a 25 kGy dose may be used to achieve an SAL of 10^{-6}. It is shown below that when Method B (from ISO/TR 13409:1996) is applied for 20 samples (10 for the bioburden determination and 10 for the verification dose experiment), from a batch size of 40, the samples fail the verification dose experiment. To increase the probability of a successful verification dose experiment, whilst at the same time substantiating a sterilization dose of 25 kGy, Method C (based on the method of Tallentire and Kowalski, set out in AAMI TIR 27:2001) is applied (see Annex A). This allows the use of a higher verification dose and it is then found that the samples pass this test, substantiating the use of a 25 kGy sterilization dose.

Procured tissue qualification

(i) Tissue type ...*Amnion (5 × 5 cm)*

(ii) Screening of tissue for transmission of disease

Age of donor ...25

Medical, social and sexual history ...*None to suggest risk of transmissible disease*

Serological tests

HIV (HIV-1,2 Ab)	...*Negative,*
Hepatitis C (HCV-Ab)	...*Negative,*
Hepatitis B (HBs-Ag)	...*Negative,*
Syphillis (VDRL)	...*Negative.*

Tissue processing and preservation qualification

(i) Description of processing technique ...*Hypochlorite*
(ii) Description of preservation technique ...*Lyophilization*
(iii) Typical microbial levels of procured tissue before processing ...*In the range of 5000–10000 cfu per tissue*
(iv) Typical bioburden levels of processed and preserved tissues ...*57 cfu per allograft product (Note 1)*

Qualification of tissue allografts for sterilization

Typical bioburden distribution (it is assumed that the Standard Distribution of Resistances, see Annex A, is valid).

Stage	Value	Comments
Stage 1		
Production batch size	40	5 × 5 cm amnion samples
Test sample size for bioburden determination	10	
Test sample size for the verification dose experiment	10	Verification dose required for SAL 10^{-1} (= 1/10)
Stage 2		
Obtain samples	20	10 for bioburden; 10 for verification dose experiment
Stage 3		
SIP	1	The whole allograft product is used.
Average bioburden	57	Bioburden results of 28, 91, 90, 30, 30, 86, 28, 64, 91, 32. Average bioburden for whole product *57 cfu* (This is less than 1000 cfu and therefore the method may be used). *Note: If a SIP<1 was taken, then the bioburden of the whole product should be calculated and should be less than 1000 cfu per allograft product for this method to be valid.*
Stage 4		
Verification dose calculation (1)	4.6 kGy	The verification dose is calculated using the method in ISO/TR 13409:1996. In this method (applicable to a Standard Distribution of Resistances only), the verification dose for a given SAL is approximated to the initial bioburden by a series of linear relationships using the parameters I and S (see below). Each linear equation is valid for a particular ten-fold domain of bioburden level, e.g. 10–100 cfu.

Stage	Value	Comments
		For a bioburden of 57 and sample size of 10, I and S values of 0.67 and 2.23 respectively are obtained from ISO/TR 13409:1996 and are given here in Annex C, Table 3. The verification dose is given by: $$\begin{aligned} \text{Dose} &= \text{I} + [\text{S} \times \log(\text{average SIP bioburden})] \\ &= 0.67 + (2.23 \times \log(57)) \\ &= 4.6\,\text{kGy} \end{aligned}$$
Stage 5		
Verification dose experiments (1)	4.5 kGy (delivered dose) 2 positives/ 10 samples	The sterility test yielded two positive tests out of ten and therefore the verification dose experiment was not successful and a sterilization dose of 25 kGy could not be substantiated.
Verification dose calculation (2)	8.7 kGy	A new verification dose was calculated using the method of Tallentire and Kowalski (see Annex A). This method takes into account how the verification dose for a Standard Distribution of Resistances (Reference microbial resistance distribution) varies with bioburden level for a given SAL (and sample size) on the assumption that an SAL of $10^{-6}$is to be achieved at 25 kGy. Application of Method 1 of ISO 11137:1995 for bioburden levels of less than 1000 cfu would yield sterilization doses of less than 25 kGy. The method of Tallentire and Kowalski assumes instead that only substantiation of a 25 kGy sterilization dose is required regardless of the bioburden level. Extrapolation of the reference distribution to produce an SAL of 10^{-6} at 25 kGy for bioburden levels of less than 1000 cfu allows the use of higher verification doses than would be predicted by Method 1 of ISO 11137:1995 and hence a greater probability of a successful verification dose experiment. For a bioburden level of 57 (i.e. between 51 and 1000), the doses corresponding to this bioburden for SAL values of 10^{-6} and 10^{-2} are found from Table 1 of ISO11137 and are designated Dose_{-6} and Dose_{-2} respectively, from which the TD_{10} is calculated as follows: $$\begin{aligned} TD_{10} &= (\text{Dose}_{-6}\,\text{kGy} - \text{Dose}_{-2}\,\text{kGy})/4 \\ &= (20.4 - 7.3)/4 \\ &= 3.27\,\text{kGy} \end{aligned}$$ *(Note: Table 1 of ISO 11137:1995 does not have a value corresponding to a bioburden of 57 and so the next highest value of 59.2 is used.)*

Stage	Value	Comments
		where TD_{10} represents the hypothetical D_{10} value for a survival curve for a Standard Distribution of Resistances which has been modified such that it is linear between log 10^{-2} and log 10^{-6} (log SAL values) when plotted against dose, with the log 10^{-6} value being set at 25 kGy. Essentially, this produces a survival curve which is more resistant to radiation than the SDR (for bioburden levels less than 1000 cfu per allograft product) and one which is appropriate to substantiation of a 25 kGy sterilization dose only. The verification dose, VD, is then calculated, as follows: $$\begin{aligned} VD &= 25\,\text{kGy} - [TD_{10}(\log SAL_{VD} + 6)] \\ &= 25 - [3.27(\log 0.1 + 6)] \\ &= 8.7\,\text{kGy (note Table 4 from AAMI gives a} \\ &\quad \text{refined value of } 8.9\,\text{kGy)} \end{aligned}$$ where SAL_{VD} is the sterility assurance level at which the verification dose experiment is to be performed, (= the reciprocal of the number of samples), in this case, 0.1.
Verification dose experiments (2)	8.5 kGy 1 positive/ 10 samples	The 10 samples are irradiated at this verification dose and tested for sterility. The sterility tests yielded one positive test out of ten and therefore the use of 25 kGy as a sterilization dose (SAL = 10^{-6}) could be substantiated (*Note however that this result does not offer the same level of protection when allowing up to 2 positives in a sample size of 100, see above*)

Conclusion

Although the tissue processing and preservation produced tissues with relatively low bioburden for which sterilization doses substantially less than 25 kGy could have been used (see example above), the tissue bank required only a method to substantiate a sterilization dose of 25 kGy. The application of the methods of ISO 13409:1996 and of Tallentire and Kowalski, which are particularly suitable for bioburden levels much less than 1000 cfu per allograft product, allowed the use of relatively high verification doses and, hence a greater probability of success. In the example chosen, the method in ISO 13409:1996 failed and hence the method of Tallentire and Kowalski was used as well. For tissue banks which prefer to use a standard 25 kGy sterilization dose, this latter method will be more efficient in that fewer verification dose experiments will fail.

3. Limited number of bone samples with very low bioburden and SDR using ISO/TR 13409:1996 to calculate the verification dose (SIP < 1)

Introduction

This method uses Method B (from ISO/TR 13409:1996) and applies it to a sample of 40 small pieces of bone.

Typically, very low bioburden levels are found after processing. In this example, very low SIP values are used so that most of the allograft product can be retained for use.

Procured tissue qualification

(i) Tissue type: *...Bone cut into 40 small pieces (chips)*

(ii) Screening of tissues donor

Age of donor ... 36

Medical, social and sexual history *...None to suggest risk of transmissible disease*

Serological tests:

HIV (HIV-1, 2 Ab)	*...Negative,*
Hepatitis C (HCV-Ab)	*...Negative,*
Hepatitis B (HBs-Ag)	*...Negative,*
Syphillis (VDRL)	*...Negative.*

Tissue processing and preservation qualification

(i) Description of processing technique *...Cut into standardized small pieces*

(ii) Description of preservation technique *...Frozen*

(iii) Typical bioburden levels of processed and preserved tissues ... 40 *cfu per allograft product*

Qualification of tissue allografts for sterilization

Stage	Value	Comments
Stage 1		
Production batch size	5	Bone cut into 40 small pieces (1 cc each) packed in flask, produced from 1donor in one processing batch.
Test sample size for bioburden determination	10	According ISO/TR 13409:1996, Table 1.
Test sample size for verification dose experiment	10	According ISO/TR 13409:1996, Table 1.
Stage 2		
Obtained samples	20	A random sample of 20 standardized product portions of 1 cc each was obtained from the production batch.
Stage 3		
SIP	0.025	Calculated from 1/40.
SIP bioburden	1	Bioburden results of 1, 0, 2, 0, 1, 2, 1, 1, 1, 1 were observed from the 10 SIP tested, for an average bioburden of 1.
Average bioburden	40	The average bioburden for the product tested was calculated as follow: 1/0.025 = 40. This is less than 1000 cfu per allograft product and therefore this method is valid.
Stage 4		
Verification dose calculation	1.3	Verification dose formula: I + (S × log (average SIP bioburden) kGy. According ISO/TR 13409:1996, table 2, the I and S values are 1.25 and 1.65 respectively. $= 1.25 + (1.65 \times \log 1)$ $= 1.25$ kGy $= 1.3$ kGy
Stage 5		
Verification dose experiment	1.3 kGy (delivered dose) 0 positive / 10 samples	The test sterility yielded 0 positive from the 10 SIPs tested. Therefore, the verification experiment was successful and no further action was necessary.
Stage 6		
Interpretation of results		The test of sterility result was acceptable, the sterilization dose of 25 kGy was confirmed.

Conclusions

Although a lower sterilization dose could be justified if the adaptation of Method 1 of ISO 11137:1995 was applied, the Tissue Bank elected to use ISO/TR 13409:1996 to substantiate a 25 kGy sterilization dose only.

Annex C

TABLES

Tables 1, 2, 3 and 4

Table 1. Microbial standard distribution of resistance (SDR).

D_{10} (kGy)	1.0	1.5	2.0	2.5	2.8	3.1	3.4	3.7	4.0	4.2
%	65.487	22.493	6.302	3.179	1.213	0.786	0.350	0.111	0.072	0.007

Davis, K.W., Strawderman, W.E. and Whitby, J.L. The rationale and computer evaluation of a gamma sterilization dose determination method for medical devices using a substerilization incremental dose sterility test protocol. J. Appl. Bact., (1984) 57, 31–50.

Table 2a. Radiation dose (kGy) required to achieve given SAL for different bioburden (cfu) having standard distribution of resistances.

Sample size (n)	SAL ($1/n$)	Bioburden															
		0.06	0.08	0.09	0.10	0.12	0.14	0.17	0.19	0.22	0.26	0.29	0.34	0.39	0.44	0.50	0.57
10	1/10																
15	1/15														1.0	1.1	1.2
20	1/20												1.0	1.1	1.2	1.3	1.4
25	1/25										1.0	1.1	1.2	1.3	1.3	1.4	1.5
30	1/30									1.0	1.1	1.2	1.3	1.4	1.5	1.5	1.6
35	1/35								1.0	1.1	1.2	1.3	1.4	1.5	1.6	1.6	1.7
40	1/40							1.0	1.1	1.2	1.3	1.4	1.5	1.6	1.6	1.7	1.8
45	1/45						1.0	1.1	1.2	1.3	1.4	1.4	1.5	1.6	1.7	1.8	1.9
50	1/50					1.0	1.1	1.2	1.2	1.3	1.4	1.5	1.6	1.7	1.8	1.9	2.0
60	1/60				1.0	1.1	1.2	1.3	1.4	1.5	1.6	1.6	1.7	1.8	1.9	2.0	2.1
70	1/70			1.0	1.1	1.2	1.3	1.4	1.5	1.6	1.7	1.7	1.8	1.9	2.0	2.1	2.2
80	1/80		1.0	1.1	1.1	1.2	1.3	1.5	1.5	1.6	1.7	1.8	1.9	2.0	2.1	2.2	2.3
90	1/90		1.1	1.1	1.2	1.3	1.4	1.5	1.6	1.7	1.8	1.9	2.0	2.1	2.2	2.3	2.4
100	1/100	1.0	1.1	1.2	1.3	1.4	1.5	1.6	1.7	1.8	1.9	2.0	2.1	2.2	2.3	2.4	2.5

Table 2a. *(Continued).*

Sample size (n)	SAL ($1/n$)	Bioburden															
		0.65	0.73	0.83	0.93	1.0	1.2	1.4	1.6	1.8	2.0	2.2	2.6	3.0	3.2	4.0	4.4
10	1/10	1.0	1.1	1.1	1.2	1.3	1.4	1.5	1.6	1.7	1.7	1.8	1.9	2.0	2.1	2.2	2.3
15	1/15	1.3	1.3	1.4	1.5	1.5	1.7	1.8	1.9	1.9	2.0	2.1	2.2	2.3	2.4	2.5	2.6
20	1/20	1.4	1.5	1.6	1.7	1.7	1.9	2.0	2.1	2.2	2.2	2.3	2.4	2.5	2.6	2.8	2.9
25	1/25	1.6	1.7	1.7	1.8	1.9	2.0	2.1	2.2	2.3	2.4	2.5	2.6	2.7	2.8	3.0	3.0
30	1/30	1.7	1.8	1.9	2.0	2.0	2.1	2.3	2.4	2.5	2.5	2.6	2.7	2.9	2.9	3.1	3.2
35	1/35	1.8	1.9	2.0	2.1	2.1	2.3	2.4	2.5	2.6	2.7	2.8	2.9	3.0	3.1	3.3	3.4
40	1/40	1.9	2.0	2.1	2.2	2.2	2.4	2.5	2.6	2.7	2.8	2.9	3.0	3.1	3.2	3.4	3.5
45	1/45	2.0	2.1	2.2	2.3	2.3	2.5	2.6	2.7	2.8	2.9	3.0	3.1	3.2	3.3	3.5	3.6
50	1/50	2.1	2.1	2.2	2.3	2.4	2.5	2.7	2.8	2.9	3.0	3.0	3.2	3.3	3.4	3.6	3.7
60	1/60	2.2	2.3	2.4	2.5	2.5	2.7	2.8	2.9	3.0	3.1	3.2	3.4	3.5	3.5	3.8	3.9
70	1/70	2.3	2.4	2.5	2.6	2.7	2.8	2.9	3.0	3.2	3.3	3.3	3.5	3.6	3.7	3.9	4.0
80	1/80	2.4	2.5	2.6	2.7	2.8	2.9	3.1	3.2	3.3	3.4	3.5	3.6	3.8	3.8	4.0	4.1
90	1/90	2.5	2.6	2.7	2.8	2.9	3.0	3.2	3.3	3.4	3.5	3.6	3.7	3.9	3.9	4.1	4.2
100	1/100	2.6	2.7	2.8	2.9	3.0	3.1	3.2	3.4	3.5	3.6	3.7	3.8	4.0	4.0	4.2	4.3

Table 2a. (*Continued*).

Sample size (n)	SAL ($1/n$)	Bioburden													
		5.0	5.4	6.0	7.0	8.0	9.0	10	11	12	13	14	15	16	17
10	1/10	2.4	2.5	2.5	2.7	2.8	2.9	3.0	3.0	3.1	3.2	3.3	3.3	3.4	3.4
15	1/15	2.7	2.8	2.9	3.0	3.1	3.2	3.4	3.5	3.6	3.7	3.7	3.8	3.8	3.9
20	1/20	3.0	3.0	3.1	3.3	3.4	3.5	3.6	3.7	3.7	3.8	3.9	4.0	4.0	4.1
25	1/25	3.2	3.2	3.3	3.5	3.6	3.7	3.8	3.9	4.0	4.0	4.1	4.2	4.2	4.3
30	1/30	3.3	3.4	3.5	3.6	3.8	3.9	4.1	4.1	4.2	4.3	4.4	4.4	4.5	4.6
35	1/35	3.5	3.6	3.6	3.8	3.9	4.0	4.1	4.2	4.3	4.4	4.4	4.5	4.6	4.6
40	1/40	3.6	3.7	3.8	3.9	4.0	4.2	4.3	4.4	4.4	4.5	4.6	4.7	4.7	4.8
45	1/45	3.7	3.8	3.9	4.0	4.2	4.3	4.4	4.5	4.6	4.7	4.7	4.8	4.9	4.9
50	1/50	3.8	3.9	4.0	4.1	4.3	4.4	4.4	4.5	4.6	4.7	4.8	4.9	4.9	5.0
60	1/60	4.0	4.1	4.2	4.3	4.4	4.6	4.7	4.8	4.9	5.0	5.0	5.1	5.2	5.3
70	1/70	4.1	4.2	4.3	4.5	4.6	4.7	4.8	4.9	5.0	5.1	5.2	5.3	5.3	5.4
80	1/80	4.2	4.3	4.4	4.6	4.7	4.9	5.0	5.1	5.2	5.3	5.3	5.4	5.5	5.6
90	1/90	4.4	4.5	4.6	4.7	4.8	5.0	5.1	5.2	5.3	5.4	5.5	5.6	5.6	5.7
100	1/100	4.5	4.6	4.7	4.8	5.0	5.1	5.2	5.3	5.4	5.5	5.6	5.7	5.7	5.8

Table 2a. (*Continued*).

Sample size (n)	SAL ($1/n$)	Bioburden														
		18	19	20	25	30	35	40	45	50	55	60	65	70	75	80
10	1/10	3.5	3.5	3.6	3.8	4.0	4.1	4.3	4.4	4.5	4.6	4.7	4.8	4.8	4.9	5.0
15	1/15	4.0	4.0	4.1	4.3	4.5	4.6	4.8	4.9	5.0	5.1	5.2	5.3	5.4	5.4	5.5
20	1/20	4.1	4.2	4.2	4.5	4.6	4.8	5.0	5.1	5.2	5.3	5.4	5.5	5.6	5.6	5.7
25	1/25	4.3	4.4	4.5	4.7	4.9	5.0	5.2	5.3	5.4	5.5	5.6	5.7	5.8	5.9	5.9
30	1/30	4.6	4.7	4.7	5.0	5.2	5.3	5.5	5.6	5.7	5.8	5.9	6.0	6.1	6.2	6.2
35	1/35	4.7	4.7	4.8	5.0	5.2	5.4	5.6	5.7	5.9	6.0	6.1	6.2	6.2	6.3	6.4
40	1/40	4.9	4.9	5.0	5.2	5.4	5.6	5.7	5.9	6.0	6.1	6.2	6.3	6.4	6.5	6.6
45	1/45	5.0	5.1	5.1	5.4	5.6	5.7	5.9	6.0	6.1	6.3	6.4	6.4	6.5	6.6	6.7
50	1/50	5.0	5.1	5.1	5.4	5.6	5.7	5.9	6.0	6.1	6.2	6.3	6.4	6.5	6.6	6.7
60	1/60	5.3	5.4	5.4	5.7	5.9	6.1	6.2	6.4	6.5	6.6	6.7	6.8	6.9	7.0	7.0
70	1/70	5.5	5.5	5.6	5.9	6.1	6.2	6.4	6.5	6.7	6.8	6.9	7.0	7.1	7.2	7.2
80	1/80	5.6	5.7	5.7	6.0	6.2	6.4	6.6	6.7	6.8	6.9	7.0	7.1	7.2	7.3	7.4
90	1/90	5.8	5.8	5.9	6.1	6.3	6.5	6.7	6.8	7.0	7.1	7.2	7.3	7.4	7.5	7.5
100	1/100	5.9	5.9	6.0	6.3	6.5	6.6	6.8	7.0	7.1	7.2	7.3	7.4	7.5	7.6	7.7

Table 2a. *(Continued)*.

Sample size (n)	SAL ($1/n$)	Bioburden											
		85	90	95	100	150	200	250	300	350	400	450	500
10	1/10	5.0	5.1	5.2	5.2	5.7	6.0	6.2	6.5	6.6	6.7	6.9	7.1
15	1/15	5.6	5.6	5.7	5.8	6.2	6.6	6.8	7.0	7.2	7.4	7.5	7.7
20	1/20	5.8	5.8	5.9	5.9	6.4	6.8	7.0	7.2	7.4	7.6	7.7	7.8
25	1/25	6.0	6.1	6.1	6.2	6.7	7.0	7.3	7.5	7.7	7.9	8.0	8.1
30	1/30	6.3	6.4	6.4	6.5	7.0	7.3	7.6	7.8	8.0	8.2	8.3	8.5
35	1/35	6.5	6.5	6.6	6.7	7.1	7.5	7.8	8.0	8.2	8.4	8.5	8.7
40	1/40	6.6	6.7	6.8	6.8	7.3	7.7	7.9	8.2	8.4	8.5	8.7	8.8
45	1/45	6.8	6.8	6.9	7.0	7.5	7.8	8.1	8.3	8.5	8.7	8.9	9.0
50	1/50	6.9	7.0	7.0	7.1	7.6	7.9	8.2	8.5	8.7	8.8	9.0	9.1
60	1/60	7.1	7.2	7.3	7.3	7.8	8.2	8.5	8.7	8.9	9.1	9.2	9.4
70	1/70	7.3	7.4	7.4	7.5	8.0	8.4	8.7	8.9	9.1	9.3	9.4	9.6
80	1/80	7.5	7.5	7.6	7.7	8.2	8.5	8.8	9.1	9.3	9.4	9.6	9.7
90	1/90	7.6	7.7	7.8	7.8	8.3	8.7	9.0	9.2	9.4	9.6	9.8	9.9
100	1/100	7.7	7.8	7.9	7.9	8.5	8.8	9.1	9.4	9.5	9.7	9.9	10.0

Table 2a. *(Continued)*.

Sample size (n)	SAL ($1/n$)	Bioburden									
		550	600	650	700	750	800	850	900	950	1000
10	1/10	7.2	7.3	7.4	7.5	7.6	7.6	7.7	7.8	7.9	7.9
15	1/15	7.8	7.9	8.0	8.1	8.2	8.2	8.3	8.4	8.5	8.5
20	1/20	8.0	8.1	8.2	8.3	8.4	8.5	8.5	8.6	8.7	8.7
25	1/25	8.2	8.4	8.5	8.5	8.6	8.7	8.8	8.9	8.9	9.0
30	1/30	8.6	8.7	8.8	8.9	9.0	9.0	9.1	9.2	9.3	9.3
35	1/35	8.8	8.9	9.0	9.1	9.2	9.3	9.3	9.4	9.5	9.6
40	1/40	9.0	9.1	9.2	9.3	9.4	9.4	9.5	9.6	9.7	9.7
45	1/45	9.1	9.2	9.3	9.4	9.5	9.6	9.7	9.8	9.8	9.9
50	1/50	9.2	9.3	9.5	9.6	9.7	9.7	9.8	9.9	10.0	10.0
60	1/60	9.5	9.6	9.7	9.8	9.9	10.0	10.1	10.1	10.2	10.3
70	1/70	9.7	9.8	9.9	10.0	10.1	10.2	10.3	10.3	10.4	10.5
80	1/80	9.9	10.0	10.1	10.2	10.3	10.4	10.4	10.5	10.6	10.7
90	1/90	10.0	10.1	10.2	10.3	10.4	10.5	10.6	10.7	10.8	10.8
100	1/100	10.2	10.3	10.4	10.5	10.6	10.6	10.7	10.8	10.9	11.0

Table 2b. Radiation dose (kGy) required to achieve an SAL of 10^{-6} for different bioburdens having standard distribution of resistances.

Bioburden	Dose	Bioburden	Dose	Bioburden	Dose
0.06	10.4	2.0	15.2	30	19.3
0.08	10.6	2.2	15.3	40	19.7
0.09	10.8	2.6	15.5	50	20.1
0.10	11.0	3.0	15.8	60	20.3
0.12	11.3	3.2	16.0	70	20.6
0.14	11.5	4.0	16.2	80	20.8
0.17	11.7	4.4	16.3	90	21.0
0.19	11.9	5.0	16.5	100	21.1
0.22	12.1	5.4	16.6	150	21.8
0.26	12.3	6.0	16.8	200	22.2
0.29	12.5	7.0	17.0	250	22.6
0.34	12.7	8.0	17.2	300	22.9
0.39	12.9	8.8	17.3	350	23.1
0.44	13.1	9.0	17.4	400	23.3
0.50	13.3	10	17.6	450	23.5
0.57	13.5	11	17.7	500	23.7
0.65	13.6	12	17.9	550	23.8
0.73	13.8	13	18.0	600	24.0
0.83	14.0	14	18.1	650	24.1
0.93	14.2	15	18.2	700	24.2
1.0	14.2	16	18.3	750	24.3
1.2	14.3	17	18.4	800	24.4
1.4	14.6	18	18.5	850	24.5
1.6	14.8	19	18.6	900	24.6
1.8	14.9	20	18.7	950	24.7
				1000	24.8

Table 3. I and S for calculation of verification dose for test sample size and bioburden level (ISO/TR 13409: 1996).

Test sample	Bioburden 1 to 10		Bioburden 11 to 100		Bioburden 101 to 1000	
size	I	S	I	S	I	S
10	1.25	1.65	0.67	2.23	−0.26	2.71
20	1.71	1.82	1.14	2.41	0.35	2.81
30	2.00	1.93	1.46	2.49	0.71	2.87
40	2.21	2.01	1.69	2.55	1.00	2.90
50	2.38	2.07	1.88	2.59	1.21	2.93
60	2.52	2.12	2.03	2.63	1.40	2.95
70	2.65	2.16	2.16	2.66	1.55	2.97
80	2.76	2.19	2.30	2.67	1.67	2.99
90	2.86	2.22	2.39	2.70	1.80	3.00

Verification dose at a given SAL $= I + (S \times \log$ (Avergare SIP bioburden)).
I = intercept.
S = slope.

Table 4. Verification doses and dose reduction factors (DRF) for an SAL of 10^{-3} using Method C (extracted from AAMI TIR 27: 2001).

Bioburden	VD (kGy)	DRF	Bioburden	VD (kGy)	DRF	Bioburden	VD (kGy)	DRF
1	4.2	4.17	40	8.6	3.29	280	8.6	2.49
2	5.2	3.97	45	8.7	3.27	300	8.6	2.46
3	5.7	3.86	50	8.8	3.25	325	8.5	2.43
4	6.1	3.79	55	8.9	3.23	350	8.5	2.40
5	6.3	3.73	60	8.9	3.21	375	8.5	2.37
6	6.6	3.69	65	9.0	3.20	400	8.4	2.34
7	6.7	3.65	70	9.1	3.19	425	8.4	2.32
8	6.9	3.62	75	9.1	3.17	450	8.4	2.30
9	7.0	3.59	80	9.2	3.15	475	8.4	2.28
10	7.1	3.57	85	9.1	3.11	500	8.4	2.26
11	7.2	3.55	90	9.1	3.08	525	8.3	2.24
12	7.3	3.53	95	9.1	3.05	550	8.3	2.22
13	7.4	3.51	100	9.0	3.01	575	8.3	2.21
14	7.5	3.50	110	9.0	2.96	600	8.3	2.19
15	7.6	3.48	120	9.0	2.91	650	8.3	2.15
16	7.6	3.47	130	8.9	2.86	700	8.2	2.14
17	7.7	3.46	140	8.9	2.83	750	8.2	2.12
18	7.8	3.45	150	8.9	2.79	800	8.2	2.09
19	7.8	3.43	160	8.8	2.76	850	8.2	2.07
20	7.9	3.42	170	8.8	2.72	900	8.1	2.05
22	8.0	3.40	180	8.8	2.68	950	8.1	2.04
24	8.1	3.39	190	8.7	2.67	1000	8.1	2.02
26	8.1	3.37	200	8.7	2.64			
28	8.2	3.36	220	8.7	2.60			
30	8.3	3.34	240	8.6	2.56			
35	8.4	3.31	260	8.6	2.52			

Annex D

Key References for the Sterilization of Tissues by Ionising Radiation

General

Advances in Tissue Banking, Volumes 1-4, (1997–2000), (Editor-in Chief, Glyn O Phillips) World Scientific, Singapore, New Jersey, London and Hong Kong (ISBNs 981-02-3190-3; 981-02-3524-8; 981-02-3872-X; 981-4287-5).

Biological Properties of Tissue Banking (1982) (Editor: R. Klen with Glyn O Phillips (English Editor)) Pergamon Press.

Dziedzic-Goclawska A (1978). Effect of radiation sterilization on biostatic tissue grafts and their constituents In "*Sterilisation by Ionizing Radiation* (Eds. Gughran WRL and Goudie AJ) Multiscience, Montreal, vol. 2, pp 156–187.

Radiation and Tissue Banking (2000), (Editor: Glyn O Phillips) World Scientific, Singapore, New Jersey, London and Hong Kong, ISBN 981-4287-7).

Bone

Akkus O and Rimnac CM (2001). Fracture resistance of gamma radiation sterilized cortical bone allografts *J Orthop Res* **19**:927–934.

Angermann P and Jepsen OB (1991). Procurement, banking and decontamination of bone and collagenous tissue allografts: guidelines for infection control. *J Hosp Infect* **17**: 159–169.

Araki N, Myoui A, Kuratsu S, Hashimoto N, Inoue T, Kudawara I, Ueda T, Yoshikawa H, Masaki N, and Uchida A (1999). Intraoperative extracorporeal autogenous irradiated bone grafts in tumour surgery. *Clin Orthop* **368**:196–206.

Burwell RG (1976). The fate of freeze-dried bone allograft. *Transplant Proc* **8**:95–111.

Cornu O, Banse X, Docquier PL, Luyckx S, and Delloye C (2000). Effect of freeze-drying and gamma irradiation on the mechanical properties of human cancellous bone. *J Orthop Res* **18**:426–431.

Dexter F (1976). Tissue banking in England. *Transplant Proc* **8**:43–48.

Dziedzic-Goclawska A, Ostrowski K, Stachowicz W, Michalik J, and Grzesik W (1991). Effect of radiation sterilization on the osteoinductive properties and the rate of remodeling of bone implants preserved by lyophilization and deep-freezing. *Clin Orthop* **272**:30–37.

Fideler BM, Vangsness CT Jr., Lu B, Orlando C, and Moore T (1995). Gamma irradiation: effects on biomechnical properties of human bone-patellar tendon-bone allografts. *Am J Sports Med* **23**:643–646.

Goertzen MJ, Clahsen H, Burrig KF, and Schulitz KP (1995). Sterilisatation of canine anterior cruciate allografts by gamma irradiation in argon. Mechanical and neurohistological properties retained one year after transplantation. *J Bone Joint Surg Br* **77**:205–212 Retracted publication.

Hilmy N, Febrida A, and Basril A (2000). Validation of radiation sterilization dose for lyphilized amnion and bone grafts. *J Cell Tissue Banking* **1**:143–147.

Horowitz M (1979). Sterilisation of homograft ossicles by gamma radiation. *J Laryngol Otol* **93**:1087–1089.

Imamaliev AS and Gasimov RR (1974). Biological properties of bone tissue conserved in plastic material and sterilized with gamma rays (clinico-experimental study). *Acta Chir Plast* **16**:129–135.

Komender J (1978). Evaluation of radiation-sterilized bone and clinical use. *Acta Med Pol* **19**:277–281.

Komender J, Komender A, Dziedzic-Goclawska A, and Ostrowski K (1976). Radiation-sterilized bone grafts evaluated by electron spin resonance technique and mechanical tests. *Transplant Proc* **8**:25–37.

Komender J, Malczewska H, and Lesiak-Cyganowska E (1978). Preserved bone in clinical transplantation. *Arch Immunol Ther Exp (Warz)* **26**:1071–1073.

Komender J, Malczewska H, and Komender A (1991). Therapeutic effects of transplantation of lyophilized and radiation-sterilised, allogeneic bone. *Clin Orthop* **272**:38–49.

Linberg JV, Anderson RL, Edwards JJ, Panje WR, and Bardach J (1980). Preserved irradiated homolgous cartilage for orbital reconstruction. *Opthalmic Surg* **11**:457–462.

Loty B, Courpied JP, Tomeno B, Postel M, Forest M, and Abelanet R (1990). Bone allografts sterilised by irradiation. Biological properties, procurement and results of 150 massive allografts. *Inst Orthop* **14**:237–242.

Loty B, Tomeno B, Evrard J, and Postel M (1994). Infection in massive bone allografts sterilised by radiation. *Int Orthop* **18**:164–171.

MacDowell S (1988). Irradiated cartilage. *Plast Surg Nurs* **8**:14–15.

Marczynski W, Tylman D, and Komender J (1997). Long-term follow up after transplantation of frozen and radiation sterilize bone grafts. *Ann Transplant* **2**:64–66.

Marquit B (1967). Radiated homogenous cartilage in rhinoplasty. *Arch Otolaryngol* **85**: 78–80.

Moreau MF, Gallois Y, Basle MF, and Chappard D (2000). Gamma irradiation of human bone allografts alters medullary lipids and releases toxic compounds for osteoblast-like cells. *Biomaterials* **21**:369–376.

Ostrowski K, Dziedzic-Goclawska A, Stachowicz W, Michalik J, Tarsoly E, and Komender A (1971). Application of the electron spin resonance technique for quantitative evaluation of the resorption rate of irradiated bone grafts. *Calcif Tissue Res* **7**:58–66.

Ostrowski K, Dziedzic-Goclawska A, Stachowicz W, and Michalik J (1974). Accuracy, sensitivity and specificity of electron spin resonance analysis of mineral constituents of irradiated tissues. *Ann NY Acad Sci* **238**:186–201.

Ostrowski K, Dziedzic-Goclawska A, Stachowicz A, and Michalik J (1991). Radiation-induced paramagnetic centers in research in bone physiopathology. *Clin Orthop* **272**: 21–29.

Ostrowski K, Kecki Z, Dziedzic-Goclawska A, Stachowicz W, and Komender A (1969). Free radicals in bone grafts sterilized by ionizing radiation. *Sb Ved Pr Lek Fak Karlovy Univerzity Hradci Kralove* Suppl.: 561–563.

Russell JL and Block JE (1999). Clinical utility of demineralized bone matrix for osseous defects, arthrodesis and reconstruction: impact of processing techniques and stud methodology. *Orthopedics* **22**:524–531.

Russell J, Scarborough N, and Chesmel K (1997). Re: Ability of commercial demineralized freeze-dried bone allograft to induce new bone formation. *J Peridontol* **68**:804–806.

Silberman F and Kairiyama E (2000). Radiation sterilization and the surgical use of bone allografts in Argentina. *Advances in Tissue Banking* **4**:27–38.

Tarsoly E, Ostrowski K, Moskalewski S, Lojek T, Kurnatowski W, and Krompecher S (1969). Incorporation of lyophilized and radiosterilized perforated and unperforated bone grafts in dogs. *Acta Chir Acad Sci Hung* **10**:55–63.

Urist MRa and Hernandez A (1974). Excitation transfer in bone. Deleterious effects of cobalt 60 radiation-sterilization of bank bone. *Arch Surg* **109**:586–593.

Wangerin K, Ewers R, and Bumann A (1987). Behaviour of differently sterilized allogenic lyophilized cartilage implants in dogs. *J Oral Maxillofac Surg* **45**:236–242.

Weintroub S and Reddi AH (1988). Influence of irradiation on the osteoinductive potential of demineralized bone matrix. *Calcif Tissue Int* **42**:255–260.

White JM, Goodis HE, Marshall SJ, and Marshall GW (1994). Sterilisation of teeth by gamma radiation. *J Dent Res* **73**:1560–1567.

Yahia LH, Drouiin G, and Zukor D (1993). The irradiation effect on the initial mechanical properties of meniscal grafts. *Biomed Mater Eng* **3**:211–221.

Zasacki W (1991). The efficacy of application of lyophilized, radiation-sterilised bone graft in orthopedic surgery. *Clin Orthop* **272**:82–87.

Zhang Q, Cornu O, and Delloye C (1997). Ethylene oxide does not extinguish the osteoinductive capacity of demineralized bone. A reappraisal in rats. *Acta Orthop Scand* **68**: 104–108.

HIV

Bedrossian EH Jr. (1991). HIV and banked fascia lata. *Ophthal Plast Reconstr Surg* **7**: 284–288.

Campbell DG, Li P, Stephenson AJ, and Oakeshott RD (1994). Sterilization of HIV by gamma irradiation. A bone allograft model. *Int Orthop* **18**:172–6.

Campbell DG and Li P (1999). Sterilization of HIV with irradiation: relevance to infected bone allografts. *Aust N Z J Surg* Jul 69, 517–521.

Fideler BM, Vangness CT Jr., Moore T, Li Z, and Rasheed S (1994). Effects of gamma irradiation on the human immunodeficiency virus. A study in frozen human bone-patelar ligament-bone grafts obtained from infected cadavera. *J Bone Joint Surg Am* **76**:1032–1035.

Hernigou P, Gras G, Marinello G, and Dormont D (2000). Inactivation of HIV by application of heat and radiation: implication in bone banking with irradiated allograft bone. *Acta Orthop Scand* **71**:508–512.

Salai M, Vonsover A, Pritch M, von Versen R, and Horoszowski H (1997). Human immunodeficiency virus (HIV) inactivation of banked bone by gamma irradiation. *Ann Transplant* **2**:55–56.

Smith RA, Ingels J, Lochemes JJ, Dutkowsky JP, and Pifer LL (2001). Gamma irradiation of HIV-1. *J Orthop Res* **19**:815–819.

Biomaterials

Al-Assaf S, Hawkins CI, Parsons BJ, Davies MJ, and Phillips BJ (1999). Identification of radicals from hyaluronan (hyaluronic acid) and cross-linked derivatives using electron paramagnetic resonance spectroscopy. *Carbohydrate Polymers* **38**:17–22.

Al-Assaf S, Meadows J, Phillips GO, Williams PA, and Parsons BJ (2000). The effect of hydroxyl radicals on the rheological performance of hylan and hyaluronan. *Int J Biol Macromol* **27**:337–348.

Andriano KP, Chandrashekar B, McEnery K, Dunn RL, Moyer K, Balliu CM, Holland KM, Garrett S, and Huffer WE (2000). Preliminary in vivo studies on the osteogenic potential of bone morphogenetic proteins delivered from an absorbable puttylike polymer matrix. *J Biomed Mater Res* **53**:36–43.

Bruck SD and Mueller EP (1988). Radiation sterilization of polymeric implant materials. *J Biomed Mater Res* **22**:133–144.

Cheung DT, Perelman N, Tong D, and Nimni ME (1990). The effect of gamma-irradiation on collagen molecules, isolated alpha-chains and crosslinked native fibers. *J Biomed Mater Res* **24**:581–589.

Deeble DJ, Phillips GO, Bothe E, Schuchmann H-P, and von Sonntag C (1991). The radiation induced degradation of hyaluronic acid. *Radiat Phys Chem* **37**:115–118.

Edwards HE, Moore JS, and Phillips GO (1977). Effects of Co-60 irradiation on chondromucoprotein. *Int J Radiat Biol* **32**:351–359.

Holy CE, Cheng C, Davies JE, and Shoichet MS (2001). Optimizing the sterilization of PLGA scaffolds for use in tissue engineering. *Biomaterials* **22**:25–31.

Nakamura Y, Ogiwara Y, and Phillips GO (1985). Free radical formation and degradation of cellulose by ionising radiations. *Polymer Photochemistry*, **6**:135–159.

Pe Myint, Deeble DJ, Beaumont, PC, Blake, SM, and Phillips GO (1987). The reactivity of various free radicals with hyaluronic acid: Steady state and pulse radiolysis studies. *Biochim, Biophy, Acta* **925**:194–202.

Phillips GO (1985). Radiation Degradation of Cellulosic Systems. *Proceedings of an International Symposium on Fiber Science and Technology*, August 20–24, Hakone, Japan, 88–90.

Phillips GO Chemical Processes Induced During Radiation Sterilisation of Cellulose. Presented at Anselme Payen Award Symposium at American Chemical Society 188th National Meeting at Philadelphia (1984). August 26–31.

Schwarz N, Redl H, Schiesser A, Schlag G, Thurnher M, Lintner F, and Dinges HP (1988). Irradiation-sterilization of rat bone matrix gelatin. *Acta Orthop Scand* **59**:165–167.

Wozniak-Parnowska W and Najer A (1978). Studies on the sterilization of pharmaceutical base materials with ionizing radiation and ethylene oxide. *Acta Microbiol Pol* **27**: 161–168.

Soft tissues

Armand G, Baugh PJ, Balazs EA, and Phillips GO (1975). Radiation protection of Hyaluronic Acid in the Solid State. *Radiation Research* **64**:573–580.

Balazs EA, Davies JV, Phillips GO, and Young M (1967). Transient intermediates in the radiolysis of hyaluronic acid. *Radiation Research* **31**:243–255.

Bumann A, Kopp S, Eickbohm JE, and Ewers R (1989). Rehydration of lyophilised cartilage grafts sterilized by different methods. *Int J Oral Maxillofacial Surg* **18**:370–372.

Cantore G, Guidetti B, and Delfini R (1987). Neurosurgical use of human dura mater sterilized by gamma rays and stored in alcohol: long term results. *J Neurosurg* **66**:93–95.

Donnelly RJ, Aparicio SR, Dexter F, Deverall PB, and Watson DA (1973). Gamma-radiation of heart valves at 4 degrees C; a comparative study using techniques of histochemistry and electron and light microscopy. *Thorax* **28**:95–101.

Edwards HE and Phillips GO (1975). Radiation protection of hyaluronic acid in the solid state radiation research. **64**:573–580.

Edwards HE, Moore JS, and Phillips GO (1978). Effects of ionising radiations on human costal cartilage and exploration of the procedures to protect the tissue from radiation damage. *Histochemical J* **62**:373–376.

Hall AN, Phillips GO, and Rassol S (1978). Action of ionizing radiations on a hyaluronate tetrasaccharide. *Carbohydrate Research* **62**:373–376.

Hinton R, Jinnah RH, Johnson C, Warden K, and Clarke HJ (1992). A biomechnical analysis of solvent-dehydrated and freeze-dried human fascia lata allografts. A preliminary report. *Am J Sports Med* **20**:607–612.

Johnson KA, Rogers GJ, Roe SC, Howlett CR, Clayton MK, Milthorpe BK, and Schindhelm K (1999). Nitrous acid pretreatment of tendon xenografts cross-linked with glutaraldehyde and sterilized with gamma irradiation. *Biomaterials* **20**:1003–1015.

Korlof B, Simoni E, Baryd I, Lamke LO, and Eriksson G (1972). Radiation-sterilization split skin: a new type of biological wound dressing. Preliminary report. *Scand J Plast Reconstr Surg* **6**:126–131.

Litwin SB, Cohen J, and Fine S (1973). Effects of sterilization and preservation on the rupture force and tensile strength of canine aortic tissue. *J Surg Res* **15**:198–206.

Maeda A, Inoue M, Shino K, Nakata K, Nakamura H, Tanaka M, Seguchi Y, and Ono K (1993). Effects of solvent preservation with or without gamma irradiation on the material properties of canine tendon allografts. *J Orthop Res* **11**:181–189.

Malm JR, Bowman FO Jr, Harris PD, Kaiser GA, and Kovalik AT (1969). Results of aortic valve replacement utilizing irradiated valve homografts. *Ann N Y Acad Sci* **30**:740–747.

Mandelcorn MS and Crawford JS (1972). Feasibility of a bank for storage of human fascia lata sutures. *Arch Opthalmol* **87**:535–537.

Martinez Pardo ME, Reyes Frias ML, Ramos Duron LE, Gutierrez Salgado E, Gomez JC, Marin MA, and Luna Zaragoza D (1999). Clinical application of amniotic membranes on a patient with epidermolysis bullosa. *Ann Transplant* **4**:69–73.

Moore JS, Phillips GO, and Rhys D (1973). Chemical Effects of ?-Irradiation of Aqueous Solutions of Chondroitin-4-Sulphate. *Int J Radiat Biol* **23**(2):113–119.

Rittenhouse EA, Sands MP, Mohri H, and Meerendino KA (1970). Sterilization of aortic valve grafts for transplantation. *Arch Surg* **101**:1–5.

Tyszkiewicz JT, Uhrynowska-Tyszkiewicz IA, Kaminski A, and Dziedzic-Goclawska A (1999). Amnion allografts prepared in the Central Tissue Bank in Warsaw. *Ann Transplant* **4**:85–90.

Welch W (1969). A comparative study of different methods of processing aortic homograft. *Thorax* **24**:746–749.

APPENDIX 3

International Atomic Energy Agency

THE IAEA PROGRAM ON RADIATION AND TISSUE BANKING

Public Awareness Strategies for Tissue Banks

August 2002

Preface

The aim of the Document is to provide guidance on organizing and running awareness compaigns and detail some promotional activities that have proved to be successful. It is not exhaustive and it cannot provide universal answers. Local conditions will dictate the appropriate approach and might also provoke innovative solutions. But it is a collection of ideas, contributed by people working against wide ranging ethnic and cultural backgrounds, which have been proved to work.

Contents

I. Public Awareness as a Component within the Total Tissue Banking System

1-Tissue Banking requires interaction between the public, the professional health care staff and the Tissue Bank. This inter-relationship is shown in the following flow chart.

2-Recognizing this integrated relationship, IAEA has addressed the following component needs:

- Public Awareness Strategies for Tissue Banks.
- International Standards on Tissue Banks
- Code of Practice for the Radiation Sterilization of Biological Tissues

3-Additionally, training programs have been identified which support the activities and Quality Management within the Tissue Bank, and the professional education of surgeons and health care personnel who use the tissues and have a role to play in promoting donor availability.

4-In this document, strategies for Public Awareness are identified. But it is important to understand that Public Awareness alone will not be successful unless it is a part of an integrated system as illustrated in Figure 1.

I. Donor Referral and Transplant Coordination Systems

5-A critical link between Tissue Banks and donor occurs within the Donor Referral and Transplant Coordination System. Public Awareness and Professional Education activities aim to increase and facilitate tissue donation within the Donor Referral and Transplant Coordination System. This System is composed of two interdependent processes: Donor Referral and Transplant Coordination.

6-These activities may not be distinct and often overlap, but in any event, the two functions need to be achieved. The Tissue Bank can either be involved in the control of the activities or contract out to another organization or individuals. This document deals with an activity, which precedes both Donor Referral and Transplant Coordination with the objective of providing information to potential donors and their families.

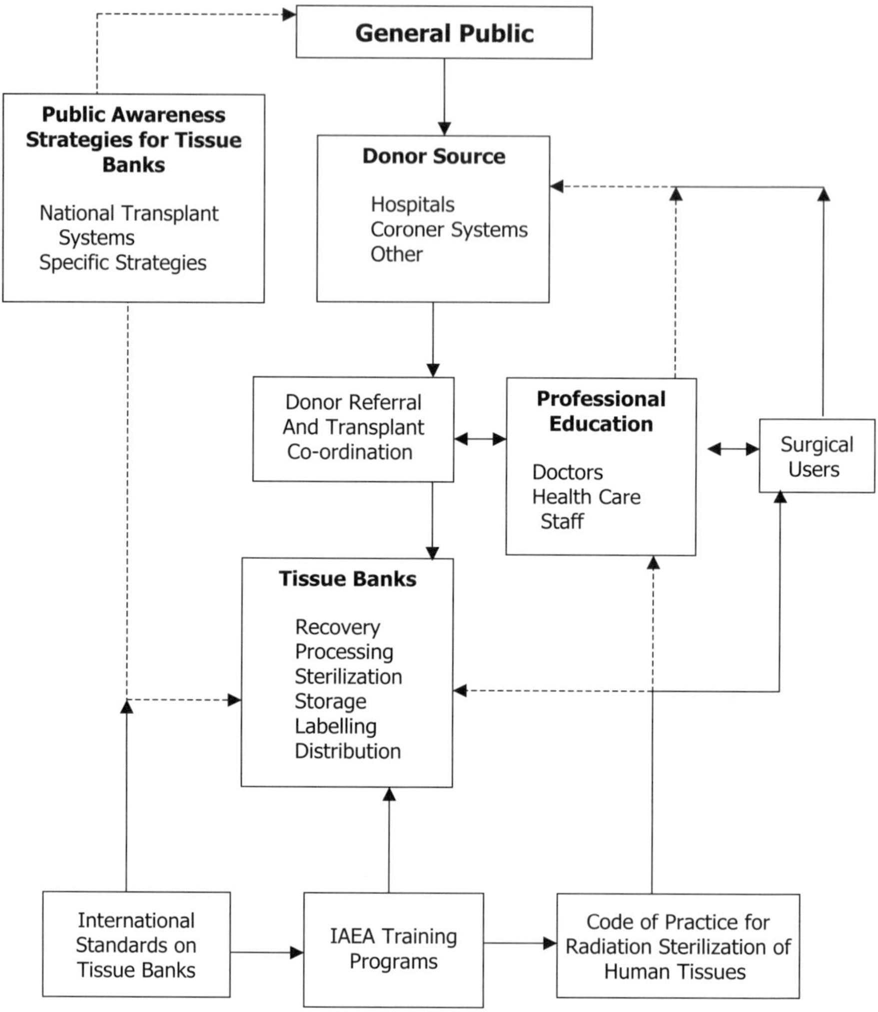

Fig. 1. A General Tissue Banking System.

a. *Donor Referral*

7-Donor Referral is the process by which the Tissue Bank is informed or notified of potential donors when a death occurs at the donor sources (hospital, coroners system, organ procurement agencies, funeral homes, other).

8-Donor referrals are made using some basic donor suitability criteria, which have been previously provided to the donor source staff as part of a Professional Education and Awareness Program.

9-Every Tissue Bank will need to establish processes to ensure suitable potential donors are identified and referred to the Tissue Bank. This notification may be made because of a mandated requirement or may be voluntary. Regardless of whether this system of referral is under the control of the Tissue Bank or not, it will require liaison with, and education of other healthcare personnel.

10-In order to establish a Donor Referral System the Tissue Bank will need to consider:

- Identification and prioritization of referral sources (these may be external or internal). General criteria on which donor suitability is based may include: age, contraindications to donation, time limits between death and donation.
- Establishment of relationships and agreements with those donor sources.
- Identification and training of donor source staff in order to participate in the identification and referral of potential donors:
  - Explain the referral and donation process and the staff members role in the process.
  - Outline timelines for referral and recovery processes.
  - Provide basic donor criteria.
  - Explain tools necessary to make referrals (phone numbers, forms, etc.)
  - Establish Professional Education that includes routine follow-up and feedback to the donor source staff.

b. *Transplant Coordination*

11-Once the donor referral is made to the Tissue Bank, the Transplant Coordination process can begin. Transplant Coordination is the responsibility of suitably qualified personnel who have been trained in performing the various elements of the Transplant Coordination process.

12-The Transplant Coordination process may include:

- Confirming the suitability of the potential donor with the referral source.
- Obtaining contact information of the next-of-kin.

- Approaching next-of-kin to discuss donation options:
  - Tissue that can be donated.
  - Uses of the donated tissue.
  - Description of the recovery, testing, processing, storage, and distribution of tissue.
  - Consent process.
  - Medical social history.
  - Services available to the donor family.
- Coordinating the recovery team.
- Performing tissue recovery.
- Completing documentation.
- Following up with family (thank you letters, donor family services, etc.).
- Following up with donor referral source (feedback on the process).

II. Planning a Public Awareness Campaign

13-Tissue Banking is the recovery, processing, sterilization, storage, labelling and distribution of tissues for transplantation. Although public awareness about all these activities might not seem to be a core activity of Tissue Banking, without donors, users and recipients, banking itself will have no value. Therefore, it is vital to communicate what Tissue Banking is, why availability of tissues for transplantation is important, its role in the community and how individuals can benefit from its existence. Finally, how its services can be accessed.

14-Some Tissue Banks have Public Awareness Programs permanently in place. This strategy can be very successful. In Thailand, for example, the promotion of the social importance of tissue donation has been introduced into the ethos of the Scout Movement which itself is a mandatory part of the education system. The Rotary Movement has also been convinced of the importance of tissue banking and promotes the principle as part of its social development policy. Religious and cultural leaders can play an important role in promoting Tissue Banking in certain communities.

15-In developed countries, for example the USA; it is the role of central Government to promote awareness amongst the public. Although the major emphasis is on organ donation it is now also being extended to tissue donation.

16-Such initiatives take time to set up and require continuing effort but the results more than justify the resources employed.

17-But persisting with a routine in communication with the public that might have been previously successful may have drawbacks. A familiar approach can lose impact. Over several years there might be demographic or cultural changes that will make the approach less effective. It is also difficult to assess the result of the effort — are people responding because of the communication or would they respond anyway? And if it is not known exactly who is responding and why, it becomes impossible to decide who is not being reached and to find ways of getting the message to them.

18-A coordinated Public Awareness Program, run over a specific time scale, will enable those operating it to:

- Set targets.
- Assess results against the targets that were set.
- Work out how many hours and the budget to be spent.
- Decide priorities.
- Decide what is possible, given staff, time and cash constraints.

19-The key to a successful Public Awareness Program is planning the communication — deciding what needs to be said, who needs to hear the message and how that message will be delivered.

III. Communication Strategy

20-Although each Tissue Bank will have to establish its own Communication Strategy taking into account its geographical area, social reality, religious beliefs and specific needs, there will be some common elements in every Communication Strategy for every Tissue Bank.

21-The following ten-point plan will provide an overview of how to develop a Communication Strategy and some of the elements that need to be considered.

1. Goals.
2. Situation Analysis.

3. Success Factors.
4. Objectives.
5. Target Audiences.
6. Selection of Media.
7. Strategic Messages.
8. Delivering Strategic Messages
9. Feedback and Evaluation.
10. Crisis Management.

1. Goals

22-Each Tissue Bank should identify the goals of its Communication Strategy and how it will achieve them. Goals may vary and might include:

- To enhance the public acceptability of allografts.
- To promote the clinical application of allografts among medical professionals.
- To ensure a high level of accessibility of allografts.
- To increase the number of tissue donors.
- To ensure the production of high quality and safe allografts.
- To maintain high ethical standards.

23-Once established, these goals would set the foundations upon which the Communication Strategy will be built.

24-The first step, however, is to evaluate the present position. The progress of any journey can best be gauged by looking back at the starting point. Just as important, it will ensure the strategy is based on current reality.

2. Situation Analysis

25-A thorough analysis of the situation upon which the Communication Strategy will be built is vital to understand the environment in which the work will take place. This will help to ensure its effectiveness. If the situation is not fully analyzed during the planning stage of the Communication Strategy, a vital component may be overlooked leading to the failure of the entire plan.

26-In order to understand the situation it might be advisable:

(a) To analyze the Strengths, Weaknesses, Opportunities and Threats (SWOT analysis) of the operation. For example:

- **Strength** The Tissue Bank is run by the Orthopedic Department whose assistants are supportive of its activities
- **Weakness** The Tissue Bank does not have access to cardiac surgeons.
- **Opportunity** The Tissue Bank's scope of activities can be widened by establishing relationships with cardiac surgeons.
- **Threat** The cardiac surgeons might decide to use imported or artificial cardiac valves.

(b) To conduct surveys (e.g. send out questionnaires to key stakeholders, etc).
(c) To interview key people (e.g. surgeons, hospital administrators, Government authorities, donor families, recipients, religious leaders, community leaders, etc).
(d) To conduct workshops with key personnel.
(e) To review the results of previous campaigns and experiences of other Tissue Banks.
(f) To analyze already available data (e.g. number of potential users, tissue demand, numbers of imported tissues, etc.).
(g) To prepare a budget so that the financial implications of developing the Communication Strategy can be fully understood.

3. Success Factors

27-From the Situation Analysis it is necessary to identify factors that will be critical to the success of the Communication Strategy. These will then become targets in the Communication Strategy. Examples:

Success Factor	Target
Low number of donations among a particular ethnic or religious group	To gain the support of these communities or religious leaders for donation of tissues

Success Factor	Target
Access to surgeons	To ensure that surgeons are aware of the safety, relative low costs and availability of allografts
Low awareness about tissue transplantation in the general public	To increase community acceptance and awareness of tissue donation by publicly recognizing the contribution of donor families

4. Objectives

28-While the Goals of a Tissue Bank will reflect its general purposes, Objectives are the means by which these Goals will be achieved.

29-Objectives that could be considered are:

- To raise awareness on Tissue Banking in the community and among medical practitioners, funding bodies and sponsors.
- To provide high quality information on the issues surrounding tissue transplantation to facilitate decision making by potential recipients, donors and their families.
- To reassure medical professionals about the safety and clinical utility of allografts.
- To publicize the availability of allografts.
- To cultivate an ethical, professional and caring image of the Tissue Bank.
- To provide donor families with a supportive communications network.
- To make tissue donation a natural consideration at the time of death.
- To form a strategic alliance with partners such as community groups, health authorities, corporations, etc. to promote tissue donation.
- To keep government authorities informed of Tissue Banking activities.
- To assist government authorities in promoting Tissue Banking.
- To assist government authorities in developing regulatory systems for Tissue Banking.
- To enlist government support for Tissue Banking.

5. Target Audiences

30-If the Communication Strategy is to be successful the audiences that need to be addressed must be identified. This means recognizing all relevant groups of people. This will help in establishing priorities within the limits of the budget or resources. It will also help in the selection of the appropriate media or techniques that will be effective with the audiences and the messages that each audience will be receptive to. But whatever the resources available the principles set out here should be followed.

31-If the audiences are not carefully selected, funds and resources will be wasted trying to reach everyone. The same message will be delivered universally. At best it will be ineffective for many groups. At worst it could be unsuitable or even objectionable.

32-Depending upon the Objectives the audiences might include:

a. *Donor Families*

33-There would be no tissue donation without the consent of donor families. Consequently donor families should be given special prominence in a Communication Strategy when an objective focuses on donors. Research indicates that most families want the option of obtaining information, even if they do not read it until well after they have made their decision. Because of their personal experience donor families are in the best position to encourage community support for tissue donation.

b. *Recipients*

34-Tissue Banks need the assistance of recipients to promote the benefits they have received from tissue donation. The provision of high quality information to surgeons for distribution to recipients may be a useful tool in gaining their support for the activities of the Tissue Bank.

c. *User Surgeons*

35-Well-informed surgeons can greatly assist the Tissue Bank by talking to their colleagues about the high quality of allografts and service supplied. They are also responsible for informing recipients. Surgeons thus need to know about the Tissue Bank's services, the kind of tissue available and their clinical usefulness. They also need to know the Tissue Bank's safety protocols and their impact on costs.

d. *Bereaved Families*

36-Effort should be made to raise community awareness of tissue donation among bereaved families.

e. *Hospital Staff*

37-Finance managers, medical directors and chief executive officers may be involved in the administration of tissue transplantation. Intensive care and specialty directors may be responsible for developing and implementing policies on tissue transplantation. They may also refer potential donors and deal with their families. They therefore need to be kept informed of all the developments and requirements of the Tissue Bank.

f. *The Media*

38-While the media is a means by which Strategic Messages are communicated to Target Audiences it is legitimate to regard it as an audience in its own right. Medical and science journalists and producers for radio and television are in a position to reflect and influence public opinion and must be appraised of the benefits of tissue transplantation, the status of tissue donation and advances in the field.

g. *Tissue Bank Staff*

39-Anecdotal evidence suggests that personal contact with donor families with the back up of a strong corporate identity would help individuals to make a commitment to donation. Tissue Bank staffs are potential ambassadors for tissue donation.

h. *Community Groups*

40-Community groups (e.g. Rotary, Churches, Scout, Scientific Societies, etc.) can be important in raising public awareness about the activities related to Tissue Banking and transplantation. They can also be supportive of these activities through spreading the word and/or fundraising.

i. *Other Transplant Groups*

41-The cooperation of other transplant groups is essential to elevate the status of tissue donation to that of organ donation.

j. *Government Departments*

42-In some countries Government departments and other regulatory authorities may set the policies for donation and transplantation programs. They may also be responsible for budget allocation and regulation of activities. For these reasons, Government departments and regulatory authorities should be kept informed about the activities of Tissue Banks and their achievements.

6. Selection of Media

43-Having agreed on the Objectives and the Target Audiences to be addressed, the communication media must be selected. This is another area where choice will be dictated by local circumstances.

44-To many people in the developed world, "the media" means the established channels of mass communication — radio, television, the press and, perhaps, cinema. However, in a far larger part of the world television is regarded as an elitist and minority media. The impact of newspapers might be restricted by low literacy, low purchasing power, distribution problems or a shortage of newsprint. Even where newspapers have few of these problems they might have to serve several language groups and so the circulations of the different editions will be small. Radio might be widespread but patchy in areas without reliable electricity.

45-Where such situations exist, public information messages have been successfully distributed by taking the message to the people by means of traveling cinemas and video shows, exhibitions and traditional or folk media.

46-However, it would be well to regularly assess the scope and influence of the various media to ensure the most effective means is being used to contact the audience selected. The media 'balance' will change if there are increases in literacy, improvements in prosperity or technological advances.

47-Political change can very quickly alter the way people receive information. Areas where controls on free expression have been relaxed have seen a huge and rapid increase in the number of newspapers published, all reflecting a wide variety of political and social attitudes. As purchasing a newspaper is a voluntary act, that is, people choose to pay for the product rather than take what is given as in radio or television, it follows that people buy a newspaper because it reflects their views.

48-This is significant because the growth of the press offers an opportunity to target specific groups in a way that is difficult with any other media.

49-In areas where controls on free expression have been introduced, individuals have used the World Wide Web to create newspapers and even run live radio stations in opposition. This creative use of the media is instructional. It is now possible to 'webcast' live video and the technology that allows this is becoming cheaper and more reliable. The 'new media' should at least be given consideration in any media communication program.

7. Strategic Messages

50-The key messages form the central core of the Communication Strategy. They should be reflected explicitly or implicitly in all communications with stakeholders so as to build within the Target Audience a broad appreciation of subjects which will ultimately lead to the fulfillment of the Objectives. The following are suggestions that could be considered as primary and subordinate Strategic Messages:

a. *Value of Tissue Transplants to Community Health*

- One donor can benefit many lives.
- Possibility of someone in the audience to benefit from a future transplant.
- Types of tissue that can be donated.
- Tissue donation can be possible even when organ donation is not.
- Advantages of tissue transplants over alternatives — e.g. cost benefits, efficacy, etc.
- Leading edge medical technology.

b. *Safety Is the First Priority*

- There is a small but finite risk associated with all biological material.
- There is comprehensive Quality Control, including irradiation of tissue.
- Need to fully inform recipients.

c. *Focus on Donor Family*

- Donor families could be important in raising community awareness.
- Donor families may seek the support of the Tissue Bank.
- Body is respected and left intact.

d. *Highly Professional and Ethical Tissue Bank*

- Leading authority in tissue donation.
- Fully accredited.
- Fees are based on the cost of producing, storing and supplying safe tissue.
- User surgeons contribute to policy development.
- Professional advice on all aspects of tissue donation and banking.

e. *Technical Aspects of Tissue Donation*

- Suitability of potential donor.
- Time frame.
- Ethical and responsible disposal of tissue.
- Restoration of the body after tissue removal.
- Administrative procedures.

f. *Technical Aspects of Tissue Transplants*

- Types and availability of tissues.
- Procedure for obtaining and using tissues.
- Procedure for sending tissues to the Tissue Bank.

8. Delivering Strategic Messages

51-Strategic Messages operate much like a Mission Statement. They reflect the value of what the Tissue Bank does, its technical and professional competence, compassion, sensitivity and ethical standards. Unlike a Mission Statement, however, Strategic Messages are not static but active. They can be used to project your values to audiences with differing needs. Finally, the Strategic Messages can be presented in different ways to make the message easily acceptable to a Target Audience.

52-The delivery of a Strategic Message is the matching of an audience, the message and the resource, or delivery vehicle. For example, the Strategic Messages for user surgeons might be:

- Safety is the first priority.

- Highly professional and ethical Tissue Bank.
- The technical aspects of tissue donation.

53-It might be decided that the most persuasive way of delivering these Strategic Messages to this group is by:

- Recipient information booklet.
- Articles in medical journals.
- Professional development of medical specialists.
- Displays or posters at medical conferences.

54-Strategic Messages might be part of a Public Awareness Campaign but they will generally be used in a different way and for a different reason. They deliver a specific message to a selected group consistently and over a long period. They aim to change attitudes and maintain that change by constant reinforcement.

55-Communication with user surgeons, for example, will always contain the Strategic Messages of safety, professionalism and technical information regardless of the main subject. As such they should be part of a Tissue Bank's continuing effort.

56-The following table shows how the three elements — Target Audience, Strategic Message and Resources can be matched to ensure success in reaching the proposed Objective. Public Awareness Campaigns are generally more focused, shorter term and aim to educate to change long-term behavior. This subject is discussed in more detail in the Public Awareness Campaign section.

Target Audience	Strategic Message (s)	Resource (s)
Donor Families	• Value of tissue transplants to community health. • Safety is the first priority.	• High quality donor information/help kit. • Establish 'Friends' to provide grief support and raise community awareness.

Target Audience	Strategic Message (s)	Resource (s)
	• Focus on the donor family. • Highly professional and ethical Tissue Bank. • Technical aspects of tissue donation.	• Quarterly newsletter. • Thanksgiving service.
Recipients	• Value of tissue transplants to community health. • Safety is the first priority. • Highly professional and ethical Tissue Bank.	• Booklet for distribution through surgeon. • Quarterly newsletter. • Thanksgiving service. • Media coverage. • Outward focused brief annual report.
User Surgeons	• Safety is the first priority. • Highly professional and ethical Tissue Bank. • Technical aspects of tissue donation.	• Recipient booklet. • Articles in medical journals. Professional development of medical specialists. • Displays/Posters at medical conferences.
Bereaved Families	• Value of tissue transplants to community health. • Focus on the donor family. • Highly professional and ethical Tissue Bank. • Technical aspects of tissue donation.	• General information on tissue donation.

Target Audience	Strategic Message (s)	Resource (s)
Media	• Value of tissue transplants to community health. • Safety is the first priority. • Focus on the donor family. • Highly professional and ethical Tissue Bank. • Technical aspects of tissue donation. • Technical aspects of tissue transplantation.	• Establish contacts. • Invite to Tissue Bank seminars. • Provide newsletters and annual report. • Invite to "Friends" events and Thanksgiving service.
Tissue Bank Staff	• Value of tissue transplants to community health. • Safety is the first priority. • Focus on the donor family. • Highly professional and ethical Tissue Bank. • Technical aspects of tissue donation. • Technical aspects of tissue transplantation. • Role in promoting activities and professionalism of Tissue Bank.	• Regular presentations to Tissue Bank seminars. • Encourage staff to join "Friends". • Provide newsletter, donor registry forms and annual report.

Target Audience	Strategic Message (s)	Resource (s)
Hospital Staff	• Safety is the first priority. • Highly professional and ethical Tissue Bank. • Technical aspects of tissue donation.	• Liaison with Tissue Bank. • In service seminars. Newsletter. • Invitation to Tissue Bank seminars. • Provide information booklets.
Community Groups	• Value of tissue transplants to community health. • Technical aspects of tissue donation.	• Seminars, presentations, promotional activities, etc.
Other Transplant Groups	• Safety is the first priority. • Focus on the donor family. • Highly professional and ethical Tissue Bank. • Technical aspects of tissue donation.	• Establish personal contact. Invite to seminars. • Market the advantages of greater collaboration. • Negotiate inclusion of tissue donation in organ donation information. • Send newsletter and annual report.
Government Departments	• Value of tissue transplants to community health. • Safety is the first priority.	• Meetings with authorities. • Provision of information.

Target Audience	Strategic Message (s)	Resource (s)
	• Highly professional and ethical Tissue Bank. • Technical aspects of tissue donation and transplantation.	• Participation in the Medical Advisory Board.

9. Feedback and Evaluation

57-There is a need for constant re-evaluation of the Communication Strategy employed in pursuing established Objectives through a feedback system. Communication Strategies are of a dynamic nature and must be modified and adapted in response to identified successes, failures or even subtle changes in the initial Objectives.

58-The outcomes from the Communication Strategy should be evaluated at regular time intervals established in the initial planning process. This will require feedback from key stakeholders using the same tools that were employed for the initial Situation Analysis.

59-The evaluation may reveal whether there have been advances in certain areas of the Communication Strategy and also other areas where the Communication Strategy has had limited success.

60-Adaptation of the Communication Strategy so as to incorporate the information obtained through feedback information and new Situation Analysis will ensure that the Communication Strategy remains effective.

10. Crisis Management

61-The success of Tissue Banks relies upon the trust and goodwill of the public as well as the confidence of medical professionals. These are based upon a positive perception of such things as the Tissue Bank's contribution to society, its procedures, the competence of its professionals, its ethical code and safety standards.

62-If, because of something that is done, something that is not done, misinformation or malicious rumor, that positive perception is damaged then years of education and promotion could be undone within days. The Tissue Bank would be facing a crisis.

10.1. Features of a Crisis

a. *Someone Is to Blame*

63-An incident that could not have been anticipated and was a result of natural forces will not usually cause a crisis for a Tissue Bank. However, if it is as a result of someone's negligence then the Tissue Bank will become the focus of public and, therefore, media attention and anger.

b. *Something Is at Stake*

64-There is no crisis if there is nothing that can be damaged by the public anger and media exposure. In the case of a Tissue Bank what is at stake might be its donor base or the cooperation of other medical professionals.

c. *Someone Finds Out*

65-A crisis only begins when it becomes public.

10.2. Usual Reaction

- Panic.
- Inaction.

66-It is tempting to think that the crisis will go away if nothing is said or done — it won't.

10.3. Result of Inaction

- Public anger grows.
- Rumor replaces fact.
- Regulatory bodies, politicians, etc, become involved.
- Confidence collapses and crisis spirals out of control.

10.4. Handle the Crisis

a. *Stop Whatever Is Causing the Problem*

67-This might be costly and inconvenient but it removes the cause of the emotion and shows the Tissue Bank to be sensitive and considerate of its public responsibilities. It can also demonstrate a commitment to safety, quality or whatever else the Tissue Bank's "brand" represents.

b. *Put Out Holding Statement*

68-Say something to show the problem has been identified, it is being dealt with, there is no cause for public alarm and, most importantly, that the Tissue Bank is a source of information on the subject. This will allow rumors to be stopped before they get into the media or into general circulation.

c. *Assemble Crisis Team*

69-Unless care is taken the crisis will take over the entire Tissue Bank. A small team must be assigned to handle the crisis while others get on with the day to day job of running things.

d. *Decide on Audiences*

70-These might be the general public, regulatory bodies, medical professionals, politicians, people living close to the building, professional bodies and associations, etc. And do not forget to inform the staff what is happening. They are an audience too!

e. *Decide What Will Be Said*

71-Separate messages will probably be needed for different audiences.

72-Your audiences will fall into one or more of three groups:

- **Passive.** They do not know.
- **Informed.** They know but are not active.
- **Active**. They know and they are taking action.

73-The purpose of communication in a crisis is to:

- Prevent the **Passive** receiving misleading or emotive information and moving from **Passive** to **Active.**

- Persuade the **Informed** audience that there is no need to take action.
- Reassure the **Active** that the crisis is being dealt with and they no longer need to become directly involved.

10.5. Planning for Crisis

74-A crisis should not catch a Tissue Bank unprepared. Almost all eventualities can be anticipated and planned for. The first step is communication.

75-If you have Tissue Banks or individuals that are not supportive of Tissue Banking, talk to them and explain what is done and why. They might never be convinced but understanding might prevent them from moving from being an informed audience to an active audience in a crisis. The second step is anticipation.

76-Decide NOW what defines a crisis for the Tissue Bank.

77-There are only a handful of things that are likely to cause problems. Work out what they are. Ask:

- What might go wrong?
- What outside events might affect us?
- What response should be made in each case?

10.6. Create a Crisis Team

78-Decide NOW who will run the crisis, who will deal with the media, Government, regulatory bodies, etc, and who will continue to run the Tissue Bank.

10.7. Identify Your Audiences

79-Decide who will need to know.

10.8. Work Out What You Will Communicate

80-What must be said to each audience.

10.9. Write It Down

81-Create a document that includes contact numbers for all the audiences as well as home, mobile and holiday numbers for key staff and 'friendly' journalists. Keep it up to date.

IV. Public Awareness Campaigns

82-Public Awareness Campaigns aim to create a climate in which the Tissue Bank's immediate goals — increasing donor registration numbers, obtaining corporate sponsorship, encouraging family discussion, etc. — become acceptable and result in increased donation.

83-Unlike Strategic Messages, which are statements of a Tissue Bank's worth and values, Public Awareness Campaigns are usually very focused. They set out to achieve a desired outcome, they often include the use of several different media to influence the Target Audience and they are finite, so the results can be measured against effort and expenditure.

84-For example, in a program to increase enrollment of university students as donors the campaign organizers would select the Target Audience — in this case both students and their families. They would decide on the messages, which would include reassuring and educating parents, persuading the young people to apply for a donor card and impressing upon them the importance of informing their families. The organizers would set a target, perhaps how many more students would carry a donor card after a specific effort over a set time period. Finally, they would decide on the communication tools to be used.

85-Given that the principal audience is the young people, the Internet might be selected together with videos. Within the university, students are a captive audience and so displays or exhibitions could be set up and lectures organized linked to the distribution of brochures.

86-If resources are available, the communication tools might be extended to include information for would-be students and their families delivered with university entrance materials; advertisements on local and university radio stations or even a donor disco; the possibilities are limited only by money, effort and the imagination of the organizing team. Examples that have already been found to work by other Tissue Banks worldwide are many and various.

IV.1. Potential Public Awareness Activities

- School Program "Teaching the Teachers" Workshop.
- Scout Program.
- Kids Club.
- Donor Registry.
- University/College Student Enrolment Program.
- Community Program.
- Corporate and Community Tissue Banks Program.
- Donor and Transplant Recipient Services.
- Drivers Licensing Bureau Program.
- Old Folks' Home.

87-There should be constant monitoring of progress throughout the campaign so that, if necessary, effort can be redirected to ensure the objectives are met.

88-Finally, there should be a careful appraisal of the results to identify what worked well, what could have worked better and what lessons have been learned.

89-To recap, a successful Public Awareness Campaign should include the following:

- An assessment of the problem or need
- The setting of realistic targets or desired outcomes.
- Assessment of resources.
- The choice of Target Audience.
- Choice of messages.
- Selection of tools.
- A distinct start — possibly a public launch.
- Constant monitoring.
- An agreed end.
- Appraisal of results.

IV.2. Tables

90-The following tables contain details of the potential Public Awareness Campaigns including their desired outcomes, messages and communications tools.

METHOD OF PRACTICE.	**School Program "Teaching the Teachers" Workshop.**
TARGET AUDIENCE	1. Primary target: • Elementary and High school teachers. 2. Secondary target: • Students and families.
DESIRED OUTCOME.	• Train teachers to educate students about organ and tissue donation. • To encourage a family discussion about donation decision.
MESSAGES.	• Overview of organ and tissue donation. • Importance of sharing your decision with your family. • Concept of giving, sharing and receiving.
TOOLS.	Two Hour Workshop: • Teacher curriculum. • Pre-Test. • Video (highlights recipients). • Brochure.
RECOMMENDATIONS.	Seek support from the education authority promoting joint programs among relevant authority.

METHOD OF PRACTICE.	**Scout Program.**
TARGET AUDIENCE.	Scouts.
DESIRED OUTCOME.	Educate scouts about donation so they can promote and discuss the donation decision with their families and the community.
MESSAGES.	"Serving Life". Provide information and promotion of donation to their community through the scouts service commitment.
TOOLS.	• Brochures/leaflets • Video (Transplant recipients). • Lecture.
RECOMMENDATIONS.	Seek scout leaders' support to implement a program with reward (badges).

METHOD OF PRACTICE.	**Kids Club.**
TARGET AUDIENCE.	Children (ages 4–12 years old) and parents.
DESIRED OUTCOME.	To promote donation discussion among the child's family, classmates and their families.
MESSAGES.	Benefits of donation and transplantation.
TOOLS.	• Videos and posters • Donor cards ("donation promoter card"). • Stickers.
RECOMMENDATIONS.	Always stress importance of child's involvement in donation discussion.

METHOD OF PRACTICE.	**Donor Registry.**
TARGET AUDIENCE.	General Public (age 18 and older).
DESIRED OUTCOME.	Develop a database to record individual donation decision to facilitate the donation process at the time of death.
MESSAGES.	Make your decision now, so your family can follow through with your wishes later.
TOOLS.	• Brochures. • Form with appropriate signatures. • Database system.
RECOMMENDATIONS.	Seek government legislation to implement and maintain a donor register.

METHOD OF PRACTICE.	**University/College Students/Enrolment Program.**
TARGET AUDIENCE.	Students and their families.
DESIRED OUTCOME.	Every student within the university / college will make a decision about donation and carry a donor card .
MESSAGES.	Educate the students about donation and the importance of making a donation decision and communicating it to their families.
TOOLS.	• Video. • Lecture. • Brochure/Donor card. • Internet. • Display / Exhibit.
RECOMMENDATIONS.	Seek support from the university or college authorities

METHOD OF PRACTICE.	**Community Program.**
TARGET AUDIENCE.	General public.
DESIRED OUTCOME.	Educate the general public about donating, the importance of making a donation decision and communicating that decision to their family.
MESSAGES.	Importance and benefits of donation and transplantation. Make a decision now, so your family can carry out your wishes later.
TOOLS.	• Media campaign • Special events • Celebrity endorsement • Displays / health fairs • Internet. • Donor Cards. • Drivers License Program (and other official identification documents). • Toll free number. • Brochure.
RECOMMENDATIONS.	Keep message simple and consistent.

METHOD OF PRACTICE.	**Corporate and Community Tissue Banks Programs.**
TARGET AUDIENCE.	• Corporations (executives, staff). • Service groups. • Community groups.
DESIRED OUTCOME.	• Educate members, staff or customers about donation • Seek sponsorship. • Make a decision now, so your family can carry out your wishes later.

METHOD OF PRACTICE.	**Corporate and Community Tissue Banks Programs.**
MESSAGES.	Benefits of donation and transplantation.
TOOLS.	• Brochures. • Video. • Internet. • Program materials with recognition of sponsorship. • Lectures. • Scholarships
RECOMMENDATIONS.	Keep message simple and consistent.

METHOD OF PRACTICE.	**Donor and Transplant Recipient Services.**
TARGET AUDIENCE.	• Donors, recipients and their families. • General public.
DESIRED OUTCOME.	• Increase donation through recognition of the donor and support of the family who generously donated. • Highlighting the improved quality of life of the recipients.
MESSAGES.	"Celebrate life".
TOOLS.	• Transplant recipient Olympic games. • Donor memorial services. • Donor recognition (day). • Donor medal / certificate. • Donor quilt.
RECOMMENDATIONS.	Enlist volunteer donor families and recipients to plan coordinate and participate.

METHOD OF PRACTICE.	**Drivers Licensing Bureau Program (or official identification document).**
TARGET AUDIENCE.	• Driver License staff. • Drivers/general public.
DESIRED OUTCOME.	• Drivers License staff consistently offers the option of a donor designation to each individual who renews or applies for Drivers License or official identification document.
MESSAGES.	• Educate the Drivers License Bureau staff about donation and importance of the donation decision and the family discussion. • Ensure Drivers License staff gives a donation brochure to individuals who have questions.
TOOLS.	• Posters (posted in the Drivers License Bureau office). • Lectures. • Videos (donor families and transplanted recipients). • Brochures (staff and public).
RECOMMENDATIONS.	Provide information/materials related to donation to Drivers License Bureau staff. Support of the Bureau staff is key in offering drivers the option of donor designation.

METHODS OF PRACTICE.	**Old Folks' Home.**
TARGET AUDIENCE.	Senior public.
DESIRED OUTCOME.	• Educate senior people to participate in promotion of program. • Promote tissue (e.g. cornea) donation.
MESSAGE.	Nobody is too old to participate in promotion of donation program.
TOOLS.	• Media campaign. • Special events. • Posters. • Brochure
RECOMMENDATIONS.	Keep message simple and consistent.

V. Using the Media

91-Most Public Awareness Programs include some attempt to involve the media. Sometimes the attempt results in an enthusiastic response from the journalists and sensitive, valuable coverage. Sometimes it results in disinterest and little or no coverage. Occasionally it results in inaccurate or sensational coverage of one unimportant aspect of the program, which misinforms the public and damages what is being attempted.

92-Many people who have occasionally had to deal with the media — medical professionals, academics, businessmen, scientists, public service workers and charities -have experienced one or more of these responses.

93-One factor that unites them all is they don't know why. Those who have had a good experience are pleased, but those who have had a bad experience are angry. Frequently both groups are mystified by the response.

94-It is true that taking the media as a whole, newspapers, radio and television, it does seems to have contradictory and conflicting needs.

95-This section of the document aims to explain why the media acts as it does and how to anticipate that response. From this it will become easier to identify the media most suitable for the Target Audience.

96-First, the media is not there to right wrongs, to shine light into dark places or to highlight those things that are important in life although it might do all of those things. It exists principally to make money and occasionally, also, to extend influence. To do this it must generate an audience. Moreover the media creates readers, viewers or listeners by identifying a target group or groups and feeding them what they want.

1. The Audience

97-A large national broadcaster will produce a range of programs to appeal to a selection of audiences. But the more media competition there is in any sector the more specific the media becomes in the audience it targets.

98-Where there is a lot of competition, typically in newspapers, both national and local, cable television and local radio, the media outlets will target a very narrow group. They will know the lifestyle of that group very well indeed and know their hopes, fears, beliefs, prejudices, drives and aspirations. They also know that people will read the newspapers and listen to programs that reflect their values and beliefs. Thus, they will provide their Target Audience with information that reflects the world as that audience sees it.

99-There are two significant points arising from this. First, it is usually a waste of time sending the same information to all sections of the media. Secondly, even when a Target Audience has been identified, the media that appeals to that Target Audience might not be interested in what you want to say.

100-For example let us suppose an objective is to persuade more 18–25 year-olds to opt to be tissue donors. Possibly the group is being targeted because it has been identified as having a general lack of awareness and interest in the subject. However, if that is the case, why should a magazine or radio station run a story or feature on something they know their readers or listeners are unaware of and probably not interested in!

2. Give Them What They Want!

102-The answer is that the information must be linked with something that the Target Audience will find interesting. This might sound like a lot of effort for no guaranteed return but trying to sell the media something they don't want is effort for no return.

3. Case Study One — Quit and Win

103-A public health organization decided to run a campaign to try and persuade young people — teenagers and early twenties — to give up smoking. The group was chosen because it was considered that although many would have been smoking for several years the habit might be easier to break and the health benefits would be easier to 'sell' and more readily recognized.

104-For economy, the campaign had to be run largely through the news columns of local newspapers and the news programs of local TV and radio rather than by advertising.

105-The campaign organizers looked at what the young people in that group valued. It was recognized that among the few things that this group felt important enough to save money for were cars and holidays.

106-A car distributor was persuaded to give a car as a first prize on the promise of publicity and several holiday companies gave holidays. The campaign became 'Quit and Win'. People pledged to give up smoking by filling in a form, signed by a friend. After three months they became eligible to take part in a free draw for a holiday. The campaign ended after six months with the final draw for the car.

107-Pictures and interviews with the happy winners were regular features in the media in months four, five and six while the car was handed over by the Minister for Health with great publicity.

108-But what of those who didn't win? A subsidiary message of the campaign was how much could be saved by not spending money on cigarettes — about the equivalent of $7 US a packet in the United Kingdom. There were other interviews at regular intervals about people who had saved for their own holidays or other consumer goods by giving up smoking.

109-There were some up-front costs. There were posters to be printed for the workplace, entry forms and administrations costs. But the value of the publicity was many times the fixed costs. More importantly, the campaign succeeded in its three aims.

- A number of people stopped smoking.
- They became role models — their success was likely to influence others.
- Giving up became a 'smart' thing to do — not something to be mocked.

4. Case Study Two — Medic Alert

110-Medic Alert is a charity that was founded by a parent whose child almost died of an allergic reaction to a food while at a playgroup. The child's allergy had been explained but the information was not passed on. Consequently, when the child became unconscious no one recognized the cause and it was only by chance that it was saved.

111-Medic Alert provides a database of the medical conditions and current treatment for hundreds of thousands of people. People at risk wear a disc bearing a personal identification number and a 24-hour emergency telephone number. It ensures that if that person is taken ill or is injured vital information can be given which might save their lives. Since its inception hundreds of lives have been saved.

112-Obviously, the more people who know about it the more can benefit. The charity decided that television was the ideal media for spreading the message.

113-They approached the producers of several popular drama series with true stories of people who would have been unwittingly killed by routine treatment when they were unconscious but at the last minute someone noticed the badge and called the emergency number. They stressed the dramatic nature of this — moments away from death.

114-The result was that Medic Alert was featured in three television series — a hospital drama and two police dramas all with an audience of several million. Very different from the first case but again, the charity recognized their product had something television producers wanted — dramatic impact.

115-The advantage of using fictional television or radio series is not only publicity but, in cases where there are ethical or religious objections, the argument itself can become part of the program story line.

5. Dealing with Journalists

116-Start by building a relationship with journalists. Getting material into a newspaper or on local television and radio is often as much about personal contact as the subject matter.

117-Each day in a newsroom hundreds of pieces of information jostle for attention. If the journalists making a decision about what to use knows and trusts the Tissue Bank and believes that what it is trying to do is a good thing they are more likely to use the information when they come across it.

118-Remember, journalists are not necessarily friends — they have a job to do. But a relationship can be built up from which both sides benefit.

119-The Quit and Win campaign was a good one but it got more publicity than it might have done because the people running it were on first name terms with a large number of news journalists and health correspondents.

6. Getting in Touch

120-The most common way of giving journalists information is the news release, mailed or e-mailed to interested journalists and news desks. Bearing in mind the previous section it should be directed to a journalist contact that has been cultivated. However, there are a few things you can do to help it further.

a. *Write an Eye-Catching Headline*

121-The headline you write is unlikely to be the headline that appears in the newspaper — the object is to make the journalist receiving it read on.

b. *Start with the Most Important Points*

122-What is actually happening? Where is it happening? Why? When? How? Answering, as many of these questions in the first paragraph will usually have the effect of ensuring the most important information comes first.

c. *Explain How It Will Benefit People*

123-Events are only news because they affect people. The event might be agreement to receive hundreds of corneas from the Tissue Bank of another country. But the effect will be the gift of sight for hundreds of people who would otherwise be blind. That makes a much more emotive and stronger story for the media.

d. *Add a Strong 'Quote' from a Senior Figure*

124-Quotations can make a story more personal and, if from a prominent person, more authoritative.

e. *Use One Side of a Standard Sheet of Paper*

125-If a news release looks long and complicated a journalist might not begin reading it. If more information is wanted they will call.

f. *End with a Contact Number*

126-Make sure someone who has authority to speak to the media is available at that number.

7. The Interview

127-It is flattering to be approached to give a media interview but anyone approached should ask themselves, honestly, if they are the right person to be interviewed. If not, who should be? Then the journalist should be asked:

a. *What Program/Publication?*

128-This will indicate the sort of audience — readers, viewers or listeners — that will receive the message.

b. *What Do You Want to Talk About?*

129-This is necessary to allow preparation of answers to anticipated questions.

c. *Are You Talking to Anyone Else?*

130-This might be the only opportunity to learn if the journalist is also talking to someone critical of Tissue Banking. Then decide, is it in the interests of the Tissue Bank to do this interview?

131-If so, prepare. Work out:

- What the journalist is likely to ask?
- What messages must be put over in the interview?

132-Remember, an interview is an opportunity to put over positive points about the Tissue Bank and what it is trying to do. Don't put an opposing point of view to be 'reasonable'. If there are two sides to the issue there will be plenty of others willing to make the opposing point of view and the journalist has probably found them.

133-Another key to preparation is being clear about what the interview should achieve. Is it to inform? Is it to encourage people to take a course of action? Is it to calm people's fears? Think of two or three main points, things that are at the heart of what must be achieved and make sure they are used. They must be delivered with enthusiasm and energy — broadcast journalists like interviews that sound good but it will also encourage a press journalist to use that as a 'quote'.

134-Do not be nervous. They need your expert knowledge. In some cases a journalist will arrive having had very little opportunity to learn about your Tissue Bank or its work. This is an opportunity to brief them and even suggest some questions they might want to ask.

135-Finally, will journalists always be open and honest about what they want from the interview? The answer is no.

136-Interviewees must try and work that out for themselves, which returns to the beginning and the audience.

- What audience is this journalist writing or broadcasting for?
- What does that audience think of the Tissue Bank and Tissue Banking in general?

137-Remember, journalists are not seekers after truth — they're seekers after stories! And that's not necessarily the same thing.

VI. Promotional Tools

138-A reference section has been compiled to illustrate how a database can be developed and provide a resource for Tissue Bank and organ transplant professionals. Through it, they can access examples of good practice, publicity, promotional and advertising materials that have proved to be successful in programs throughout the world. It is by no means exhaustive. Users may access information via the IAEA website or by contacting the relevant institutions that have contributed to that database.

139-The information has been categorized as follows: Public Education, Professional Education, Donor Appeal and Donor Management. The material is further grouped into the following sub-categories: fliers; posters; stickers; audio-visual aids; newsletter; calendar themes, etc.

Index

Page numbers followed by f indicate figures; those followed by t indicate tables.

B

E

F

G

J

K

L

Q

R

S

X

Y

Z